APPLIED PHARMACOLOGY

for the

Veterinary Technician

Boyce P. Wanamaker, DVM, MS

Program Director
Veterinary Technology Program
Columbia State Community College
Columbia, Tennessee

Christy L. Pettes, LVMT, ART, CPHQ

Veterinary Medical Technician
Lewisburg, Tennessee

Second Edition

with 141 illustrations

W.B. SAUNDERS COMPANY

A Harcourt Health Sciences Company
St. Louis   London   Philadelphia   Sydney   Toronto

W. B. SAUNDERS COMPANY
A Harcourt Health Sciences Company

11830 Westline Industrial Drive
St. Louis, Missouri 63146

Editor-in-Chief: John A. Schrefer
Editorial Manager: Linda L. Duncan
Senior Development Editor: Teri Merchant
Project Manager: Deborah L. Vogel
Production Editor: Sarah E. Fike
Design Manager: Bill Drone
Cover Designer: Kathi Gosche

Library of Congress Cataloging-in-Publication Data

Wanamaker, Boyce P.
    Applied pharmacology for the veterinary technician / Boyce P. Wanamaker, Christy L.
Pettes. —[2nd ed].
        p. cm.
    Includes bibliographical references (p.).
    ISBN 0–7216–8577–3
    1. Veterinary pharmacology.   I. Pettes, Christy L. II. Title.

    SF915.W36 2000
    636.089′57—dc21

                                                                    99-049766

Applied Pharmacology for the Veterinary Technician   ISBN 0–7216–8577–3

Last digit is the print number: 9   8   7   6   5   4   3   2   1

This book is dedicated to
Tippy, Mammy, Megan, and the other dogs of my past and future
for their unwavering loyalty, affection, and companionship.

Doris and Preston, my parents,
for a lifetime of encouragement, discipline, and love.

Karen, my wife,
for her emotional support and editorial assistance.

The students with whom I have had the pleasure
to share knowledge through the years.

B.W.

Dedicated to my husband, Lee,
and my children, Wayne and Amelia Joy,
for their patience with me
during the many months I worked on this book.

I would like to thank
Ray Wakefield, DVM,
Doug Balthaser, DVM, and
John Collier, DVM,
for their ideas and the resources they contributed to my research.
Most of all I thank God
for answering my prayers and helping me to finish my work.

C.P.

Preface

Applied Pharmacology for the Veterinary Technician is designed for both the graduate technician and the student. As a teaching and reference book, its purpose is to help veterinary technicians to become familiar with the many veterinary pharmacologic agents, their uses, adverse side effects, and dosage forms. We feel it is very important for the technician to understand the uses of pharmacologic agents and to have the ability to provide client education under the supervision of the attending veterinarian. A key feature to this publication is a format intended to provide easy and quick access to chapter information. Each chapter is introduced with learning objectives, a chapter outline, and key terms with simple definitions. "Technician's Notes" throughout the text provide helpful hints and important points we feel technicians should be aware of to avoid errors and increase their efficiency.

Features of the second edition of *Applied Pharmacology* include a realignment of the chapters to allow a smoother transition from one to another, updated information on new products and laws, and a section on neutraceuticals. Chapters 1, 2, and 3 remain in their original sequence and establish the fundamental principles that apply to the chapters that follow. Chapters 4 through 11 have been rearranged to cover the organ systems in a sequential manner before moving on to chapters on anti-infectives, antiparasitics, anti-inflammatory agents, and others. Summaries of new drug laws such as the Animal Medicinal Drug Use Clarification Act (AMDUCA) and the Animal Drug Availability Act have also been added. A section on the growing area of neutraceutical use is another of the many new features of this edition. Finally, expanding the number of questions and answers at the end of the chapters and the number of dosage calculations throughout the text make this second edition a valuable tool for pharmacology education.

Our intent in writing this book has been to combine the comprehensiveness of a veterinary pharmacology textbook with the coverage of pharmacologic fundamentals needed by veterinary technicians. No longer will veterinary technician educators have to draw from two sources for this type of coverage. The scope and organization of the information in this book should make it a useful reference for the practicing technician as well.

Boyce P. Wanamaker, DVM, MS
Christy L. Pettes, LVMT, ART, CPHQ

Contents

Chapter 10

DRUGS USED IN OPHTHALMIC AND OTIC DISORDERS, 179

Chapter 11

DRUGS USED IN SKIN DISORDERS, 191

Chapter 12

ANTI-INFECTIVE DRUGS, 205

NOTICE

Pharmacology is an everchanging field. Standard safety precautions must be followed, but as new research and clinical experience broaden our knowledge, changes in treatment and drug therapy become necessary or appropriate. The editors of this work have carefully checked the generic and trade drug names and verified drug dosages to ensure that the dosage information in this work is accurate and in accord with the standards accepted at the time of publication. Readers are advised, however, to check the product information currently provided by the manufacturer of each drug to be administered to be certain that changes have not been made in the recommended dose or in the contraindications for administration. This is of particular importance in regard to new or infrequently used drugs. It is the responsibility of the treating physician, relying on experience and knowledge of the patient, to determine dosages and the best treatment for the patient. The editors cannot be responsible for misuse or misapplication of the material in this work.

THE PUBLISHER

General Pharmacology

LEARNING OBJECTIVES

After studying this chapter, you should be able to:

1. Define terms relating to general pharmacology
2. List common sources of drugs used in veterinary medicine
3. Outline the basic principles of pharmacotherapeutics
4. Define the difference between prescription and over-the-counter drugs
5. Describe the events that occur after a drug is administered to a patient
6. List and describe the routes of administration of drugs
7. Define biotransformation, and list common chemical reactions involved in this process
8. List routes of drug excretion
9. Discuss in basic terms the mechanisms by which drugs produce their effects in the body
10. Discuss the different names that a particular drug is given
11. List the items that should be on a drug label
12. List the steps and discuss the processes involved in gaining approval for a new drug
13. List the government agencies involved in the regulation of animal health products
14. Describe reasons for dispensing rather than prescribing drugs in veterinary medicine
15. Discuss the primary methods of drug marketing

KEY TERMS

Adverse drug reaction An undesirable response to a drug by a patient; it may vary in severity from mild to fatal.

Agonist A drug that brings about a specific action by binding with the appropriate receptor.

Antagonist A drug that inhibits a specific action by binding with a particular receptor.

Compounding Any manipulation (e.g., diluting or combining) to produce a dosage-form drug other than that manipulation provided for in the directions for use on the labeling of the approved drug product.

Drug A substance used to diagnose, prevent, or treat disease.

Efficacy The extent to which a drug causes the intended effects in a patient.

Extralabel use The use of a drug that is not specifically called for on the Food and Drug Administration (FDA)-approved label.

Half-life The amount of time (usually expressed in hours) that it takes for the quantity of a drug in the body to be reduced by 50%.

Manufacturing The bulk production of drugs for resale outside of the veterinarian-client-patient relationship.

Metabolism (biotransformation) The biochemical process that alters a drug from an active form to a form that is inactive or that can be eliminated from the body.

Parenteral The route of administration of injectable drugs.

Partition coefficient The ratio of the solubility of substances (e.g., gas anesthetics) between two states in which they may be found (e.g., blood and gas or gas and rubber goods).

Prescription (legend) drug A drug that is limited to use under the supervision of a veterinarian because of potential danger, difficulty of administration, or other considerations. The legend designating a prescription drug states, "Caution: Federal law restricts this drug to use by or on the order of a licensed veterinarian."

Regimen A program for administering a drug that includes the route, the dose (how much), the frequency (how often), and the duration (for how long) of administration.

Residue An amount of a drug still present in animal tissues or products (e.g., meat, milk, or eggs) at a particular point (slaughter or collection).

Veterinarian-client-patient relationship The set of circumstances that must exist between the veterinarian, the client, and the patient before dispensing prescription drugs is appropriate.

Withdrawal time The amount of time that it takes for a drug to be eliminated from animal tissue or products after use of that drug has been stopped.

INTRODUCTION

Veterinary technicians are an essential part of the efficient health care delivery team in veterinary medicine. One of the important roles that veterinary technicians carry out is administration of **drugs** to animals on the order of a veterinarian. Because this role may have serious consequences on the outcome of a case, it is mandatory that technicians have a thorough knowl-edge of the types and actions of drugs used in veterinary medicine. They should have an understanding of the reasons for using drugs, called *indications,* and the reasons for not using drugs, called *contraindications* (pharmacotherapeutics); what happens to drugs once they enter the body (pharmacokinetics); how drugs exert their effect (pharmacodynamics); and how adverse drug reactions are manifested (toxicity). Because veterinarians dispense a large amount of drugs, technicians must also be well versed in the components of a valid veterinarian-client-patient relationship, the importance of proper labeling of dispensed products, and client education on the proper use of the products to avoid toxicity or residue. Finally, technicians should have a basic understanding of the laws that apply to drug use in veterinary medicine and the concept of the marketing of veterinary drugs. In short, veterinary technicians need a working knowledge of the science of veterinary pharmacology.

DRUG SOURCES

The traditional sources of drugs were plant (botanical) and mineral. Plants have long been a source of drugs. The active components of plants that are useful as drugs include alkaloids, glycosides, gums, resins, and oils. The names of alkaloids usually end in *-ine,* and the names of glycosides end in *-in* (Williams and Baer, 1990). Examples of alkaloids include atropine, caffeine, and nicotine. Digoxin and digitoxin are examples of glycosides. Bacteria and molds (e.g., *Penicillium)* produce many of the antibiotics (penicillin) and anthelmintics (ivermectin) in use today. Animals once were important as a source of hormones, such as insulin, and as a source of anticoagulants, such as heparin. Today, most of the hormones are synthesized in a laboratory. Mineral sources of drugs include the electrolytes (sodium, potassium, and chloride); iron; selenium; and others. Laboratories are now one of the most important sources of existing drugs because chemists have found methods of reproducing the drugs isolated from plant and animal sources. Advances in recombinant deoxyribonucleic acid (DNA) technology have also made it possible to produce animal and human products (e.g., insulin) in bacteria in large quantities.

PHARMACOTHERAPEUTICS

Veterinarians are challenged with assessing a patient to determine a diagnosis and arrive at a plan of treatment. If the plan of treatment includes the use of drugs, the veterinarian must choose an appropriate drug and a drug regimen. The choice of a drug is determined by using one or more of the broadly defined methods called *diagnostic, empirical,* or *symptomatic.* The diagnostic method involves the use of an assessment of a patient, including a history, physical examination, laboratory tests, and other diagnostic procedures, to arrive at a specific diagnosis. Once the diagnosis is determined, the causative microorganism or altered physiologic state is revealed to allow the choice of the appropriate drug. The empirical method calls on the use of practical experience and common sense to make the drug choice. In other instances, drugs are chosen to treat the symptoms or signs of a disease if a specific diagnosis cannot be determined. In veterinary medicine, the comparative cost of a drug may also be an important consideration in choosing an appropriate drug. Once the drug to be used in the treatment has been determined, the next step for the veterinarian is to determine the plan for administering the drug. This plan, called a **regimen,** includes details about the following:

The route of administration
The amount to be given (dosage)
How often to give the drug (frequency)
How long to give the drug (duration)

Every drug has the potential to cause harmful effects if given to the wrong patient or according to the wrong regimen. Some medications have greater potential for causing harmful outcomes than others. According to the FDA, when a drug has potential toxicity or must be administered in a way that requires trained personnel, that drug cannot be approved for animal use except under the supervision of a veterinarian. In such a case, the drug is classified as a **prescription drug** and must be labeled with the following statement: "Caution: Federal law restricts the use of this drug to use by or on the order of a licensed veterinarian." This statement is sometimes referred to as the *legend,* and the drug is called a *legend (prescription) drug.* Labels that state "for veterinary use only" or "sold to veterinarians only" do not designate prescription drugs. Technicians should be aware that prescription drugs have often been approved by the FDA for use in specific species or for specific diseases or conditions. Veterinarians have some discretion to use a drug in ways not indicated by the label if they take the responsibility for the outcome of this use. Using a drug in a way not specified by the label is called **extralabel use.**

Federal law and sound medical practices dictate that prescription drugs not be dispensed indiscriminately. Before prescription drugs are issued or extralabel use is undertaken, a valid **veterinarian-client-patient relationship** must exist. For this relationship to exist, certain conditions must be met. These include but are not limited to the following:

The veterinarian has assumed responsibility for making clinical judgments about the health of the animal(s) and the need for treatment, and the client has agreed to follow the veterinarian's instructions.

The veterinarian has sufficient knowledge of the animal(s) to issue a diagnosis. The veterinarian must have recently seen the animal and be acquainted with its husbandry.

The veterinarian must be available for follow-up evaluation of the patient.

Drugs that do not have enough potential for toxicity or that do not require administration in special ways do not require the supervision of a veterinarian for administration and are called *over-the-counter* drugs because they may be purchased directly without a prescription. Drugs that have the potential for abuse or dependence by people have been classified as *controlled substances.* Careful records of the inventory and use of these drugs must be maintained, and some of these drugs must be kept in a locked storage area.

When a drug and its regimen have been determined, veterinary technicians are often directed to administer the drug through verbal or written orders. Technicians have several important responsibilities in carrying out these orders:

1. Making sure that the correct drug is being administered
2. Administering the drug by the correct route and at the correct time
3. Carefully observing the animal's response to the drug
4. Questioning any medication orders that are not clear
5. Accurately creating and affixing labels to medication containers
6. Explaining administration instructions to clients
7. Recording appropriate information in the medical record

Technicians should be aware that even when the correct drug is administered in a correct manner, an unexpected adverse reaction may occur in a patient. All **adverse reactions** should immediately be reported to the veterinarian.

PHARMACOKINETICS

Pharmacokinetics is the complex sequence of events that occurs after a drug is administered to a patient (Figure 1-1). Once a drug is given, it is available for absorption into the bloodstream and delivery to the site where it will exert its action. After a drug is absorbed, it is distributed to various fluids and tissues of the body. It is not enough for the drug simply to reach the desired area, however. It must also accumulate in that fluid or tissue at the required concentration to be effective. Because the body immediately begins to break down and excrete the drug, the amount available to target tissues becomes less and less over time. The veterinarian must then administer the drug repeatedly and at fixed time intervals to maintain the drug at the site of action in the desired concentration. Some drugs are administered at a high dose (loading dose) until an appropriate blood level is reached, and then the dosage is reduced to an amount that replaces the amount lost through elimination. Other drugs are dosed at the replacement level throughout the regimen. Underdosing leads to less-than-effective levels in tissue, and overdosing may lead to toxic levels (Figure 1-2). Drug levels can be measured in blood, urine, cerebrospinal fluid, and other appropriate body fluids to help a veterinarian determine whether an appropriate level of the drug is being achieved. The cost of

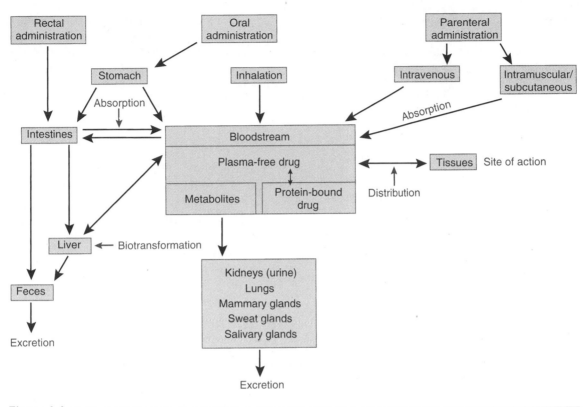

Figure 1-1

Outline of the possible sequence of events that a drug may follow in an animal's body.

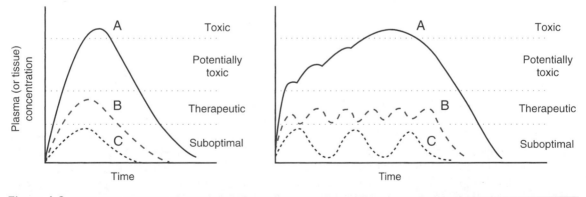

Figure 1-2

The effect of dose on the effects of a drug. (From Jenkins, W.L.: In Ettinger, S.J. [ed.]: Textbook of Veterinary Internal Medicine, Diseases of the Dog And Cat. Philadelphia, W.B. Saunders, 1983, p. 322.)

this procedure, however, usually restricts its use to research settings.

The primary factors that influence blood concentration levels of a drug and a patient's response are thus:

1. The rate of drug absorption
2. The amount of drug absorbed
3. The distribution of the drug throughout the body
4. Drug metabolism or biotransformation
5. The rate and route of excretion

These factors are explored after the discussion of the routes by which drugs may be administered.

ROUTES OF ADMINISTRATION

A drug is of no use unless it can be delivered to a patient in a form and at a site that is appropriate. The way in which a drug is administered to an animal patient is influenced by several factors:

The pharmaceutical form of the drug available
The physical or chemical properties (irritation) of the drug
How quickly the onset of action should occur
Restraint or behavioral characteristics of the patient
The nature of the condition being treated

The routes of administration of drugs to animal patients are discussed next.

Oral

A common method of administering drugs in veterinary medicine is the oral route. Medications given by this route may be placed directly in the mouth or given by a tube passed through the nasal passages (nasogastric tube) or through the mouth (orogastric tube). The mucosa of the digestive tract is a large absorptive surface area with a rich blood supply. Drugs given by this route are not absorbed as quickly, however, as drugs administered by injection, and their effects are subject to species (e.g., ruminants versus animals with a simple stomach) and individual differences. Many factors may influence the absorption of drugs from the digestive tract, including the pH of the drug, the solubility (fat versus water), the size and shape of the molecule, the presence or absence of food in the tract, the degree of gastrointestinal (GI) motility, and disease processes. *This route is not suitable for animals with vomiting or diarrhea.* Drugs given by this route generally produce a longer-lasting effect than those given by injection.

Parenteral

Drugs that are given by injection are called **parenteral** drugs. There are many different routes for injection of a drug:

1. Intravenous (IV)
2. Intramuscular (IM)
3. Subcutaneous (SC)
4. Intradermal (ID)
5. Intraperitoneal (IP)
6. Intra-arterial (IA)
7. Intra-articular
8. Intracardiac
9. Intramedullary
10. Epidural/subdural

Drugs given by the intravenous route produce the most rapid onset of action, accompanied by the shortest duration. Medications that are irritating to tissue are generally given by this route because of the diluting effect of the blood. Intravenous medications should also be administered slowly to lessen the possibility of a toxic or allergic reaction. Unless a product is specifically labeled for intravenous use, it should never be given by this route, and oil-based drugs and those with suspended particles (i.e., those that look cloudy or thick) should generally not be given intravenously because of the possibility of embolism. Special care should be taken to ensure that irritating drugs are injected into the vein and not around it to avoid causing phlebitis.

The intramuscular route of administration produces a slower onset of action than the intravenous route but usually a longer duration of action. The onset of action by this route can be relatively fast with a water-based form (aqueous) or slower with other diluents (vehicles), such as oil, or forms such as microfine crystals. When an injectable drug is placed in a substance that delays its absorption, it may be referred to as a *depot* preparation.

Altering the molecule of the drug itself can also influence the onset or duration of its action. The onset of action is usually inversely related to the duration of action. Irritating drugs should not be given by the intramuscular route, and back pressure should always be applied to the syringe plunger before intramuscular administration of a drug to ensure that the injection is not into a blood vessel.

The subcutaneous route has been called *hypodermoclysis* in some texts. It produces a slower onset of action than the intramuscular route but a slightly longer duration. Irritating or hyperosmotic solutions (i.e., those with more suspended particles than body fluid) should not be given by this route. Quantities of medication that are appropriate for the species or individual being treated should be used to avoid possible dissection of the skin from underlying tissue, which could lead to death and loss (sloughing) of that skin on the surface of the skin and not in the subcutaneous space by avoiding inserting the syringe needle all the way through the skin. Adding an enzyme called *hyaluronidase* to a drug given subcutaneously may speed its absorption.

The intradermal route involves injecting a drug into the skin. This route is used in veterinary medicine primarily for testing for tuberculosis and allergic conditions.

The intraperitoneal route is used to deliver drugs into the abdominal cavity. The onset and duration of action of drugs given by this route are variable. This route is used to administer fluids, blood, and other medications when the normal routes are not available or are not practical. Problems such as adhesions of abdominal organs and puncture of abdominal organs may result from using this method.

The intra-arterial route involves injecting a drug directly into an artery. This route is seldom used intentionally but may happen by mistake. Administration of drugs into the jugular vein of a horse must be made with caution to avoid injection into the underlying carotid artery. Intracarotid injection into an animal results in a high concentration of the drug delivered directly to the brain, and seizures or death could result.

The intra-articular route consists of injecting a drug directly into a joint. This method is used primarily to treat inflammatory conditions of the joint. Extreme care must be exercised to ensure that sterile technique is used when performing an intra-articular injection. This route is not normally used by technicians.

The intracardiac route is used to inject through the chest wall directly into the chambers of the heart. This provides immediate access to the bloodstream and ensures that the drug is delivered quickly to all tissues of the body. This method is often used in cases of cardiopulmonary resuscitation and in euthanasia.

The intramedullary route is another seldom-used route in veterinary medicine. It involves injection of the substance directly into the bone marrow. The femur and the humerus are the bones that are usually used. It is used most often to provide blood or fluids to animals with very small or damaged veins or for animals with very low blood pressure.

When spinal anesthesia is used, the drugs may be injected in the epidural or subdural space. The epidural space is outside the dura mater (meninges) but inside the spinal canal. The subdural space is inside the dura mater. Injection of drugs into the subdural space (cerebrospinal fluid) is also called the *intrathecal route*. These methods of drug delivery are usually carried out by a veterinarian.

Inhalation

Medications may be delivered to a patient in inspired air by converting a liquid form into a gaseous form through the use of a vaporizer or nebulizer. Examples of drugs that may be given by this route include anesthetics, antibiotics, and bronchodilators.

Topical

Drugs that are topically administered are placed on the skin or on mucous membranes. Drugs are generally absorbed more slowly through the skin than through other body membranes. The rate of absorption may be increased or facilitated by placing the drug in a vehicle such as dimethyl sulfoxide (DMSO). Medication may also be applied to the mucosa of the oral cavity (sublingual), the rectum (suppositories), the uterus, the vagina, the mammary glands, the eyes, and the ears. In horses, caustic materials may be applied topically to inhibit the growth of exuberant granulation tissue (proud flesh).

Transdermal drug administration is a form of topical administration that involves using a patch applied to the skin to deliver a drug through the intact skin directly into the blood. This method is most commonly used to provide an analgesic in a slow, continuous manner.

DRUG ABSORPTION

Before drugs can reach their site of action, they must pass across a series of cellular membranes that make up the absorptive surfaces of the sites of administration. The degree to which a drug is absorbed and reaches the general circulation is called *bioavailability*.

The **manufacturing** process can have a significant effect on physical and chemical characteristics of drug molecules that influence their bioavailability. Because of manufacturing differences, the generic form of a drug may differ somewhat from a trademark form in overall efficacy. Bioavailability is often demonstrated by the use of a blood level curve (Figure 1-3). Some of the factors that affect the absorption process include the following (Upson,1988):

    The mechanism of absorption
    The pH and ionization status of the drug
    The absorptive surface area
    The blood supply to the area
    Solubility of the drug
    The dosage form
    The status of the GI tract
    Interaction with other medications

Drugs pass across cellular membranes by three common methods. Passive absorption (transport) occurs by simple diffusion of a drug molecule from an area of high concentration on one side of the membrane to an area of lower concentration on the other side. This method requires no expenditure of energy by the cell. The drug may pass through small pores in the cell membrane or may dissolve into the cell membrane on one side, pass through the membrane, and exit the other side. For example, a disintegrated tablet or capsule results in a high concentration of the drug in the GI tract, and this concentration then passes

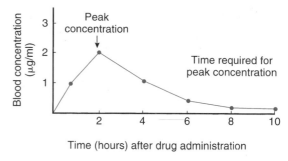

Figure 1-3

The blood level of a drug varies with the passage of time.

through the cellular membranes of the intestinal villi and adjacent capillaries into the lesser concentration of the bloodstream. Alternatively, a drug may passively cross a membrane through the help of a carrier.

Some small drug molecules, such as electrolytes, may simply move with fluid through pores in cell membranes. Active transport of drugs across cell membranes moves molecules from an area of lower concentration to an area of higher concentration and requires that the cell use energy. This is the usual mechanism for the absorption of sodium and potassium and other electrolytes. In pinocytosis, a third method of passive transport, cells engulf drug molecules by invaginating their cell membrane to form a vesicle that then breaks off from the membrane in the interior of the cell. The method of absorption that occurs in a particular situation depends on whether the drug is fat-soluble or water-soluble, the size and shape of the drug molecule, and the degree to which the drug is ionized.

Many drugs can pass through a cell membrane only if they are non-ionized (i.e., not positively or negatively charged). Most drugs exist in the body in a state that has both ionized and non-ionized forms. The pH of a drug and the pH of the area in which the drug is located can determine the degree to which a drug becomes ionized and thus absorbed. Weakly acidic drugs that are placed in an acidic environment do not ionize readily and therefore are absorbed well, and the absorption of basic drugs is favored in an alkaline environment. If a drug is placed in an environment in which it readily ionizes, such as a mildly acidic drug in an alkaline environment or a mildly alkaline drug in an acidic environment, it does not diffuse and may become trapped in that environment.

The greater the absorptive surface of the area in which a drug is placed, the more that absorption is facilitated. One of the largest absorptive surfaces in the body is found in the small intestine because the efficient design of the villi maximizes surface area per unit of space.

At any site of drug administration, the greater the blood supply to the area, the faster the absorption of the drug. Drugs are absorbed from an intramuscular site at a faster rate than from a subcutaneous site because of the proportionately larger blood supply to muscle. Initiating the flight-or-fight response increases blood flow to muscle but decreases blood flow to the intestines. Heat and massage also increase blood flow to an area. Poor circulation, as may occur in shock or cardiac failure, decreases blood flow, as does cooling or elevation of a body part. These factors can then positively or negatively influence drug absorption.

Another important factor that determines the rate at which drugs pass across cell membranes is the solubility of a drug. The lipid (fat) solubility of a drug tends to be directly proportional to the degree of drug non-ionization, and the non-ionized form is, as previously stated, the form that is usually absorbed. The degree of lipid solubility of a drug is often expressed as its lipid **partition coefficient.** A high lipid partition coefficient indicates enhanced drug absorption.

Drug absorption rates often depend on the formulation of the drug. Various inert ingredients such as carriers (vehicles), binding agents, and coatings are used to prepare dosage forms. These substances have major roles in the rate at which the formulations dissolve. *Depo* and *spansule* are terms that are associated with prolonged- or sustained-release formulations in veterinary medicine. Subcutaneous implants containing growth stimulants that break down slowly and release their products for prolonged periods are used in some situations.

When drugs are given by the oral route, the condition of the GI tract can have a major influence on the rate and extent of drug absorption. Factors such as the degree of intestinal motility, the emptying time of the stomach, irritation or inflammation of the mucosa (e.g., gastritis or enteritis), damage or loss of villi (e.g., viral diseases), the composition and amount of food material, and a change in intestinal microorganisms all can affect the rate and extent to which medications are absorbed. Another consideration concerning drugs that are absorbed from the GI tract is the first-pass effect (see Figure 1-6, p. 12). This refers to the fact that substances are absorbed from the GI tract into the portal venous system, which delivers the drug to the liver before it enters the general circulation. In some instances, a drug is then metabolized in the liver to altered forms, which may make it inactive or less active.

Combining some drugs with other drugs or with certain foods can negatively affect drug absorption. The availability of tetracycline is reduced if it is administered with milk or milk products. Antacids may reduce the absorption of phenylbutazone or iron products. Technicians should always consult appropriate references about potential interactions before administering new drugs.

DRUG DISTRIBUTION

Drug distribution is the process by which a drug is carried from its site of absorption to its site of action. Drugs move from the absorption site into the plasma of the bloodstream, out of the plasma into the interstitial fluid surrounding cells, and from the interstitial fluid into the cells, where they combine with cellular receptors to create an action. An equilibrium is soon established between these three compartments as the drug moves out of the blood into the tissue and then out of the tissue back into the blood (Figure 1-4). How well a drug is distributed throughout the body depends on several factors, which are addressed next.

The rate of movement of drug molecules from one of the previously listed compartments to the other is proportional to the difference between the amount of drug in each of the areas. The difference between the amount of drug in two compartments is called the *concentration gradient,* and the greater the gradient (difference), the greater the tendency of the drug to move from the area of greater concentration to the area of lesser concentration.

A drug in the plasma comes into contact with various proteins (e.g., albumin) and either binds with

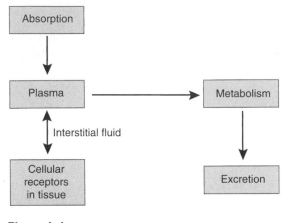

Figure 1-4 ─────────────────

Drug distribution establishes an equilibrium between the amount of drug at the site of absorption, the amount in the plasma, and the amount at the cellular receptor sites.

these proteins or remains free. When a drug is bound to a protein, it becomes inactive and is unavailable for binding with cell receptors or for metabolism. Bound drug may be considered to be a storage site of a drug because bound drug eventually frees itself from the protein. Low levels of plasma proteins may occur in malnutrition or in certain diseases and reduce plasma binding.

Drugs that are highly lipid-soluble tend to move readily out of the plasma and into the interstitial fluid, and drugs that are in the non-ionized form follow a similar pattern. Once a drug is in a tissue, it may become bound or stored there. Tissues such as fat, liver, kidney, and bone may act as storage sites of drugs such as barbiturates, inhalation anesthetics, and others. When a drug moves out of the storage tissue back into the blood, it may produce an exaggerated or prolonged effect because of the additive effect if additional doses of the drug are given.

Barriers that exist in particular tissues tend to retard the movement of all or certain classes of drugs into them. The exact nature of these barriers has not been well explained in the literature. The placenta acts as a barrier to some drugs that could be toxic to a fetus and permits the passage of others. Anesthetics that do not excessively depress a fetus thus must be chosen when a cesarean section must be performed. The so-called blood-brain barrier is generally less perme-able to all drugs, although it becomes relatively permeable to many antibiotics when it is inflamed. The eye also has a barrier that impedes some drugs from diffusing into its tissues.

Disease processes can interfere with drug distribution. Antibiotics usually do not diffuse well into abscesses or exudates. Heart failure and shock can reduce normal blood flow to tissues and thus impede drug distribution. Kidney failure (uremia) can alter the plasma binding of some drugs, such as furosemide and phenylbutazone, and liver failure can cause a reduction in the amount of protein (albumin) available for protein binding.

Reptiles have a renal-portal system that can distribute potentially toxic levels of a drug to the kidney if the drug is injected into the posterior one-third of the body.

BIOTRANSFORMATION

Biotransformation, or **metabolism,** is the body's ability to change a drug chemically from the form in which it was administered into a form that can be eliminated from the body. Most biotransformation occurs in the liver as a result of the action of microsomal enzymes found in liver cells. These enzymes induce chemical reactions that render a drug water-soluble, allowing its subsequent elimination in the urine. Once a drug has been biotransformed, it is called a *metabolite*. Metabolites are usually inactive but in some cases may be more active. A few highly lipid-soluble drugs are incorporated into bile and eliminated through the biliary system. Some biotransformation does occur in other tissues such as the kidney, lung, and nervous system.

The four chemical reactions induced by microsomal enzymes in the liver to biotransform drugs are:

Oxidation—a loss of electrons
Reduction—a gain of electrons
Hydrolysis—splitting of the drug molecule with the addition of a water molecule to each of the split portions
Conjugation—the addition of glucuronic acid to the drug molecule; when glucuronic acid is attached to a drug molecule, the drug becomes much more water-soluble

Many factors can alter drug metabolism, including species, age, nutritional status, tissue storage, and

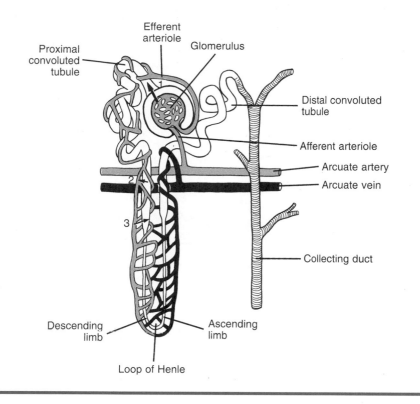

Proximal convoluted tubule

Efferent arteriole

Glomerulus

Distal convoluted tubule

Afferent arteriole

Arcuate artery

Arcuate vein

Collecting duct

Descending limb

Ascending limb

Loop of Henle

Figure 1-5

The kidneys eliminate or conserve drug metabolites by glomerular filtration (1), tubular reabsorption (2), and tubular secretion (3).

health status. Cats have limited ability to metabolize aspirin, narcotics, and barbiturates because of reduced ability to form glucuronic acid. Young animals usually have poor ability to biotransform drugs because their liver enzyme systems are not fully developed. Old animals have a decreased capacity to biotransform because they have impaired ability to synthesize the needed liver enzymes. Malnourished animals have fewer protein raw materials available to manufacture enzymes for biotransformation, and animals with liver disease are not able to process the raw materials available for enzyme production. Drugs that are in storage compartments, such as fat or plasma proteins, are not available for metabolism.

DRUG EXCRETION

Most drugs are metabolized by the liver and then eliminated from the body by the kidneys via the urine. They can, however, be excreted by the liver (bile),

mammary glands, lungs, intestinal tract, sweat glands, salivary glands, and skin. It is very important to know the route of excretion of drugs because alterations or diseases of that organ can cause a reduced capacity to excrete the drug, and toxic accumulations may result. For example, the anesthetic agent ketamine can cause serious central nervous system depression in cats with urinary obstruction because this drug is excreted by the kidneys.

The kidneys excrete drugs by two principal mechanisms. The first of the methods is called *glomerular filtration*. A glomerulus and its corresponding tubule make up the individual functional unit of the kidney called a *nephron*. A glomerulus acts like a sieve to filter drug molecules (metabolites) out of the blood into the glomerular filtrate, which is then eliminated as urine (Figure 1-5). The second mechanism that the kidneys use to excrete drugs is called *tubular secretion*. Kidney tubule cells secrete metabolites out of the capillaries surrounding the tubule and into the glomeru-

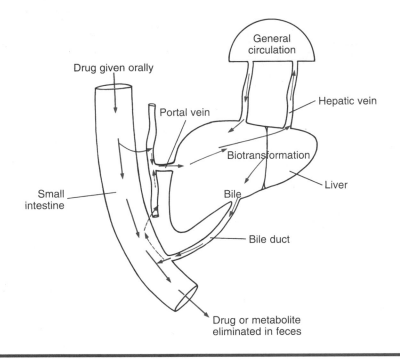

Figure 1-6

Drugs or their metabolites in the intestine may be eliminated in the feces or absorbed/reabsorbed for a pass through the liver.

lar filtrate, which becomes urine as it exits the kidneys. In some instances, drug molecules may be reabsorbed out of the glomerular filtrate and back into the blood by *tubular reabsorption.*

It is important that the nephrons (glomerulus and corresponding tubule) be healthy and have an adequate blood supply to do an effective job of excreting metabolites. The lower urinary tract (bladder and urethra) must also be functioning normally for the filtered or secreted metabolites to be eliminated. If any part of this system from the glomerulus to the urethra is compromised or diseased, toxic levels of drug may accumulate.

The liver excretes drugs by first incorporating them into bile, which is eliminated into the small intestine. In the small intestine, the drug may then become a part of the feces and be eliminated from the body, or it may be reabsorbed into the bloodstream (Figure 1-6).

Some drugs or their metabolites may pass directly out of the blood and into the milk via the mammary glands. This is an important consideration because of the potential effects of the drug on the nursing offspring or the effects of the drug on people who drink the milk. Quantities of drug remaining in animal products when consumed are called **residues.** Residues found in milk, eggs, or meat products are potentially dangerous to people because of the following:

People may be allergic to the drug.
Prolonged exposure to antibiotic residues can result in resistant strains of bacteria.
Residue of some drugs may cause cancer in humans.

Drugs that convert readily between a liquid and a gaseous state (gas anesthetics) may be eliminated from the blood via the lungs. These gas molecules move out of the blood and into the alveoli of the lungs to be eliminated in expired air.

Drugs that are given orally and are not absorbed readily out of the intestinal tract may pass through that

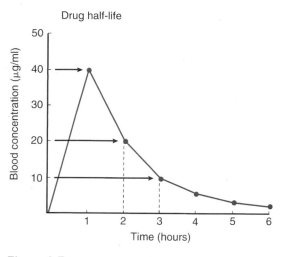

Drug half-life

Figure 1-7

This graph illustrates a drug half-life of 1 hour.

tract and be eliminated through the feces. As mentioned previously, some drugs are excreted through the bile into the intestinal tract, and a few may be actively secreted across the intestinal mucosa into the intestine for elimination.

Some drugs are eliminated through sweat and saliva, although these routes usually are not clinically important.

The rate of drug loss from the body can be estimated by calculating the drug's half-life. The **half-life** is the time required for the amount of the drug in the body to be reduced by one half (Figure 1-7).

PHARMACODYNAMICS

Pharmacodynamics is the study of the mechanisms by which drugs produce physiologic changes in the body. Drugs may enhance or depress the physiologic activity of a cell or tissue. Drug molecules combine with components of the cell membrane or with internal components of the cell to cause alterations in cell function. The way in which drugs combine with structures (receptors) on or in a cell can be compared to a lock-and-key model. The geometric match of a drug molecule and a cellular receptor must be exact

for the appropriate action to occur (Figure 1-8). The tendency of a drug to combine with a receptor is called *affinity,* and the degree to which the drug binds with its receptor helps to determine drug efficacy. A drug with a high level of affinity and efficacy causes a specific action and is an **agonist.** A drug with less affinity and efficacy is a partial agonist. A drug that blocks another drug from combining with a receptor is an **antagonist.** The combining of a drug and its receptor causes a particular drug action, and the result of this interaction produces a particular drug effect. Examples of drug effect include stimulation, depression, irritation, and cell death. Sometimes a drug replaces a substance that is missing or is in short supply in the body.

A dose-response curve displays the relationship between the dose of a drug and the response achieved. The dose-response curve shows that as increasing doses of a drug are given, an increase in response occurs until a maximum response or plateau is achieved. *No drug produces a single effect.* Low doses of a narcotic may be used to treat diarrhea, higher doses may be used for pain relief, and even higher doses may depress the respiratory system. The *potency* of a drug is described as the amount of a drug needed to produce a desired response and is represented by a position along the dose-response curve.

The **efficacy** of a drug represents the degree to which a drug produces its desired response in a patient. Once the efficacy level of a drug is reached, increasing the dose does not improve the effect.

The *therapeutic index* is the relationship between a drug's ability to achieve the desired effect compared with its tendency to produce toxic effects. The therapeutic index is expressed as the ratio between the LD_{50} and the ED_{50} and quantitates the drug's margin of safety. The LD_{50} is the dose of a drug that is lethal to 50% of the animals in a dose-related trial. The ED_{50} is the dose of a drug that produces the desired effect in 50% of the animals in a dose-related trial. The index is calculated as follows:

$$\text{Therapeutic index} = LD_{50}/ED_{50}$$

The larger the number produced by dividing the LD_{50} by the ED_{50}, the greater the safety. Drugs with a

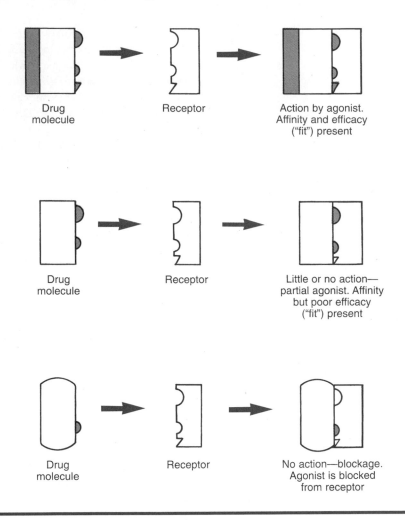

Drug molecule → Receptor → Action by agonist. Affinity and efficacy ("fit") present

Drug molecule → Receptor → Little or no action—partial agonist. Affinity but poor efficacy ("fit") present

Drug molecule → Receptor → No action—blockage. Agonist is blocked from receptor

Figure 1-8

Drug molecules must combine with specific cellular receptors to exert their effects.

narrow margin of safety (low therapeutic index) must be administered with caution to avoid toxic or fatal effects. The drugs used to treat cancer often have a low therapeutic index.

An **adverse drug reaction** is an undesirable response to a drug and can be mild to life threatening. Adverse reactions can be related to the characteristics of the drug itself, the quality or purity of the drug, and the dose of the drug administered. Phenobarbital is potentially toxic to the liver, and amphotericin B may damage the kidneys. Drugs can have carriers or vehicles that are toxic to some individuals. Some adverse reactions are allergic and can cause a range of reactions from dermatitis to anaphylactic shock. Drugs can cause changes in the skin that make it very sensitive to sunlight. This type of reaction is called *photosensitivity.*

Other types of adverse responses include abortion, liver or kidney damage, infertility, vomiting or diarrhea, and cancer. An unusual or unexpected reaction is called an *idiosyncratic drug reaction.* All adverse reactions should be reported to the drug manufacturer or the FDA. If the report is made to the drug company, the company is obligated to report the incident to the FDA.

DRUG NAMES

During the course of its testing, development, and marketing, a drug may have several names assigned. These multiple names can be a source of confusion. For practical purposes, drugs are given the following names:

1. *Chemical*—the name that describes the molecular structure of a drug. These names are scientifically very accurate but complex and are impractical to use in clinical settings.
2. *Code or laboratory*—the name given to a drug by the research and development investigators. It is used for communications between the research teams. It includes abbreviations and code numbers.
3. *Compendial*—the name listed in the *United States Pharmacopoeia (USP)*. The *USP* is the legally accepted compendium that lists drugs and standards for their quality and purity.
4. *Official*—usually the same as the compendial or generic name.
5. *Proprietary or trade*—the name chosen by the manufacturing company. When it is registered, it is the exclusive property of the company. A name that is short and easily recalled is usually picked for the proprietary name. This name is protected by federal copyright and trade name laws. On drug container labels, in package inserts, and in drug references, the proprietary name can be distinguished by a superscript R with a circle around it after the name.
6. *Generic*—the common name chosen by the company. It is not the exclusive right of the company. It may be the same as the official or compendial name. These are drugs with patents that have expired or were never patented.

The following illustration points out the use of the name categories: Ketaset, Ketaject, Ketavet, and Vetalar are proprietary names for ketamine, which is the generic and compendial name for 2-(*o*-chlorophenyl)-2-methyl-aminocyclohexanone (chemical name).

Code or laboratory names for this drug include Cl-581 and Cl-369 (Webb and Aeschbacher, 1993).

In textbooks and other scholarly works, generic names begin with a lowercase letter, and proprietary names begin with a capital letter. This practice is followed throughout this text—for example: ketamine (Ketaset).

DRUG LABELS

The Center for Veterinary Medicine of the FDA requires that drug container labels list the following items (Webb and Aeschbacher, 1993):

Drug names (both generic and trade names)
Drug concentration and quantity
Name and address of the manufacturer
The controlled substance status
The manufacturer's control or lot number
The drug's expiration date

The labeling is also required to list instructions for use of the drug and warnings of possible adverse effects of the drug. Because the label on the container usually has limited space, many manufacturers list this added information in an insert. An insert is a small folder that is placed in the box with the drug container or provided as a tear-off portion of the label.

The trade name is usually placed first on a drug label and is scripted in bold letters (Figure 1-9). The generic name typically follows the trade name in smaller print. The label must display the concentration (strength) of a drug and the total quantity in the container. Drug strength is often expressed as milligrams or units per dosage unit (mg/ml, mg/capsule, and so forth). Some drugs are sold in different concentrations with similar labels, and underdosing or overdosing can result. When the same drug is marketed in different strengths with similar labels, some companies use different sizes of bottles for the different strengths and display the concentration in bold print. Atropine and xylazine are examples of drugs marketed in different concentrations for large and small animals.

The label must include the name and address of the manufacturer of the drug. This is important in order to

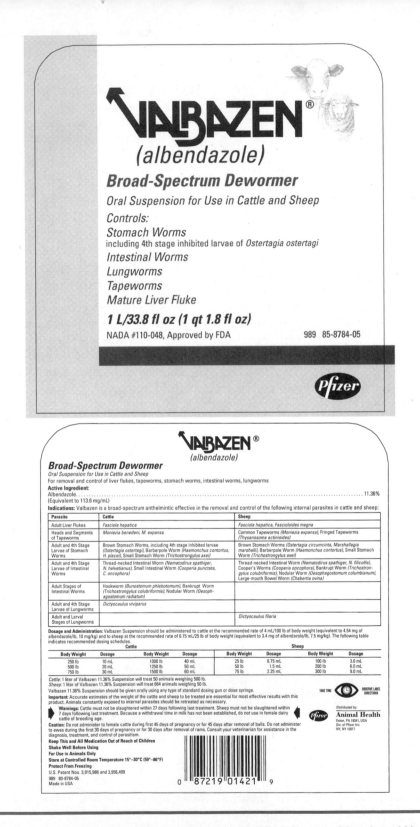

Figure 1-9

A label showing the components of a drug label as required by the FDA. (Courtesy Pfizer Animal Health.)

be able to know who to contact if adverse drug reactions occur or if other problems with the drug arise.

Drugs that have potential for abuse by humans are controlled under the Comprehensive Drug Abuse Prevention and Control Act of 1970. The Drug Enforcement Administration places drugs into categories or schedules according to their potential for abuse and requires that the label of a container for a controlled substance be identified with a capital C followed by a Roman numeral identifying which of the five categories is appropriate. This labeling must be placed in the upper right-hand side of the container label.

Drug labels are required to list an expiration date for the product. This is to ensure that dispensed drugs have the safety and efficacy that was intended. Drugs are tested during development to determine the effective shelf life and the proper storage conditions. Some drugs must be stored under refrigeration, and others must be stored in light-resistant (amber) containers to make sure that the shelf life is not shortened. *Storage instructions on the label should be followed carefully to validate the expiration date.*

All drugs must have a lot or batch number on the label. The purpose of the lot number is to allow the manufacturer to know the exact time and date of production of the product as well as the quality and quantity of the ingredients used. The lot number is determined by the manufacturer and may consist of numbers or numbers and letters.

Another feature that is often found on a drug label but not required by FDA is the national drug code (NDC) number. The NDC is a 10-digit number that identifies the manufacturer or distributor, the drug formulation, and the package size.

Drugs that are intended for animals that may be consumed by humans must have the appropriate **withdrawal time** listed on the insert or label.

DEVELOPMENT AND APPROVAL OF NEW DRUGS

The federal government requires that before any new animal health product can be marketed, it must be proved through rigorous testing that it is both safe and efficacious. This testing requires the expenditure of much time and money. It has been estimated that on average 7 to 10 years of testing is required at a cost of $15 to $20 million to the manufacturer to get a new animal drug on the market. The steps in this process are outlined in Figure 1-10.

The development of new animal health products begins in the research and development department of the manufacturing company. The company, through its research and development department, wants to ensure that the drug is not only safe and effective for animals but also safe for the environment and the people who will consume products from animals treated with the product. The company wants to be certain that a market is available for the product, that it will be able to produce it at a cost that is reasonable for consumers, and that it will be able to make a profit from its sales.

REGULATORY AGENCIES

The three agencies of the United States government that regulate animal health products include the FDA, the Environmental Protection Agency (EPA), and the United States Department of Agriculture (USDA). The FDA regulates the development and approval of animal drugs and feed additives through its Center for Veterinary Medicine, the EPA regulates the development and approval of animal topical pesticides, and the USDA regulates the development and approval of biologics (vaccines, serums, antitoxins, and similar products).

The Food Animal Residue Avoidance Databank

The Food Animal Residue Avoidance Databank (FARAD) is a project sponsored by the USDA Extension Service that provides a repository of residue avoidance information and educational materials. FARAD provides expert advice concerning the avoidance of drug residues in an effort to achieve its goal of producing "safe foods of animal origin." FARAD produces a compendium of FDA-approved drugs that provides information about withholding times for milk and preslaughter withdrawal times for meat. The information in this compendium is available on-line (www.farad.org), and additional direct telephone ac-

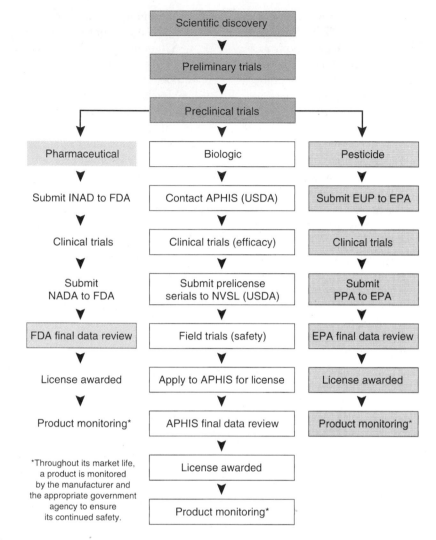

Figure 1-10

A flow chart of the animal health product approval process. *INAD,* Investigational New Animal Drug; *FDA,* Food and Drug Administration; *APHIS,* Animal and Plant Health Inspection Service; *NVSL,* National Veterinary Services Laboratory; *USDA,* United States Department of Agriculture; *EUP,* Experimental Use Permit; *EPA,* Environmental Protection Agency; *PPA,* Pesticide Permit Application. (From Etchison, K. [ed.]: The path to approval: How research discoveries become federally licensed products. Top. Vet. Med. 4[1]:13, 1993.)

cess is provided for situations in which the on-line information is not sufficient.

STEPS IN THE DEVELOPMENT OF A NEW DRUG

Preliminary Trials. When a new drug or product shows potential for development by a company, it is first subjected to a series of preliminary trials. The company wants to know whether the product will actually perform as expected, whether it has potential harmful side effects, and whether it will be profitable to market. If these concerns are satisfactorily answered, testing begins. First the product is tested on simple organisms such as bacteria, yeasts, or molds in a laboratory. Computer models may also be used to simulate animal models at this time.

Preclinical (Animal Safety) Trials. If the preliminary trials prove satisfactory, the next step involves preclinical trials. These trials are usually carried out using laboratory animals to determine information about appropriate doses of the drug. A few target (intended species) animals may be used as well. If the results of the preclinical trials are satisfactory, the company then notifies the appropriate government agency that a new drug is under investigation. It does this by filing an Investigational New Animal Drug (INAD) application with the FDA. If the product is a pesticide, it files for an Experimental Use Permit (EUP) with the EPA. If a biologic is involved, the company contacts the Animal and Plant Health Inspection Service of the USDA.

Clinical Trials. By this time, the manufacturer has compiled enough information to decide whether the product should be tested in the target species. The tests must prove that the drug is safe and effective. Potential toxic and adverse side effects must be determined. Tissue residue and withdrawal time information must be accumulated if the product will be used in food-producing animals. Possible toxicity to pregnant animals is determined, along with information about the potential production of birth defects (teratogenesis). Shelf life studies must also be conducted to establish expiration date data. Results of the studies are validated through the use of statistical analysis.

Submit a New Animal Drug Application. If the manufacturing company decides to market the drug,

it then must file a New Animal Drug Application (NADA) with the FDA. Procedures for pesticides and biologics are similar.

Final Review by the FDA. Volumes of research are submitted to the FDA, EPA, or USDA for review. If the appropriate agency validates the information, approval and a license for manufacture are granted.

Product Monitoring. As long as a product is marketed, it is constantly monitored by the company and the government to ensure its continuing safety and efficacy.

The *Green Book*. The *Green Book* is a list of all animal drug products that have been approved by the FDA for safety and effectiveness. This list was first published in 1989 as a cooperative, non-profit effort between the USDA and Virginia Polytechnic Institute and State University. It is funded through an inter-agency agreement between the USDA and the FDA. Monthly updates are made to the list, and the entire list is published each January. The *Green Book* is available electronically at the FDA-CVM World Wide Web site (http://www.fda.gov/cvm/fda/greenbook/greenbook.html).

FEDERAL LAWS RELATING TO DRUG DEVELOPMENT AND USE

In 1906, Congress passed the first legislation regulating the manufacture, use, and sales of drugs. Table 1-1 provides a list of the major acts of legislation passed before the 1990s and the significance of each.

THE ANIMAL MEDICINAL USE CLARIFICATION ACT

In 1994, Congress passed the Animal Medicinal Drug Use Clarification Act (AMDUCA). This legislation made extralabel use of approved veterinary drugs legal under certain well-defined conditions. The act came about as a result of lobbying efforts by the AVMA and other groups in response to the FDA tightening its policies concerning extralabel use of veterinary drugs. Previously, veterinarians had been permitted to use any drug as long as it could be legally obtained, used according to sound professional practice, and left no

TABLE I-I Federal Laws Regulating the Use of Pharmaceuticals

Date	Legislation	Summary
1958	Food additives amendment	Regulation of substances added to food for human consumption. Delaney clause provided that no additive may be added if it causes cancer in humans or animals.
1962	Kefauver-Harris amendment	Provided for safety and effectiveness of drugs by strict control of manufacturing companies.
1968	Animal drug amendment	Provided regulations for new animal drugs.
1970	Comprehensive drug abuse and control act	Placed controlled substances into schedules according to their potential for abuse. Called for registration of veterinarians.

residue in food products (Coppoc, 1996). However, public concerns over food safety issues related to residues of substances such as diethylstilbestrol, chloramphenicol, and antibiotics caused the FDA to issue Compliance Policy Guidelines (CPGs) that made extralabel use illegal. Even though the FDA would not routinely prosecute veterinarians for extralabel use after the issuance of the CPGs, practitioners were nonetheless placed in the position of breaking federal law to meet their obligations to animals and their owners. AMDUCA allows veterinarians to legally select the most efficacious drug for their patients. The AVMA issued an AMDUCA *Guidance Brochure* in 1998. The brochure outlines requirements of the act and provides and algorithm for determining when extralabel use is appropriate.

COMPOUNDING OF VETERINARY DRUGS

FDA-approved drugs are labeled for specific therapeutic uses in defined species. Since veterinarians must treat a variety of animal species that may vary greatly in size, it is not always possible to use an approved drug for every clinical situation, therefore veterinarians may need to dilute or combine (compound) existing medications. For example, it may be in the best interest of a horse to combine more than one drug in a single syringe to minimize the number of injections. It also may be essential to dilute an injectable agent to obtain an appropriate concentration for a bird or mouse or to prepare an antidote (e.g., sodium sulfate) that is not commercially available. None of these activities would be permitted under a strict interpretation of FDA regulations, which traditionally have not distinguished the act of diluting or combining drugs from manufacturing. Any alteration of a drug by a veterinarian or his or her employee that changes the concentration of the active ingredient, the preservatives, or the vehicles results in a new animal drug subject to the FDA approval process (Davidson, 1997). Recognizing the difficulties imposed by these regulations, the FDA issued a Compliance Policy Guide (608.400) in 1996 to better define the conditions under which compounding would be permitted. Those conditions include, but may not be limited to, (1) the identification of a legitimate veterinary medical need; (2) a need for an appropriate regimen for a particular species, size, gender, or medical condition of the patient; (3) no approved animal or human drug that when used as labeled will treat the condition, and (4) too long a time interval for securing the drug to treat the condition.

THE VETERINARY FEED DIRECTIVE

Congress established the Veterinary Feed Directive (VFD) as a part of the Animal Drug Availability Act of 1996. The VFD established a new category of drugs "as an alternative to prescription status" for certain antimicrobial animal feed additives. Before this directive, all commercially available animal drugs for use in medicated feeds were available on an over-the-counter basis. The VFD therefore provides the FDA Center of Veterinary Medicine (CVM) greater control over the use of some new animal feed additives.

The use of VFD drugs requires a valid veterinarian-patient-client relationship and the issuance of a VFD form by a veterinarian. The animal producer must secure the VFD form from the veterinarian and present it to a feed mill to receive the medicated feed.

DISPENSING VERSUS PRESCRIBING DRUGS

Although most physicians prescribe drugs, most veterinarians dispense them. The primary reason why veterinarians maintain a pharmacy in their hospitals is that drug sales represent an important source of income. Food animal practitioners in particular use profit from drug sales to supplement their income because it may be difficult for them to charge sufficiently for their time. Another reason veterinarians dispense drugs from their hospitals is that human pharmacies usually do not stock veterinary drugs. A few drugs are available only from human pharmacies, and others are used so infrequently that veterinarians find it more practical and economical to write a prescription for them.

MARKETING OF DRUGS

Pharmaceutical products are purchased by veterinarians from various sources. Some products are purchased directly from the manufacturer by telephone or mail, and others are obtained from sales representatives (detail persons) who call on the veterinary clinics. Distributors (wholesalers) are companies that buy products from many different manufacturers and then resell the products to veterinarians through sales representatives or by phone. Generic drug companies sell generic products under their own label, usually by mail order.

Most of the pharmaceutical manufacturers are large companies that have separate divisions; one division sells products to veterinarians only, and the other sells over-the-counter products. It should be noted that the statement "sold to graduate veterinarians only" on a drug label does not mean that the product is a prescription drug; it only indicates a sales policy of the company. In a few instances, the same product is sold under different labels to veterinarians only and to over-the-counter markets. Some feed stores and cooperatives are able to sell over-the-counter products (similar to products sold by veterinarians) to consumers at prices lower than veterinarians can charge because of the quantity purchasing power of the stores. This can be a source of tension between veterinarians and the retail markets.

REFERENCES

Davidson, G.: Pharmacy update: New FDA policy gives clear guidance for compounding. Vet. Tech. 18(3):195-201, 1997.

Coppoc, G.L. (1996, Spring). Extralabel drug use and compounding in veterinary medicine: http://www.vet.purdue.edu/depts/bms/courses/clinph/cmpdextr.htm

Upson, D.W.: General principles. In Upson, D.W. (ed.): Handbook of Clinical Veterinary Pharmacology. Dan Upson Enterprises, Manhattan, KS, 1988.

Webb, A.I., Aeschbacher, G.: Animal drug container labels: A guide to the reader. J.A.V.M.A. 202:1591-1599, 1993.

Williams, B.R., Baer, C.: Introduction to pharmacology. In Williams, B.R., Baer, C. (eds.): Essentials of Clinical Pharmacology in Nursing. Springhouse Corporation, Springhouse, PA, 1990.

■ Review Questions

1. Define the following terms:
   a. Agonist _____
   b. Contraindication

   _____

   c. Efficacy _____
   d. Over-the-counter drug

   _____

   e. Prescription drug

   _____

   f. Receptor _____
   g. Therapeutic index

   _____

   h. Withdrawal time

   _____

   i. Veterinarian-client-patient relationship

   _____

2. List four sources of drugs used in veterinary medicine.

   _____

3. What are four components of a drug regimen?

   _____

4. Discuss the conditions that must be met before a valid veterinarian-client-patient relationship can be shown to exist. _____

5. Discuss the responsibilities of a veterinary technician in the administration of drug orders.

   _____

6. Describe the sequence of events that a drug undergoes from administration to excretion.

   _____

7. List 11 possible routes for administering a drug to a patient and discuss the advantages and/or disadvantages of each. _____

8. List some of the factors that influence drug absorption. _____

9. Most biotransformation of drugs occurs in which of the following?
   a. Kidney
   b. Liver
   c. Spleen
   d. Pancreas

10. Most drug excretion occurs via which of the following?
    a. Kidneys
    b. Liver
    c. Spleen
    d. Intestine

11. Drugs usually produce their effects by combining with specific cellular_____.

12. The drug name that is chosen by the manufacturer and that is the exclusive property of that company is called _____.

13. What are six items that must be on a drug label?

    _____

14. What are three government agencies that regulate the development, approval, and use of animal health products? _____

15. Why do many veterinary clinics dispense rather than prescribe most of the drugs that they use?

    _____

16. Describe the marketing of animal health products.

    _____

17. All FDA-approved veterinary drugs are listed in the publication entitled

    _____.

18. What is the purpose of FARAD?

    _____

19. Extralabel veterinary drug use was made legal (under prescribed circumstances) by what act of Congress?

    _____

20. Define compounding.

    _____

Routes and Techniques of Drug Administration

LEARNING OBJECTIVES

After studying this chapter, you should be able to:

1. Be familiar with the many types of drug forms available
2. Know and understand the five rights for administering medication
3. Understand the types of syringes and needles available and know their common uses
4. Correctly read doses in a syringe
5. Know the techniques for administering medications, the common routes, and how to document the administration
6. Know what is involved in preparing a prescription and documenting the medical record
7. Understand U.S. Drug Enforcement Administration (DEA) requirements for keeping inventory and dispensing controlled substances

KEY TERMS

Counterirritant An agent that produces superficial irritation intended to relieve some other irritation.

Cream A semi-solid preparation of oil, water, and a medicinal agent.

Elixir A hydroalcoholic liquid containing sweeteners, flavoring, and a medicinal agent.

Emulsion A medicinal agent consisting of oily substances dispersed in an aqueous medium with an additive to stabilize the dispersion.

Liniment A medicine in an oily, soapy, or alcoholic vehicle to be rubbed on the skin to relieve pain or to act as a counterirritant.

Ointment A semi-solid preparation containing medicinal agents for application to the skin or eyes.

Parenteral Administration by a route other than the alimentary canal (e.g., intramuscular, subcutaneous, intravenous).

Speculum An instrument for dilating a body orifice or cavity to allow visual inspection.

Suspension A preparation of solid particles dispersed in a liquid but not dissolved in it.

DOSAGE FORMS

Drugs are manufactured in many different forms. Some drugs are prepared in several different forms, but others may be available in only one type of preparation. These preparations are designed to provide a convenient means of administering a drug to a patient. Drug preparations are designed for oral administration, **parenteral** injection, inhalation, or topical application.

The most common type of preparation is for oral administration. These drugs are generally easy to administer, have long shelf lives, and are manufactured uniformly with respect to drug content. Tablets are the most commonly used oral form. They may be scored or unscored (Figure 2-1). A scored tablet can be easily broken to provide a smaller dose. Some tablets, which generally contain drug types that may be irritating to the stomach or destroyed by gastric juices, may be enteric coated. Capsules are containers made of gelatin and glycerin. They contain a powder drug form or occasionally a liquid (Figure 2-1). An advantage of capsules is that the drug, which may have an unpalatable taste, does not come in contact with the oral mucosa during administration. Capsules cannot provide a smaller dose than for what they were manufactured.

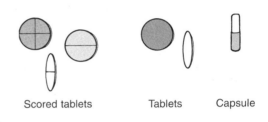

Scored tablets   Tablets   Capsule

Figure 2-1

Tablets and capsules are the most common forms of oral medications.

Boluses are large rectangular tablets. These are used to provide large animals (e.g., cattle, horses, and sheep) with a larger dose that may be easily swallowed. Liquid preparations for oral administration may be found in several different forms (e.g., mixtures, emulsions, syrups, and elixirs). Mixtures are aqueous solutions or **suspensions** for oral administration. Because of the separation of contents, a suspension should always be shaken well prior to use in order to provide a uniform dose. Syrups, often used as cough remedies, contain the drug and a flavoring in a concentrated solution of sugar in water or other aqueous liquid. **Elixirs** usually

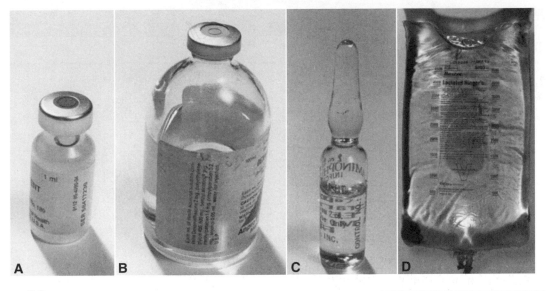

Figure 2-2

Parenteral medications are supplied in single-dose vials *(A)*, multidose vials *(B)*, ampules *(C)*, and large-volume bottles or bags used for intravenous administration *(D)*.

are a hydroalcoholic liquid containing sweeteners, flavoring, and a medicinal agent. **Emulsions** consist of oily substances dispersed in an aqueous medium with an additive to stabilize the dispersion.

Two types of dosage forms are available for parenteral administration: injections and implants. Injections may be supplied in single-dose vials, multidose vials, ampules, or large-volume bottles to which an intravenous infusion set may be attached (Figure 2-2). Vials are bottles sealed with a rubber diaphragm. They can contain a single dose or several doses. Once a single-dose vial has been opened, it must be discarded after one use or dose. Multidose vials contain preservatives that enable them to have longer shelf lives, and they may be used for more than one dose. Ampules contain a single dose of medication in a small glass container with a thin neck, which is usually scored so that it can be snapped off. Some drugs are unstable in solution and need to be reconstituted with sterile water or other diluent and used immediately for injection (Procedure 2-1).

TABLE 2-1 Species and Commonly Used Needle Gauges	
Species	**Needle Gauge**
Swine	16, 18
Cattle	16, 18
Horses	16, 18, 20
Dogs	20, 21, 22, 25
Cats	22, 25
Small exotics	23, 25, 27

Syringes and needles are used for parenteral administration of drugs (Box 2-1). These must be clean and sterile, and the needles must be sharp. Drugs to be given by injection should not be stored in syringes for any length of time before administration, because some drugs may absorb into the syringe, resulting in an inadequate dose. Table 2-1, above, lists commonly used

Text continued on p. 31

Procedure 2-1

Reconstitution of a Medication

MATERIALS NEEDED

Syringe of adequate size for the amount of diluent with a needle attached
70% isopropyl alcohol
Cotton swab

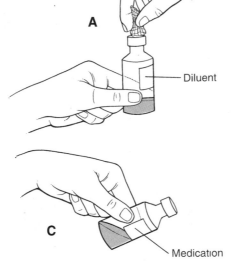

A

Diluent

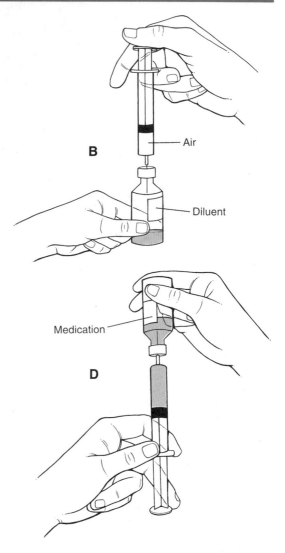

B — Air

Diluent

Medication

C

D

Medication

Figure 2-3

PROCEDURE

1. Clean the rubber diaphragm of the medication vial and the diluent vial with an alcohol swab (Figure 2-3, A).
2. Remove the needle cap and pull back on the plunger to fill the barrel with air equal to the desired amount of diluent. Inject the air into the vial of diluent to create positive pressure and to ease withdrawal (Figure 2-3, B). Invert the diluent vial and withdraw the desired amount of diluent.
3. Inject the diluent into the medication vial and withdraw the syringe and needle. Shake the vial to mix well (Figure 2-3, C).

4. Positive pressure may be created in the freshly mixed medication vial before withdrawing the desired amount of medication. Once the medication has been withdrawn (Figure 2-3, D), label the syringe, if needed, or administer the drug to the patient. After withdrawing the patient's medication, dispose of the vial or store it according to the label.

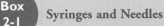

Box 2-1	Syringes and Needles

Syringes

Syringes are available in various sizes and styles. The most commonly used sizes are 3, 6, 12, 20, 35, and 60 ml. Syringes are available with or without a needle attached. The tip of the syringe where the needle attaches can be one of four types: Luer-Lok tip (Figure 2-4, *A*), slip tip (Figure 2-4, *B*), eccen-

tric tip (Figure 2-4, *C*), or catheter tip (Figure 2-4, *D*). Each type of tip has its own advantages and disadvantages and is often chosen because of personal preference. A complete syringe consists of a plunger, barrel, hub, needle, and dead space (Figure 2-5). The dead space is the area in which fluid remains when the plunger is completely depressed.

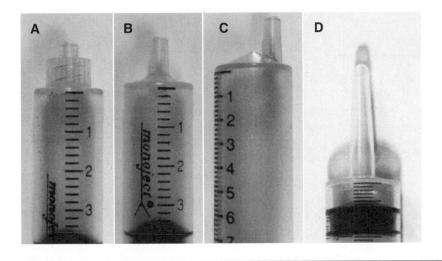

Figure 2-4

Syringes are available with different tips such as Luer-Lok tip *(A)*, slip tip *(B)*, eccentric tip *(C)*, and catheter tip *(D)*. (Courtesy Sherwood Medical, St. Louis, MO.)

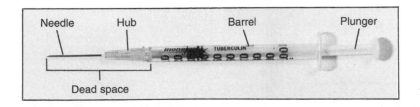

Figure 2-5

The parts of a needle and syringe. (Courtesy Sherwood Medical, St. Louis, MO.)

Continued

> **Box 2-1**   Syringes and Needles—cont'd

Tuberculin Syringe

A tuberculin syringe (Figure 2-6) holds up to 1 ml of medication. It usually is available with a 25-gauge or smaller needle attached. This syringe is commonly used for injections of less than 1 ml and for small patients.

Multidose Syringe

A multidose syringe (Figure 2-7) is commonly used for large animals when several animals require the same injection. It allows the user to set the dose and give it repeatedly until the barrel is empty of medication. This type of syringe may be disassembled and disinfected for reuse.

Insulin Syringe

An insulin syringe (Figure 2-8) is usually supplied with a 25-gauge needle, and unlike other syringes, it has no dead space. The syringe is divided into units instead of milliliters and should be used only for insulin injection.

Figure 2-6

A tuberculin syringe with needle attached. (Courtesy Sherwood Medical, St. Louis, MO.)

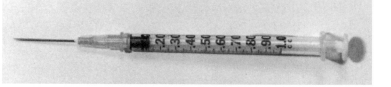

Figure 2-7

A multidose syringe.

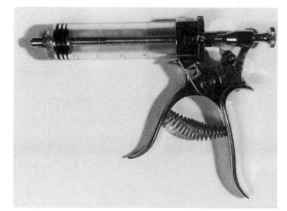

Figure 2-8

An insulin syringe with needle attached. (Courtesy Sherwood Medical, St. Louis, MO.)

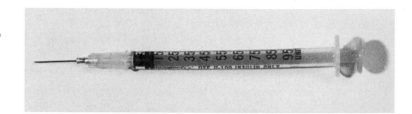

Box 2-1	Syringes and Needles—cont'd

Figure 2-9, *A* to *H,* shows examples of syringes with medication and how to read the amount of medication in each syringe.

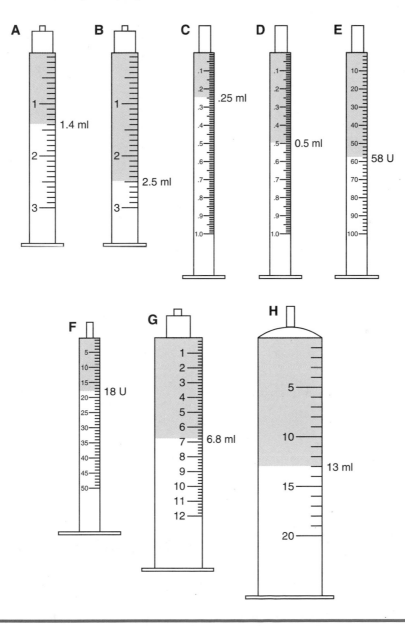

Figure 2-9

Examples of how to read amounts of medication contained in a syringe.

Continued

Box 2-1   *Syringes and Needles—cont'd*

Needles

Needles are available in various sizes and styles, but all needles have the following three parts: hub, shaft, and bevel (Figure 2-10). Needle sizes vary by gauge and by length. The gauge refers to the inside diameter of the shaft: the larger the gauge number, the smaller the diameter. The length of the needle is measured from the tip of the hub to the end of the shaft. Lengths longer than 1 inch are usually used in large animals and occasionally for biopsy. The bevel is the angle of the opening at the needle tip. It is often helpful when performing venipuncture to have the beveled side of the needle facing up before inserting the needle into the patient.

Bleeding needles (Figure 2-11) are 3 inches long, are large gauge (16 to 14 gauge), and are usually used for obtaining blood from cattle and swine. These needles are made of stainless steel and are reusable after proper cleaning and disinfection. Biopsy needles (Figure 2-12) are used for obtaining bone marrow or soft tissue and organ specimens. These needles vary in size and styles.

Figure 2-10

A needle consists of three parts—hub, shaft, and bevel.

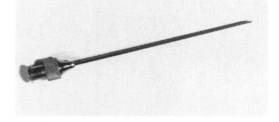

Figure 2-11

A 3-inch stainless steel bleeding needle.

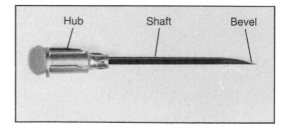

Figure 2-12

A stainless steel biopsy needle.

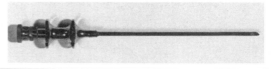

needle gauges and the species in which they are used to inject medication.

Implants are very hard, sterile pellets that contain a medicinal agent. The pellets are inserted under the skin, where they dissolve very slowly. Growth hormones are commonly manufactured in this form for use in cattle.

Topical medications are available in several forms. **Liniments** are medicinal preparations intended to be rubbed on the skin as a **counterirritant** or to relieve pain. Lotions are liquid suspensions or solutions with soothing substances to be applied to the skin. An **ointment** is a semi-solid preparation containing medicinal agents to be applied to the skin or eyes. **Creams** are semi-solid preparations of oil, water, and a medicinal agent; the water evaporates after application and leaves the drug and a thin oily film on the skin. Dusting powders are mixtures of drugs in a powder form to be applied topically. These powders may have adsorbent (cornstarch) or lubricant (talcum) properties. Aerosols are drugs incorporated in a suitable solvent and packaged under pressure with a propellant. Dusting powders and aerosols are common forms for some topical insecticides and wound dressings.

Microencapsulation is a drug form that stabilizes substances commonly considered unstable. When the drug's active ingredients are microencapsulated, a protective environment is formed against harmful substances and improves the stability of the product. Microencapsulation completely masks the flavor of the drug, allowing an animal to receive the drug without being able to taste or smell the ingredients.

DRUG PRESERVATIVES AND SOLVENTS

In addition to the active ingredient, many drugs contain organic or inorganic agents as additives or pharmaceutic aids. These inactive (or inert) ingredients facilitate tableting, improve solubility, or increase stability. Although the amount of inert ingredients is usually small, they can cause adverse effects or a patient may be sensitive to the ingredients or may smell the ingredients.

Parenterally administered drugs often contain chemical preservatives to prevent destruction and loss of potency through oxidation or hydrolysis. Drugs that are sensitive to ultraviolet light are usually contained in amber bottles to prevent light penetration. They may also contain buffer systems to decrease changes in hydrogen ion concentration. Multidose vials often contain preservatives to prevent microbial contamination and to help prevent deterioration of the drug formulation and the possibility of causing iatrogenic bacterial or fungal infections when administered. Because the amount of preservative in the formulation is at an optimal concentration, it is very important that any dilutions of these drug formulations be used immediately. Dilution of the drug decreases the effectiveness of the preservatives. Although most drugs are water-soluble, some may need additives to increase solubility. Glycols are one example of additives used to increase solubility. Because ethylene glycols are too toxic, propylene and polyethylene glycols are generally used for this purpose.

DRUG ADMINISTRATION

Administration of drugs for therapeutic purposes is initiated by a veterinarian. The role of the technician is to administer the drug to the patient on the order of a veterinarian. When doing this, a technician must always follow the "five rights":

Right patient
Right drug—check label three times before administering the drug
Right dose
Right route
Right time and frequency

By following these rules, a technician can efficiently and effectively medicate a patient.

ORAL MEDICATIONS

The most common forms of drug therapy are tablets and capsules. These are easily administered (Procedure 2-2) and are sometimes used in conjunction with other drug forms.

Procedure 2-2

Oral Administration of Tablets or Capsules for Dogs and Cats

MATERIALS NEEDED

Medication in tablet or capsule form
Pilling gun (optional) (Figure 2-13)

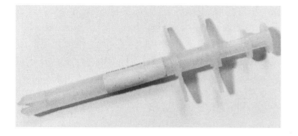

Figure 2-13 ━━━━━━━━

Example of a small-animal pilling gun.

PROCEDURE

1. Hold the animal's upper jaw with one hand and apply pressure against the upper premolars to cause the mouth to open.
2. Push the medication over the tongue of the animal with the other hand or the pilling gun (Figure 2-14).

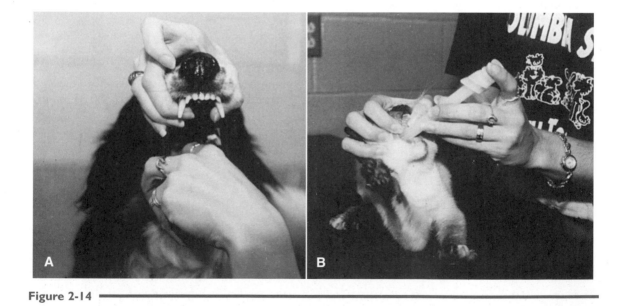

Figure 2-14 ━━━━━━━━

Procedure 2-2

Oral Administration of Tablets or Capsules for Dogs and Cats—cont'd

3. Close the animal's mouth.
4. Initiate swallowing by blowing into the animal's nose or rubbing its throat (Figure 2-15).

TECHNICIAN'S NOTES

Coating the tablet or capsule with a palatable substance such as Cat Lax, peanut butter, or canned food may help in pilling difficult animals.

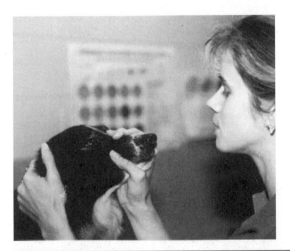

Figure 2-15

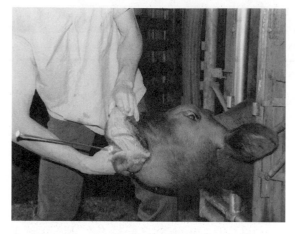

Figure 2-16 ━━━━━━━

A balling gun used to administer a bolus to large animals.

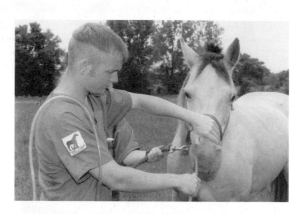

Figure 2-18 ━━━━━━━

A large-animal stomach tube may be used to administer liquid medications to cattle or horses.

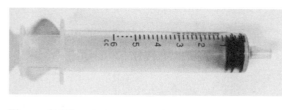

Figure 2-17 ━━━━━━━

A syringe without a needle may be used to administer oral liquid medication.

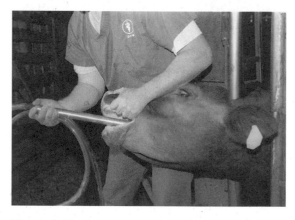

Figure 2-19 ━━━━━━━

A Frick speculum can be used to facilitate passage of the stomach tube through the mouth of cattle.

In large animals, a balling gun (Figure 2-16) is used to administer boluses. With proper restraint, this is usually not too difficult.

Liquid oral medications may be administered to small animals through a syringe with the needle removed (Procedure 2-3 and Figure 2-17) or in some instances through an orogastric or nasogastric tube. Most liquid medications are made palatable to ease administration. Oral liquid medications are commonly used in exotics and may be administered through the drinking water or an orogastric tube. In large animals, a stomach tube is usually used for administering oral liquid medications (Figure 2-18). In cattle, the stomach tube is passed through a Frick **speculum** (Figure 2-19).

Procedure 2-3

Oral Administration of Oral Liquid Medication with a Syringe for Dogs and Cats

MATERIALS NEEDED

Syringe with the needle removed or oral dose syringe
Oral medication in liquid form

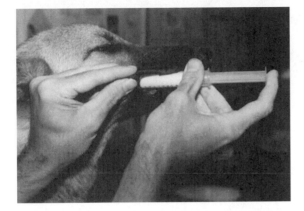

Figure 2-20

PROCEDURE

1. Fill syringe with the calculated amount of medication.
2. Tilt the animal's head up slightly.
3. Insert the tip of the syringe into the animal's cheek pouch (Figure 2-20).
4. Administer the medication slowly.

> **TECHNICIAN'S NOTES**
> Attachment of a J-12 Teat Infusion Cannula (Jorgenson Laboratories) is handy for administering oral liquid medications.

PARENTERAL MEDICATIONS

Parenteral administration, or injection, of liquid medications may be used alone or in conjunction with other forms of medication. Some conditions are unfavorable for oral administration, and some drugs are available only for parenteral administration. There are 10 routes for parenteral administration of drugs (see Chapter 1). The most common routes for injection are intramuscular, subcutaneous, and intravenous (Figures 2-21 to 2-23). A technician must be aware of the proper route of administration for each drug. The routes of administration are usually listed on the drug label or package insert. Complications may occasionally develop after parenteral administration of a drug. If any complications are observed, they should immediately be reported to the veterinarian. Some of these complications are irritation, necrosis, or infection of the injection site. Allergic reactions to the medications may also occur. Care should be taken when administering intramuscular injections to avoid nerve damage or inadvertent injection into a vein or artery. The most common complications of intraperitoneal injections are damage to the abdominal viscera and peritonitis.

Proper administration involves knowing what equipment is needed, how to calculate the dose, and the proper method for withdrawing and administering the medication (Procedure 2-4).

IV administration allows rapid, effective drug administration (Procedure 2-5). The most common uses of IV therapy are maintaining and restoring fluid and electrolyte balance, administering drugs, transfusing blood, and delivering parenteral nutrition. IV admin-

Text continued on p. 40

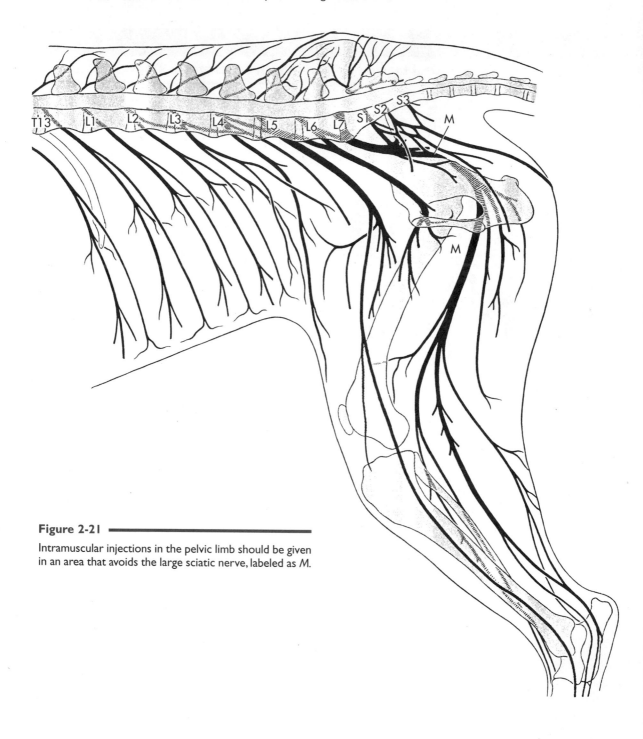

Figure 2-21 ━━━━━━━━━━━

Intramuscular injections in the pelvic limb should be given
in an area that avoids the large sciatic nerve, labeled as *M*.

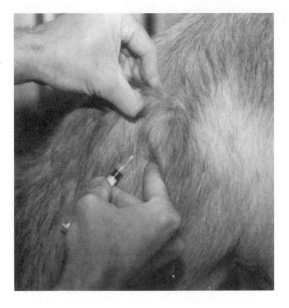

Figure 2-22 ━━━━━━━━━━━━━━━━
Subcutaneous injection.

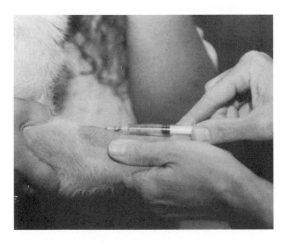

Figure 2-23 ━━━━━━━━━━━━━━━━
Intravenous injection.

Procedure 2-4

Parenteral Administration of Medications—Intramuscular or Subcutaneous

MATERIALS NEEDED

Syringe and needle (Figure 2-24)
Parenteral medication
Cotton swabs
70% isopropyl alcohol

PROCEDURE

1. If the syringe is not supplied ready-to-use, firmly attach the needle to the syringe.
2. Swab the bottle's rubber diaphragm with cotton that is saturated with alcohol.
3. Remove the needle cap, insert the needle at an angle into the rubber diaphragm, and withdraw the calculated amount.

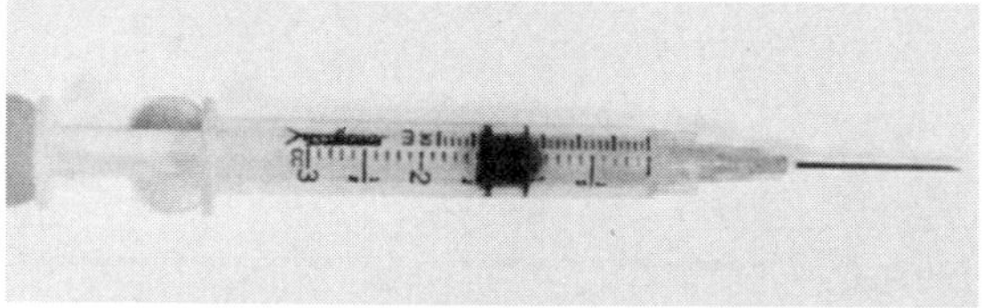

Figure 2-24

(Courtesy Sherwood Medical, St. Louis, MO.)

4. Hold the syringe with the needle pointing upward and remove the large air bubbles by briskly tapping the barrel of the syringe.
5. Release the air bubbles by slightly pushing on the syringe plunger. Carefully replace the needle cap if the medication is not to be given immediately. *Avoid contamination.*
6. Swab the injection site with another cotton swab that is saturated with alcohol.
7. Insert the needle in the appropriate site, and pull slightly on the plunger. If no blood is seen, inject the medication and remove the needle from the site. Blood indicates that a vessel has been entered; withdraw the needle and continue with the same procedure at a different site.
8. Massage the injection site to aid distribution and decrease pain.
9. Properly dispose of the syringe and needle.

TECHNICIAN'S NOTES

Injecting multidose vials with air sometimes allows easier withdrawal of the medication.

Procedure 2-5

Parenteral Administration of Medication—Intravenous Direct Bolus

MATERIALS NEEDED

Syringe containing calculated dose with needle attached

Cotton swabs

70% isopropyl alcohol or surgical scrub

Butterfly catheter (scalp vein needle, Figure 2-25)—optional

Syringe containing 3 ml of flushing solution (e.g., heparinized saline: 500 IU sodium heparin in 250 ml of normal saline)

Tape (optional)

PROCEDURE WITHOUT CATHETER

1. Clip the area over the venipuncture site, if desired.
2. Prepare the area with alcohol swabs or surgical scrub.
3. Have the restraint person hold pressure on the vein or use a tourniquet.
4. Perform venipuncture with the medication syringe and needle; if blood enters the hub of the needle, the venipuncture is successful.

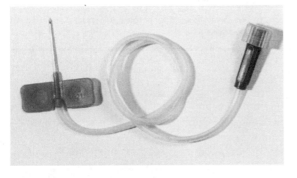

Figure 2-25
Butterfly catheter.

5. Release pressure from the vein, and proceed to inject the medication over the recommended time interval.
6. Remove the needle, and apply pressure to the site to stop bleeding.
7. A bandage made of tape and cotton may be applied if needed.

PROCEDURE WITH A BUTTERFLY CATHETER

Proceed with steps 1 through 3 described in the previous section.

1. Remove the cap from the catheter tubing and needle cover.
2. Perform venipuncture with the catheter; if it is successful, blood will return into the catheter tubing.
3. Release pressure from the vein, and allow the blood to fill the catheter tubing.
4. Remove the needle from the medication syringe, and attach the syringe hub to the catheter tubing.
5. Administer the medication at the recommended time interval.
6. Remove the needle from the syringe containing the flushing solution; remove the medication syringe from the catheter and attach the syringe containing the flushing solution.
7. Flush the catheter with 1 to 2 ml of solution to ensure that all medication is administered.
8. Remove the catheter and apply pressure to the site to stop bleeding.
9. A bandage may be applied as described earlier.
10. Properly dispose of all syringes and needles.

> **TECHNICIAN'S NOTES**
>
> Watch for swelling at the injection site; it may signal extravascular injection. Notify the veterinarian immediately if this occurs.

Procedure 2-6

Administration by Bolus with an Indwelling Intravenous Catheter

MATERIALS NEEDED

Syringe containing flushing solution (about 3 ml)
70% isopropyl alcohol
Cotton swabs
Syringe with medication and attached needle

PROCEDURE

1. Clean the cap of the indwelling catheter with an alcohol swab.
2. Insert the needle of the syringe containing the flushing solution into the catheter cap (use the smallest-gauge needle possible to help prevent a leak in the catheter cap).
3. Gently aspirate to determine correct placement of the catheter (blood entering the hub shows proper placement).
4. Inject half of the flushing solution into the catheter; observe the area over the vein for swelling.
5. Remove the syringe and needle, and carefully replace the cap to prevent contamination.
6. Insert the needle of the syringe containing the medication into the catheter cap, and inject the medication over the recommended time interval.
7. Remove the syringe and needle from the catheter.

8. Flush the catheter with the remaining flushing solution.
9. Observe the area for swelling and look for signs of discomfort; report any abnormal observations to the veterinarian.
10. Properly dispose of syringes and needles.

TECHNICIAN'S NOTES

Some hospitals may require using two syringes with flushing solution, instead of using the same syringe and needle for both flushes. Keep additional male adapter plugs (catheter caps) (Figure 2-26) in stock to replace a leaky cap.

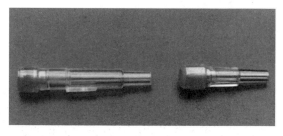

Figure 2-26

Examples of a male adapter plug. (Manufactured by Abbott Laboratories.)

istration is also used when the medication is contraindicated for other routes of administration. Sites for IV administration include the cephalic, jugular, lateral saphenous, and occasionally the femoral veins. Long-term IV therapy is best achieved with the cephalic or jugular veins.

In some cases, an animal may need repeated IV injections. The veterinarian may choose to place and maintain an indwelling IV catheter to lessen vein damage and pain for the animal (Procedures 2-6 and 2-7).

If the patient is receiving IV fluids, the Y injection site (Figure 2-28) located on the IV tubing may be used to administer medications by direct bolus (Procedure 2-8).

When medications are to be administered contin-

Procedure 2-7

Administration of Intravenous Fluids

MATERIALS NEEDED

Indwelling catheter (Figure 2-27)
Tape
70% isopropyl alcohol or surgical scrub
Infusion set
IV fluids
Clippers

PROCEDURE

1. Remove the IV tubing from the container and the protective covering from the medication bottle or bag.
2. Remove the covering of the diaphragm of the medication bag or bottle.
3. Close the clamp on the IV tubing. Remove the cap of the IV tubing spike, and insert it into the diaphragm of the medication bag or bottle.
4. Squeeze the drip chamber to allow fluid to collect in the chamber. Fill to the designated line or about half full.
5. Remove the protective cap from the end of the IV tubing, and slowly open the roller clamp to allow the fluid to clear the tubing of air. Replace the protective cap, and hang the medication bag or bottle on the IV pole near the patient.

6. Clip and prepare the chosen site for catheter placement.
7. After successful catheter placement, cap the catheter, wipe away any blood, and quickly tape in place.
8. Remove the catheter cap and the protective cap of the IV tubing and insert the end of the tubing directly into the end of the catheter, or if desired, a needle may be placed on the end of the tubing and inserted into the catheter cap.
9. Open the clamp to begin a slow drip, and lower the medication bag or bottle below the IV site to confirm correct placement.
10. Return the bottle or bag to the IV pole and set at desired flow rate.
11. Tape the tubing to the patient at the catheter site.

TECHNICIAN'S NOTES

1. Mark the fluid level and time on tape placed on the bag with a permanent marker (tape can be used on bottles); continue this procedure each time the patient is checked.
2. If any medications are added to the fluids, write the medication, time, and amount on the medication bag or tape.
3. Tape the catheter cap to the bag or bottle so that it will be ready when needed.

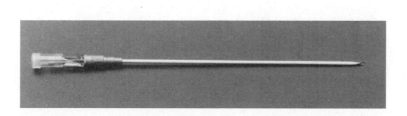

Figure 2-27

A 14-gauge indwelling catheter. (ABBOCATH is a registered trademark of Abbott Laboratories.)

Procedure 2-8

Administration By Bolus Using the Y Injection Site

MATERIALS NEEDED

Syringe with medication and the needle attached
Cotton swabs
70% isopropyl alcohol

PROCEDURE

1. Close the clamp on the infusion set.
2. Clean the Y injection site (Figure 2-28) with an alcohol swab.
3. Insert the needle of the medication syringe into the Y injection site.
4. Inject the medication over the recommended time interval.
5. Remove the medication syringe and needle.
6. Open the clamp on the infusion set. Allow enough fluid to flow through the infusion set to ensure that all medication is received; then return to the desired flow rate.
7. Properly dispose of the syringe and needle.
8. NOTE: No flushing solution is required for this procedure.

TECHNICIAN'S NOTES

To check for proper placement of the IV catheter, remove the bag of fluids from the IV pole and hold the bag and tubing below the level of the catheter (do not close the clamp on the infusion set). If blood returns into the tubing, the catheter is properly placed. Return the bag to the IV pole and continue fluid administration.

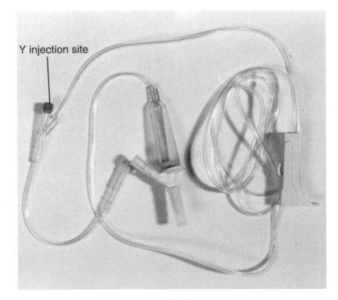

Figure 2-28
Intravenous set with Cair clamp and Y injection site.

uously and for a long period, the IV tubing needs to be changed after a 24- to 48-hour period. The medication bottle or bag needs to be replaced as often as necessary to facilitate care of the patient. It is also recommended that the indwelling IV catheter be replaced after 72 hours. If the catheter is not used continuously, it should be flushed with heparinized saline every 8 to 12 hours.

A simplex IV set is used to administer medications or fluids intravenously to large animals (Figure 2-29). This administration set may be disinfected and reused.

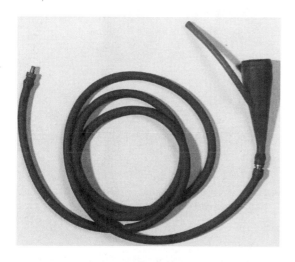

Figure 2-29 ━━━━━━
A large-animal intravenous set.

Disposable IV sets and large-volume fluid bags are available for large animals requiring longer IV therapy.

In pediatric patients and small exotics, IV medications may be administered by intraosseous cannulation. This route may also be used in larger patients when rapid administration of fluids or drugs is necessary and a vein is not readily available. Large volumes of fluid may be administered by this route if needed.

In some veterinary hospitals, continuous IV administration may be facilitated by using an infusion pump. After determining the required flow rate, the technician sets the infusion pump to deliver a constant amount of solution per minute or hour. To determine the pump settings, the technician considers the total amount of solution to be given and the time interval over which it must be infused. Because different infusion pumps have their own set of operating instructions, a technician must follow the manufacturer's guidelines to ensure adequate functioning of the infusion pump.

INHALATION MEDICATIONS

In veterinary medicine, inhalation is primarily used in maintenance anesthesia. The medication is vaporized in an anesthesia machine and delivered through an endotracheal tube, anesthesia mask, or induction chamber (Figures 2-30 to 2-32). Medications may occasionally be nebulized to treat an upper respiratory tract problem, or oxygen may be delivered in this manner to a dyspneic patient.

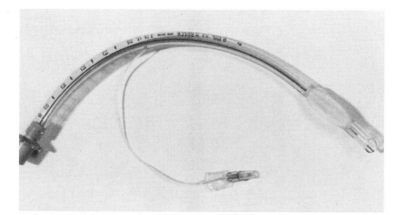

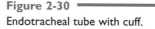

Figure 2-30 ━━━━━━
Endotracheal tube with cuff.

Figure 2-31

A small-animal anesthesia mask.

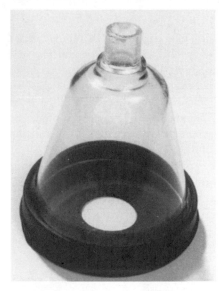

Figure 2-32

A small-animal induction chamber.

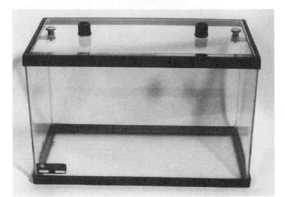

Figure 2-33

Ointment is applied to the dog's eye on the lower palpebral border.

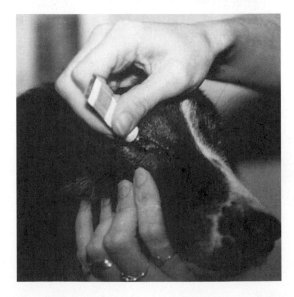

TOPICAL MEDICATIONS

The topical route of drug administration involves applying drugs to various body surfaces. Topical preparations typically provide local rather than systemic effects. Before applying topical skin medication, it is important to clip hair from the area to facilitate easier application and better absorption. It is important for the technician to observe the area after treatment and to report any adverse reactions. Client education for skin medications should involve not only the frequency of application but also the amount to be applied. Many owners seem to apply too much, a practice that is unnecessary and can be very costly with some medications.

Ophthalmic drugs can be administered to the eyes as solutions or ointments. Because of the eyes' ability to remove foreign substances rapidly, ophthalmic preparations are usually applied several times a day. Application frequency depends on the disease or disorder, the drug, and the type of formulation. When applying ophthalmic preparations, rest the hand holding the medication on the animal's head above the eye to be medicated (Figure 2-33). Drops should be placed on the inner canthus of the eye. When using an ointment, apply a small strip along the lower palpebral border. Avoid touching the eye with the applicator tip to prevent contamination of the medication container. When teaching a client how to apply eye medications, point out that the applicators have blunt tips to avoid injuring the eye if the tip does touch the eye.

Drugs applied topically to the ears are for local effect, to soften earwax and ease its removal, or to treat a superficial infection or ear mites. To aid the effectiveness of otic medication, the ears should be cleaned before medicating. Clients must be shown how to clean the ears properly and how to apply the ear medication. Explain the ear's anatomy to reassure the owner that it is difficult to reach the eardrum when swabbing the ear clean.

MEDICATION ORDERS

In a veterinary hospital, most medication orders are written or verbal. A written order may be in prescription form or noted in the medical record. Verbal orders are given directly to the technician by the veterinarian. When filling an order, the technician must be familiar with frequently used abbreviations used in drug therapy. Appendix A lists common abbreviations used in veterinary medicine. The technician must know the patient being treated, the drug needed for therapy, the dose required, the route of administration, and the frequency of administration. This information is described by the medication order. After the medication is administered to the patient, a notation should be made in the medical record describing when, what, how, and by whom the medication was administered. Any observations of the patient's progress should also be noted in the medical record (Figure 2-34). If the medication order is a prescription (Figure 2-35) to be filled for administration at home by the owner, the order should be dated and noted in the medical record (Figure 2-36). If the owner visits the hospital to refill a prescription, the medical record should be retrieved and presented to the veterinarian for approval of the refill. The same format as described earlier should be followed for dispensing the medication.

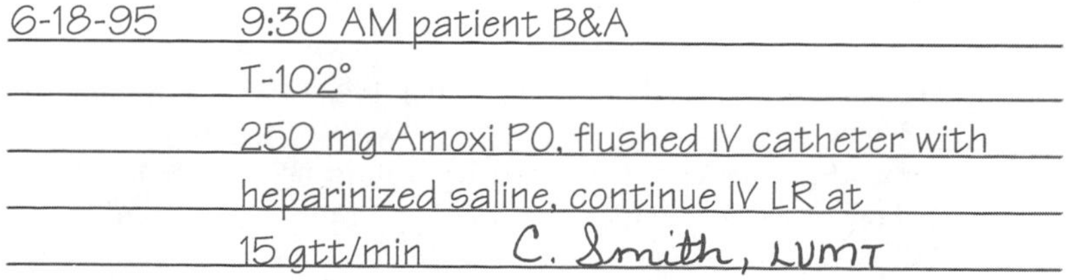

6-18-95   9:30 AM patient B&A
           T-102°
           250 mg Amoxi PO, flushed IV catheter with
           heparinized saline, continue IV LR at
           15 gtt/min   C. Smith, LVMT

Figure 2-34
After administering a medication to a patient, a notation should be made in the patient's medical record.

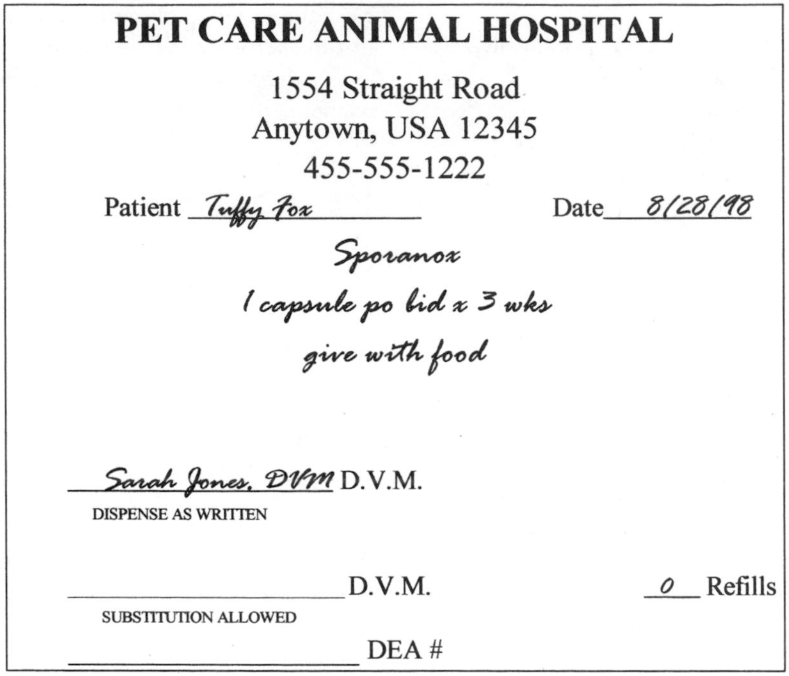

PET CARE ANIMAL HOSPITAL

1554 Straight Road
Anytown, USA 12345
455-555-1222

Patient _Tuffy Fox_   Date___8/28/98_

Sporanox
1 capsule po bid x 3 wks
give with food

Sarah Jones, DVM D.V.M.
DISPENSE AS WRITTEN

_____ D.V.M.   _0__ Refills
SUBSTITUTION ALLOWED

_____ DEA #

Figure 2-35

Sample prescription order.

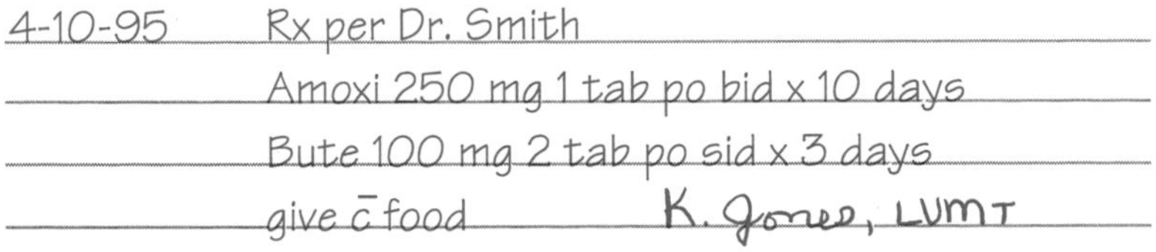

4-10-95   Rx per Dr. Smith
            Amoxi 250 mg 1 tab po bid x 10 days
            Bute 100 mg 2 tab po sid x 3 days
            give c̄ food   K. Jones, LVMT

Figure 2-36

Prescriptions should be written in the patient's medical record.

CONTROLLED SUBSTANCES

Some medications are labeled controlled substances because of their ability to become habit-forming to humans. The DEA requires that the upper right corner of the original container show a code containing a capital C, for controlled, followed by a Roman numeral of one of the five schedules that are defined by the Code of Federal Regulations. Because of the potential for these drugs to be abused, the DEA requires that these drugs be kept in an unmovable, locked area and that an inventory log showing amounts on hand and amounts used be kept (Figure 2-37). Each time a controlled drug is administered or dispensed to a patient, it must be documented in the controlled substance inventory log in addition to the patient's medical record. This documentation should include the following: (1) date, (2) owner's name, (3) patient's name, (4) drug name, (5) amount administered or dispensed, and (6) the names of the technician and

Drug: diazepam

Patient		Owner		Beginning		Administered		On hand		Initials
Toby	:	Smith	:	5 ml	:	0.2 ml	:	4.8 ml	:	BD/JC
Prissy	:	Potts	:	4.8 ml	:	0.15 ml	:	4.65 ml	:	LW/RW
Gilbert	:	Pettes	:	4.65 ml	:	0.5 ml	:	4.15	:	LW/RW
T.J.	:	Curtis	:	4.15 ml	:	0.2 ml	:	3.95	:	BD/JC

Figure 2-37

Example of a controlled substance inventory log.

veterinarian dispensing the drug. If dispensed, the dispensing label must bear the following warning: "Caution: Federal law prohibits the transfer of this drug to any person other than the patient for whom it was prescribed" (Webb and Aeschbacher, 1993). A list of the most common controlled substances used in veterinary medicine is available in Appendix D.

CLIENT EDUCATION

Technicians should be familiar with all drugs administered and dispensed. It is often the technician's duty to inform clients about how medication should be administered, why it has been prescribed, and any adverse reactions that may occur. The technician should consult the veterinarian about any questions that he/she is not able to answer. If necessary, written information about the medication should be available for the client to refer to at home.

REFERENCE

Webb A.I., Aeschbacher, G.: Animal drug container labels: A guide to the reader. J.A.V.M.A. 202:10, 1993.

■ Review Questions

1. What are the most common dosage forms of oral medications? _____

2. What should be documented in the medical record when a medication is given? _____

3. What information is required when prescribing a controlled substance? _____

4. What are the five rights for administering medication? _____

5. Describe the difference between an insulin syringe and a tuberculin syringe. _____

6. Why do some drugs require reconstitution before administration? _____

7. What role does a technician have in the dispensing of medication? _____

8. Why do ophthalmic drugs require frequent application? _____

9. Why is clipping the hair usually necessary before application of topical medication? _____

Practical Calculations in Pharmacology

LEARNING OBJECTIVES

After studying this chapter, you should be able to:

1. Develop an understanding of the systems of measurement
2. Understand how to perform conversions using the metric system and other systems of measurement
3. Know how to perform dosage calculations
4. Understand how to prepare percent concentrations

KEY TERMS

Equivalent weight 1 g molecular weight (from periodic chart) divided by the total positive valence of the material.
Milliequivalent $1/1000$ of an equivalent weight; a term used to express the concentration of electrolytes in a solution.

Molarity (M) The number of moles of a substance (solute) found in 1 L of solution.
Normality (N) Denotes a solution containing 1 g equivalent weight of solute in 1 L of solution; a normal solution.

INTRODUCTION

Veterinary technicians are often called on to prepare and administer medications to animal patients. A veterinarian's orders may call for administration of a specific number of milligrams or units of the medication (dose). The technician must then determine the quantity (in milliliters, tablets, and so forth) of the preparation that contains the appropriate dose. In other instances, the technician may be called on to calculate the dose based on a dosage rate (found in the insert or in reference books) and the animal's weight. In either case, an error in calculation can seriously affect the health of a patient. This chapter deals with the background information and applications necessary to accurately carry out a veterinarian's medication orders.

MATHEMATICS FUNDAMENTALS

It is assumed that the student using this text has a basic understanding of fractions and decimals. With these fundamentals as a background, the concepts of percent, ratio, and proportion should be reviewed before moving to the practice problems.

Percent is defined as parts per hundred. Percent is a fraction with the percent as the numerator and 100 the denominator (e.g., 5% = $5/100$). Percents may be written as decimals, fractions, and whole numbers.

Example 1: Decimal: 0.3%
  (three-tenths percent [$3/10 \div 100$])
  Fraction: $1/5$%
  (one-fifth percent [$1/5 \div 100$])
  Whole number: 5%
  (five percent [$5 \div 100$])

Percent may be changed to fractions or decimals.

Example 2: Change to a fraction:
  5% = $5/100$ = $1/20$
  Change to a decimal: .05
  5% = $5/100$ = 100 $\overline{)5.00}$ = 0.05

Note that a percent can be changed to a decimal quickly by dropping the percent sign and moving the decimal two places to the left.

Example 3: 5% = 0.05

A *ratio* is a way of expressing the relationship between a number, quantity, substance, or degree between two components. In reality, ratios are fractions with the first number in the ratio the numerator and the second number the denominator. The numbers may be placed side by side and separated by a colon or set up as a numerator/denominator (e.g., 1:5 or $1/5$). In mathematics, a ratio may be expressed as a quotient, a fraction, or a decimal; see the following:

Example 4:
  1 ÷ 5, $1/5$, 5 $\overline{)1.0}$ = 0.2

A *proportion* shows the relationship between two ratios. When setting up a proportion, the two ratios are usually separated by an = (equal) sign.

Example 5: $8:16 = 1:2$ or $\dfrac{8}{16} = \dfrac{1}{2}$

The proportions above read eight is to sixteen as one is to two. The two inner numbers in the first example (16 and 1) are called the means, and the two outer numbers (8 and 2) are called the extremes. In a true proportion the product of the means equals the product of the extremes ($16 \times 1 = 16$; $8 \times 2 = 16$). This fact makes the proportion a useful mathematical tool. When a part of the problem is unknown, X can be substituted for the unknown part in the proportion and the equation solved for X. Care must be used to ensure that the proportion is set up correctly and that the same units of measure are on both sides of the equation.

Example 6: $8:16 = 1:X$ or $\dfrac{8}{16} = \dfrac{1}{X}$

$$8X = 16$$
$$X = 2$$

Example 7: To convert 0.2 g to milligrams:

$$1000 \text{ mg}:1 \text{ g} = X \text{ mg}:0.2 \text{ g} \text{ or } \dfrac{1000 \text{ mg}}{1 \text{ g}} = \dfrac{X \text{ mg}}{0.2 \text{ g}}$$
$$X = 200 \ (1000 \times 0.2)$$

SYSTEMS OF MEASUREMENT

The first step in the successful calculation of doses is to develop an understanding of the units of measurement used to carry out the calculations. These units are components of the following three separate systems:

1. The metric system
2. The apothecary system
3. The household system

All three systems are expressed in the fundamental units of weight, volume, and length. Technicians should be able to convert values within each system and between the three systems.

THE METRIC SYSTEM

The fundamental units of measurement in the metric system are the gram (weight), the liter (volume), and the meter (length). Gram is abbreviated *g* or *gm,* liter is abbreviated *L* or *l,* and meter is abbreviated *m.* The utility of the metric system is that all units are powers of the fundamental units. Prefixes are used in combination with the fundamental units to denote smaller or larger quantities. Table 3-1 illustrates the units of measurement for the biologic sciences.

The units that are used most commonly in dosage calculations include the gram, the kilogram (kg, 1000 g), the milligram (mg, $\frac{1}{1000}$ g), and the milli-

TABLE 3-1 Units of Measure for the Biologic Sciences

Weight	Volume	Length	Multiple Power of 10
Gram (g)	Liter (L)	Meter (m)	1
Kilogram (kg)	Kiloliter (kl)	Kilometer (km)	1000
Decigram (dg)	Deciliter (dl)	Decimeter (dm)	$\frac{1}{10}$
Centigram (cg)	Centiliter (cl)	Centimeter (cm)	$\frac{1}{100}$
Milligram (mg)	Milliliter (ml)	Millimeter (mm)	$\frac{1}{1000}$
Microgram (μg)	Microliter (μl)	Micrometer (μm)	$\frac{1}{1,000,000}$
Nanogram (ng)	Nanoliter (nl)	Nanometer (nm)	$\frac{1}{1,000,000,000}$
Picogram (pg)	Picoliter (pl)	Picometer (pm)	$\frac{1}{1,000,000,000,000}$

liter (ml, $\frac{1}{1000}$ L). It should be noted that a milliliter is equivalent to the quantity of water contained in 1 cubic centimeter (cc), which is also equivalent to 1 g of weight. Therefore, we may say that for practical purposes, 1 ml = 1 cc = 1 g.

On occasion, the microgram (μg) may be used. (It should be noted that this unit may also be abbreviated as *mcg*.) Care should be taken to differentiate this abbreviation from *mg,* which looks very similar when written orders are used.

CONVERSION BETWEEN METRIC UNITS

The most fundamental way to convert between metric units is to multiply the units given by the conversion factor involving the units desired. If the desired conversion is from milligrams (mg) to grams (g), the number of milligrams given should be multiplied by the factor 1 g/1000 mg since 1 g = 1000 mg. The steps involved in this conversion would be:

1. Write down the number of milligrams to be converted to grams.
2. To the right of that number write down the number of milligrams in 1 g, with the milligrams as the denominator. (The numerator should always contain the unit to which you want to convert.)
3. Multiply the two numbers together.

Example 1: Convert 3000 mg to grams.

1. **3000 mg**

2. **3000 mg** $\dfrac{1\ g}{1000\ mg}$

3. **3000 mg** $\times \dfrac{1\ g}{1000\ mg} = 3\ g$

Figure 3-1 illustrates the stairstep method to convert from one unit to another within the metric system. When converting measurements in the metric system by using the stairstep method, divide by 10 for each step up to the desired measurement and multiply by 10 for each step down to the desired measurement.

You may also think of converting measurements with this method by remembering that for each step up, the decimal point is moved to the left one place. For each step down, the decimal point is moved to the right one place.

Example 2: 500 ml = _____ L

To convert milliliters to liters requires three steps upward; therefore, divide 500 by 10 three times (or 500 ÷ 1000). This moves the decimal point to the left three places, and the answer is 500 ml = 0.5 L.

Example 3: 2 g = _____ mg

To convert grams to milligrams, go down three steps; therefore, multiply 2 by 10 three times (or 2 × 1000). This moves the decimal point to the right three places, and the answer is 2 g = 2000 mg.

A second method for making conversions in the metric system can be called the "arrow" method. When using this method it must be remembered which units of measure are larger. As an example, conversions between the commonly used units of kilogram, grams, milligrams, and micrograms are illustrated in the following text.

When considering these units it is known that a kilogram is 1000 times larger than a gram (g), a gram is 1000 times larger than a milligram (mg), and a milligram is 1000 times larger than a microgram (mcg). This relationship can be abbreviated using the greater than symbol (>):

$$kg > g > mg > mcg$$

Many times the technician will have to calculate the amount of a drug to give when the supply on hand is not in the same units as the order. For example, the order is for 0.3 g of drug A and the supply on hand is 150 mg tablets. Before we can determine how many tablets to give, we must convert 0.3 g to milligrams. Since we know that 1 g = 1000 mg, we could change 0.3 g to milligrams by multiplying 0.3 g with $\dfrac{1000\ mg}{g}$ (0.3 × 1000 = 300 mg). The decimal point was moved three places to the right (0.3 → $3{,}0{,}0{,}$).
                                             $^{1\ 2\ 3}$
The conversion could have been made very quickly

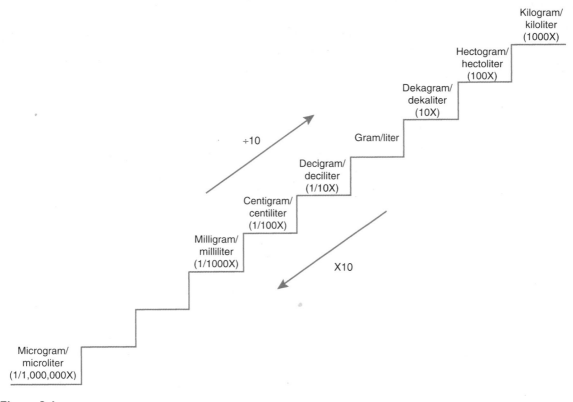

Figure 3-1

The stairstep method for converting within the metric system. For each step up the stairs, divide the given amount by 10; for each step down the stairs, multiply the given amount by 10.

by simply moving the decimal point three places to the right. To know which direction to move the decimal, determine which way the arrow is pointing (e.g., kg > **g** > **mg** > mcg).

Any time the conversion is between two adjacent units in the relationship of kg > g > mg > mcg, the decimal point will be moved three places.

The steps for converting grams to milligrams using this method are as follows.

1. Write down the order first, using the units called for **(0.3 g)**.
2. Write down the equivalent units (on hand) needed next to the order units (0.3 g = ___ **mg**).
3. Place an arrow between the two units with the closed part of the arrow pointing toward the smaller unit **(g > mg)**.

4. Move the decimal point three places in the direction the arrow points (0.3 g → 3_100_1 mg).

In the previous problem it would take two of the 150 mg tablets to fill the 300 mg order.

If the order had been for 300,000 mcg of drug A and the supply on hand had been 150 mg tablets, we would need to convert micrograms to milligrams by using the following steps:

1. Write the order (300,000 **mcg**).
2. Write down the equivalent units needed next to the order units (300,000 mcg = ___ **mg**).
3. Place an arrow between the two units with the closed part of the arrow pointing toward the smaller units **(mcg < mg)**.

4. Move the decimal three places in the direction the arrow points $(300 \text{ mg} \leftarrow 300{,}0_{1}0_{2}0_{3} \text{ mcg})$.

In this problem, it would take two of the 150 mg (150,000 mcg) tablets to provide the 300,000 mcg order.

More problems for converting within the metric system are provided at the end of this chapter.

THE APOTHECARY AND HOUSEHOLD SYSTEMS

The apothecary and household systems of measurement are older systems than the metric system. The apothecary system is seldom used, but the household system is used in giving clients instructions about dosage.

Box 3-1   Weight Equivalents

1 kg = 1000 g = 2.2 lb
1 g = 1000 mg
1 mg = 1000 μg = 0.001 g
65 mg = 1 gr
1 μg = 0.001 mg = 0.000001 g
1 lb = 453.6 g = 0.4536 kg = 16 oz
1 oz = 28.35 g

Box 3-2   Volume Equivalents

1 L = 1000 ml = 1 qt (946.4 ml)
500 ml = 1 pt (473 ml) = 2 cups
   (equivalent to 1 lb of water)
15 ml = 1 Tbsp
5 ml = 1 tsp
30 ml = 1 oz
240 ml = 1 cup/glass
4 ml = 1 dram
1 ml = 15 gtt/min*

*The number of drops/minims in 1 ml depends on the size of the dropper. With a standard-size dropper, 1 ml equals 15 drops.

The units most often encountered in the apothecary system are the minim, abbreviated *m* or *min;* the dram, abbreviated *dr;* the ounce, abbreviated *oz;* and the grain, abbreviated *gr.* A minim is equal to 1 drop, a dram is equal to 4 ml, an ounce is equal to 30 ml, and a grain is equal to 65 mg (64.8, sometimes rounded off to 65). When writing quantities relating to grains, the symbol *gr* should be placed before the number, and common fractions are used when appropriate (e.g., gr ⅟₅₀). The apothecary pound (12 oz) is not used when calculating doses; instead, the avoirdupois pound (16 oz) is used.

The units commonly used in the household system include the drop, abbreviated *gtt;* the tablespoon, abbreviated *T* or *Tbsp;* and the teaspoon, abbreviated *t* or *tsp.* One drop is equivalent to 1 min, 1 Tbsp is equivalent to 15 ml, and 1 tsp is equivalent to 5 ml. The pint, quart, and gallon are other units sometimes encountered. Boxes 3-1 and 3-2 illustrate equivalent values useful in dosage calculations. Problems converting within and between the apothecary and household systems are found at the end of the chapter.

DOSAGE CALCULATIONS

The quantity of drug that is to be delivered to a patient is called the *dose.* A dosage rate expressed in milligrams per kilogram (or milligrams per pound) is multiplied by the animal's weight in kilograms (or pounds) to determine the dose. The dose is then divided by the amount (concentration) of the drug in the pharmaceutic form (tablet, solution, and so forth) to determine the actual amount of the pharmaceutic form to administer. The formula for dosage calculation that should be committed to memory is:

$$\text{Dose} = \frac{\text{Animal's weight} \times \text{dosage rate}}{\text{Concentration of drug}}$$

Example 1: If a 20-kg dog is to be given amoxicillin at the rate of 10 mg/kg and injectable amoxicillin with a concentration of 100 mg/ml is available, the dosage calculation would be as follows:

$$\text{Dose} = \frac{20 \text{ kg} \times 10 \text{ mg/kg}}{100 \text{ mg/ml}} = \frac{200 \text{ mg}}{100 \text{ mg/ml}} = 2 \text{ ml}$$

Note that in the first step of the calculation, kilograms cancel out to leave only milligrams in the numerator; in the second step, milligrams cancel out to leave milliliters. If 100-mg amoxicillin tablets are available, the formula becomes:

$$\text{Dose} = \frac{20 \text{ kg} \times 10 \text{ mg/kg}}{100 \text{ mg/tablet}} =$$

$$\frac{200 \text{ mg}}{100 \text{ mg/tablet}} = 2 \text{ tablets}$$

Because most scales used to weigh animals for drug dosage calculation provide the weight in pounds, a conversion must be made from pounds to kilograms. To do this, divide the weight in pounds by 2.2.

Example 2: The dog in the previous problem weighed 44 lb, and 44 divided by 2.2 equals 20 kg. To convert kilograms to pounds (if the dose is provided in milligrams per pound), multiply the weight in kilograms by 2.2 (e.g., 20 kg × 2.2 = 44 lb).

If the order to the technician is to "give a dog 300 mg of amoxicillin," then the ordered amount is simply divided by the concentration of the drug to determine the amount to administer.

Example 3: If the order is to give a dog 300 mg of amoxicillin (concentration 100 mg/ml), the calculation would be:

$$\frac{300 \text{ mg}}{100 \text{ mg/ml}} = 3 \text{ ml}$$

It should be noted that most drugs used to treat neoplasms are dosed according to the total body surface area of the patient. Body surface area is correlated with the weight of the animal. A table is available in Chapter 16 (Table 16-2) for converting an animal's weight to surface area in square meters (sq M or m²). In these cases, the formula for dosage calculation becomes:

$$\text{Dose} = \text{mg/m}^2 \text{ (from insert)} \times \text{m}^2 \text{ (from table)}$$

Dosage calculation problems are provided at the end of this chapter.

SOLUTIONS

To understand dosage calculation problems as well as how to prepare dilutions of substances (e.g., formalin and dextrose), a technician must have a basic understanding of solutions. *Solutions* are mixtures of substances that are not usually chemically combined with each other. Solutions are made up of a dissolving substance, called the *solvent,* and a dissolved substance, called the *solute.* Not all substances form solutions with each other; those that form solutions are called *miscible,* and those that do not are called *immiscible.* A solution is said to be *saturated* if it contains the maximum amount of solute at a particular temperature and pressure. Under some circumstances, a solution can become supersaturated. Mixtures of substances in which the solute is made up of very large particles are called *suspensions.* The particles in suspensions settle out on standing, and the mixture must be agitated before it is administered. True solutions do not settle out, and they remain mixed without agitation. All parts of solutions contain equal parts of the solute.

When dealing with solutions, it is important to know the amount of solute in the solvent or to be able to measure it. The amount of solute dissolved in the solvent is referred to as the *concentration* of the substance. Concentrations may be expressed in a number of ways, including the following:

1. Parts
2. Weight per volume (w/v) for liquids
3. Volume per volume (v/v) for liquids
4. Weight per weight (w/w) for solids

Solutions can be described in terms of parts without any reference to units of measurement. The parts simply refer to the relationship between the solvent and the solute. For example, instructions may call for a 1-to-30 (1:30) dilution of a disinfectant.

One unit that describes the relationship of parts is called *parts per million* (ppm). Parts per million is equal to 1 mg of a solute in a kilogram or liter of solvent. One part per million is also equivalent to 1 μg in a gram or milliliter. Upson (1988) reports that 1 ppm is equivalent to 1 minute in approximately 2 years or 1 oz of sand in approximately 31 tons of cement. Parts per billion is a unit that is occasionally used. It is equivalent to 1 μg in a kilogram or liter or 1 nanogram in a gram or milliliter.

The most common way of expressing drug concentrations when the solute is a solid and the solvent is a liquid is weight per volume (w/v). For example, the concentration of most pharmaceutic preparations is expressed as milligrams per milliliter (mg/ml); the concentration for Ketaset is 100 mg/ml. The weight-per-weight (w/w) and the volume-per-volume (v/v) solutions are not used as often in veterinary pharmaceutic preparations as the w/v preparations.

PERCENT CONCENTRATIONS

The term *percent concentration* may be used when describing w/v, w/w, or v/v concentrations. Percent (percentage) means parts of solute per 100 parts of the solution. Percent w/v means the number of grams of solute in 100 ml of solution; percent w/w describes the number of grams of solute in 100 g of solution; and v/v expresses the number of milliliters of solute in 100 ml of the solution.

A 100% solution (w/v) contains 100 g of solute per 100 ml of solution. Another way to say this is that it contains 1 g (1000 mg) of solute per 1 ml of solution (1000 mg/ml). To convert from a percent solution to mg/ml, multiply the percentage by 10 (e.g., a 5% Lasix solution contains 50 mg/ml). To convert milligrams per milliliter to a percent, divide the milligrams per milliliter by 10 (e.g., a Lasix solution containing 50 mg/ml is a 5% solution). Sometimes the term called *milligrams percent* (mg%) is encountered. This term is used to refer to the number of milligrams in 100 ml of solution. It is an expression of concentration but not of percent concentration (g/100 ml). A more accurate description of what is meant by mg% would be milligrams per deciliter (mg/dl), because a deciliter is equal to 100 ml.

A 100% solution (w/w) contains 100 g of solute in 100 g of solution. A 5% solution (w/w) of sodium chloride would contain 5 g of sodium in 100 g of the solution. To make this preparation, weigh out 5 g of sodium chloride and mix it with 95 g of water.

A 100% solution (v/v) would simply be pure drug or chemical. A 10% solution would contain 10 ml of the chemical in 100 ml of solution. When preparing a w/v solution or v/v solution, the desired amount of solute is added to a container and enough solvent is added to create the desired volume. This process is called *diluting up,* or it may be said that you *q.s.* to the desired volume. The abbreviation *q.s.* means to add a "quantity sufficient" to arrive at the desired volume. For example, to make 100 ml of a 10% formalin solution, place 10 ml of formaldehyde (100% formalin) in a container and q.s. to 100 ml (10 ml formalin + 90 ml distilled water).

CALCULATIONS INVOLVING CONCENTRATIONS

To determine the amount of solute needed to make a desired amount of solution, the following formula may be used:

$$\text{Grams of solute to q.s. to desired volume} = \frac{\% \times \text{desired volume}}{100}$$

Example 1: How many grams of sodium chloride are needed to make 1 L of 0.9% sodium chloride?

Answer: $\text{Grams needed} = \frac{0.9 \times 1000 \text{ ml}}{100} = 9 \text{ g}$

Nine grams of sodium chloride would be added to a container and diluted up to 1000 ml.

When the amount of solute and the volume of solution are known, the percent solution may be found as follows:

$$\text{Percent solution} = \frac{\text{grams of solute} \times 100}{\text{volume of solution}}$$

Example 2: What percentage is a solution containing 9 g of sodium chloride?

Answer: $\frac{\text{Percent}}{\text{solution}} = \frac{9 \times 100}{1000} = \frac{900}{1000} = 0.9\%$

To solve problems involving a change in concentration of the solution, the following formula may be used:

Volume one × concentration one =
volume two × concentration two

Example 3: How would you prepare 100 ml of a 5% dextrose solution from a 50% dextrose solution?

Answer: $V1 \times C1 = V2 \times C2$
$100 \times 5 = V2 \times 50$
$500 = 50V2$
$10 = V2$

This formula demonstrates that you would take 10 ml of the 50% dextrose solution and q.s. it to 100 ml to prepare the 5% solution.

Another formula that may be used to solve problems in which a change in concentration is involved is as follows:

$$\frac{\text{Desired strength}}{\text{Available strength}} = \frac{\text{amount to use}}{\text{amount to make}}$$

Example 4: In solving the foregoing problem, the desired strength is 5%, the available strength is 50%, the amount to make is 100 ml, and the amount to use is the unknown.

Answer: $\dfrac{5}{50} = \dfrac{x}{100}$
$50x = 500$
$x = 10 \text{ ml}$

MILLIEQUIVALENTS

When electrolytes are involved, the concentration of a solution is often expressed in terms of **milliequivalents** (mEq). One milliequivalent is equal to $\frac{1}{1000}$ of an equivalent. An equivalent is equal to (for practical applications) 1 g molecular weight divided by the total positive valence of the material in question (Blankenship and Campbell, 1976). The concentration of an electrolyte solution is expressed as milliequivalents per liter (mEq/L), which can be calculated when the concentration of the solution is known by using the following formula:

$$\text{mEq/L} = \frac{\text{mg/dl} \times 10}{\text{eq wt}}$$

Example 1: How many milliequivalents per liter are found in a sodium chloride solution that contains 700 mg/dl?

Answer: $\text{mEq/L} = \dfrac{700 \times 10}{58.5} = 119.66$

The number of milligrams per deciliter can also be calculated when the number of milliequivalents per liter is known by manipulating the previous formula as follows:

$$\text{mg/dl} = \frac{\text{mEq/L} \times \text{eq wt}}{10}$$

Example 2: How many milligrams per deciliter are contained in a solution that has 119.66 mEq/L?

Answer: $\text{mg/dl} = \dfrac{119.66 \times 58.5}{10} =$

$\dfrac{7000}{10} = 700 \text{ mg/dl}$

CALCULATIONS INVOLVING IV FLUID ADMINISTRATION

Calculations for determining the volume of fluid to administer are covered in Chapter 15. The rate at which to run intravenous fluids (in drops per minute) can be determined by dividing the volume of fluids to be administered by the time in minutes over which they are to be administered and then multiplying that number by the number of drops per milliliter delivered by the administration set being used.

$$\frac{\text{Volume of infusion (ml)}}{\text{Time of infusion (min)}} \times$$
$$\text{drop factor (gtt/ml)} = \text{drops per minute}$$

The drip rate in drops per minute can be divided by 60 to determine the rate in drops per second, a number that is easier to work with when actually adjusting the flow.

Example 1: Give 480 ml of lactated Ringer's solution to Dog A over a 4-hour period using a standard 15 gtt/ml administration set:

$$\frac{480 \text{ ml}}{240 \text{ min}} = \frac{2 \text{ ml}}{\text{min}} \times \frac{15 \text{ gtt}}{\text{ml}} = \frac{30 \text{ gtt}}{\text{min}} \times \frac{1 \text{ min}}{60 \text{ sec}} = \frac{1 \text{ gtt}}{2 \text{ sec}}$$

Giving one drop every 2 seconds will obviously deliver 60 drops in a minute.

CALCULATIONS FOR CONSTANT RATE INFUSION PROBLEMS

Sometimes medications given by intravenous infusion need to be given at a dose that is delivered at a constant rate over a period of time. The dosage is often ordered in micrograms per kilogram per minute. The following example problem illustrates a method for solving these problems. Short-cut formulas are used by some clinicians.

Example 1: A 44 lb dog in acute heart failure is ordered to receive 10 mcg/kg/min of dopamine. You will add a 200 mg vial of dopamine to a 1 L bag of D5W solution (0.2 mg/ml). At what rate in drops per minute will you administer this solution to deliver the correct dosage?

Step 1: Convert to the same units. The dose is expressed in mcg/kg so the patient's weight must be converted from pounds to kilograms, and the drug concentration must be expressed in mcg/ml.

$$44 \text{ lbs} \times \frac{1 \text{ kg}}{2.2 \text{ lb}} = \frac{44 \text{ kg}}{2.2} = 20 \text{ kg}$$

$$\frac{0.2 \text{ mg}}{1 \text{ ml}} \times \frac{1000 \text{ mcg}}{1 \text{ mg}} = \frac{200 \text{ mcg}}{1 \text{ ml}}$$

Step 2: Determine the number of mcg/min.

$$20 \text{ kg} \times \frac{10 \text{ mcg}}{\text{kg/min}} = \frac{200 \text{ mcg}}{\text{min}}$$

Step 3: Determine the number of ml's per minute.

$$\frac{200 \text{ mcg}}{1 \text{ min}} \times \frac{1 \text{ ml}}{200 \text{ mcg}} = \frac{1 \text{ ml}}{1 \text{ min}}$$

Step 4: Determine the number of drops per minute using a mini-drip (60 gtt/ml) administration set.

$$\frac{1 \text{ ml}}{\text{min}} \times \frac{60 \text{ gtt}}{1 \text{ min}} = \frac{60 \text{ gtt}}{1 \text{ min}} \text{ or } 1 \text{ gtt/sec}$$

REFERENCES

Blankenship, J., Campbell, J.B.: Solutions. In Blankenship, J., Campbell, J.B. (eds.): Laboratory Mathematics: Medical and Biological Applications. Mosby, St. Louis, 1976.

Upson, D.W.: General principles. In Upson, D.W. (ed.): Handbook of Clinical Veterinary Pharmacology, 3rd ed. Dan Upson Enterprises, Manhattan, KS, 1988.

Review Questions

PROBLEMS USING RATIOS AND PROPORTIONS

RATIOS

1. Express ¼ as a ratio and as a decimal.
2. Express 0.75 as a ratio and as a fraction.
3. Express 0.004 as a ratio and as a fraction.
4. Express 1:80 as a fraction and as a decimal.
5. Express 9⁄1000 as a ratio and as a decimal.
6. Express 1:32 as a fraction and as a decimal.

PROPORTIONS (SOLVE FOR X)

1. 25:X = 5:10

2. $\dfrac{4}{5} = \dfrac{X}{10}$

3. ½:100 = X:500

4. $\dfrac{¼}{X} = \dfrac{20}{400}$

5. Convert 0.2 g to milligrams using a proportion

$$\frac{1000 \text{ mg}}{1 \text{ g}} = \frac{X \text{ mg}}{0.2 \text{ g}}$$

6. If a drug concentration is labeled 5 ml = 250 mg, how many mg are in ¾ ml?

$$\frac{250 \text{ mg}}{5 \text{ ml}} = \frac{X}{¾ \text{ ml}}$$

7. How much bleach would you use to prepare 1000 ml of a 1:32 solution?

$$1:32 = X:1000$$

8. How much bleach would you use to prepare 1 gallon (3784 ml) of a 1:32 solution?

$$1:32 = X:3784$$

9. If you are to give a horse 1 ml per 250 lb of body weight of an anthelmintic, how many ml would you give to a horse that weighs 1250 lb?

$$\frac{1}{250} = \frac{X}{1250}$$

10. If a 10 lb dog gets one-fourth of a tablet of an antibiotic, how many tablets will a 50 lb dog get?

$$¼:10 = X:50$$

PROBLEMS USING THE METRIC SYSTEM

1. 150 mg = _____ g
2. 2 L = _____ ml
3. 2250 mg = _____ g
4. 5 g = _____ mg
5. 3000 ml = _____ L
6. 2 kg = _____ g
7. 0.5 kg = _____ g
8. 5000 mg = _____ kg
9. 1.25 mg = _____ g
10. 0.004 g = _____ mg
11. 2050 μg = _____ mg
12. How many grams would you administer if the veterinarian ordered 10 mg of acepromazine?

_____

13. If the medical order is 0.5 L of sodium chloride 0.9%, how many milliliters would be administered?

_____

14. How many liters would you administer to the patient if the order called for 750 ml to be administered?

_____

15. If the veterinarian orders 300 μg of vitamin B_{12}, how much is this in milligrams?

_____

16. If the order is 2.5 mg of vitamin B_{12}, how many micrograms are administered?

_____

■ **Review Questions—cont'd**

PROBLEMS USING THE APOTHECARY AND HOUSEHOLD SYSTEMS

1. 1.5 qt = _____ pt
2. 12 pt = _____ gal
3. 3 tsp = _____ Tbsp
4. 3 qt = _____ cups
5. 12 cups = _____ pt
6. 2 oz = _____ Tbsp
7. 1 gal = _____ oz
8. 1 pt = _____ oz
9. 6 pt = _____ qt

PROBLEMS COMBINING BOTH SYSTEMS

1. 1 pt = _____ ml
2. 2 Tbsp = _____ ml
3. 15 ml = _____ cc
4. 2 cups = _____ oz
5. 6.5 ml = _____ pt
6. 125 ml = _____ tsp
7. 1.5 oz = _____ ml
8. 15 kg = _____ lb
9. 250 ml = _____ pt
10. 5 oz = _____ ml
11. 35 lb = _____ kg

PROBLEMS MEASURING ORAL MEDICATIONS

1. The order is 500 mg of amoxicillin; tablets on hand are 250 mg. How many tablets will be administered?
   _____

2. The order is 15 mg of prednisone; tablets on hand are 10 mg (scored). How many tablets will be administered? _____

3. The order is 960 mg of SMZ-TMP; tablets on hand are 240 mg. How many tablets will be administered?
   _____

4. The order is 0.5 mg of Centrine; tablets on hand are 0.2 mg. How many tablets will be administered?
   _____

5. The veterinarian prescribes 15 mg of prednisone every other day for 10 days. The tablets on hand are 10 mg. How many tablets will be administered? How many tablets will be dispensed?
   _____

6. The veterinarian prescribes 100 mg of cephalexin twice a day (b.i.d.) for 10 days. You have 100-mg tablets on hand; how many will be dispensed?
   _____

7. The veterinarian prescribes Albon for Coccidia. Your patient is a puppy weighing 8 lb and needing treatment for 21 days. The dosage for Albon is 25 mg/lb loading dose and 12.5 mg/lb maintenance dose to be given once daily (s.i.d.). The drug is supplied at 250 mg/5 ml. How many milligrams does your patient need for a loading dose? _____
   A maintenance dose?
   _____
   How many mg/ml are there in Albon?
   _____
   How many milliliters does your patient need for a loading dose? _____
   A maintenance dose?
   _____
   How many milliliters will be dispensed?
   _____

8. The veterinarian prescribes 250 mg phenylbutazone b.i.d. for 5 days for your patient; tablets on hand are 100 mg scored. How many tablets will be administered? _____
   How many tablets will be dispensed?
   _____

9. The veterinarian prescribes chloramphenicol, 250 mg three times daily (t.i.d.) for 7 days, for your patient. The tablets on hand are 1 g scored. How many tablets will be given? _____
   How many will be dispensed?
   _____

10. The veterinarian prescribes 2.5 mg of acepromazine t.i.d. for 3 days; tablets on hand are 5 mg scored. How many tablets will be administered?

    _____

    How many will be dispensed?

    _____

11. The veterinarian prescribes aminophylline to be given three times daily for 14 days to a 15-lb dog. The dose for aminophylline is 10 mg/kg. How many kg does your patient weigh? _____
    How many milligrams does your patient need to be administered? _____
    Because the tablets on hand are 100 mg scored, how many tablets will the patient be administered?

    _____

    How many tablets will be dispensed?

    _____

12. The veterinarian orders mebendazole and Combot to deworm a 1000-lb horse via a nasogastric tube. The dose for mebendazole is 30 ml/250 lb body weight, and the dose for Combot is 0.5 oz/100 lb body weight. How many milliliters of mebendazole and Combot are needed? _____

13. A farmer has 10 calves weighing approximately 100 lb each. A microscopic fecal examination reveals Coccidia. The veterinarian chooses to treat all 10 calves with Corid powder (20% amprolium) by drenching daily for 10 days. To make a drench solution, mix 3 oz of Corid powder in 1 qt of water (1 oz of powder = 3.5 Tbsp). The dose of Corid for drenching is 1 oz of solution per 100 lb of body weight. How much solution should be mixed to drench these 10 calves for 10 days?

    _____

14. Doxycycline has been chosen as treatment for a 1-kg Amazon parrot at the rate of 25 mg/kg b.i.d. for 7 days. The tablets on hand are 50 mg scored. How many tablets will be given for each treatment?

    _____

    How many tablets will be dispensed?

    _____

15. The veterinarian orders doxylamine succinate to treat a 200-lb foal. The dosage to be administered is 1 mg/lb/day, divided into three doses and given orally. The vial is labeled 11.36 mg/ml. How many milligrams will be given at each treatment?

    _____

    How many milliliters of medication will be needed for treatment for 1 day? _____

PROBLEMS MEASURING PARENTERAL MEDICATIONS

1. The veterinarian orders prednisone, 20 mg intramuscularly (IM). The vial is labeled 50 mg/ml. How many milliliters will be administered?

    _____

2. The veterinarian orders Cortisate-20 at 2 mg/lb to be administered IV. Your patient weighs 37 lb. The vial of Cortisate-20 is labeled 20 mg/ml. How many milliliters will be administered?

    _____

3. The veterinarian orders phenylbutazone to be administered to a 1500-lb horse at a dose of 5 mg/kg intravenously (IV). The vial is labeled 200 mg/ml. How many milliliters will be administered?

    _____

4. The veterinarian orders penicillin G procaine for a 25-lb dog to be administered at a dose of 40,000 U/kg IM. The vial is labeled 300,000 U/ml. How many milliliters will be administered?

    _____

5. The veterinarian orders cephalothin sodium to be administered every 8 hours IM to a 23-lb dog. The dosage to be given is 50 mg/kg/day. The vial is labeled 1 g/10 ml. How many milligrams will be administered for the day? _____
    How many milliliters will be administered at each treatment? _____

6. A 78-lb dog is to be administered ampicillin trihydrate at a dose of 5 mg/lb subcutaneously (SC). The antibiotic has been reconstituted, and the concentration is 200 mg/ml. How many milliliters will be administered to the patient? _____

■   Review Questions—cont'd

7. A microscopic fecal examination reveals a *Giardia* infection in a 500-g African gray parrot. The veterinarian chooses to treat the infection with metronidazole injectable at a dosage of 30 mg/kg daily for 3 days. How many milligrams will the parrot receive at each treatment? _____

8. A 45-lb dog is to be treated for lymphosarcoma with vincristine sulfate, 1 mg/ml. The dose is 0.5 mg/m². How many square meters of body surface area does this patient have? _____
How many milligrams will the patient be administered?

_____

How many milliliters?

_____

9. The veterinarian orders lincomycin HCl for a 500-lb Yorkshire boar. The dosage to be administered is 5 mg/lb/day IM for 5 days. The medication on hand is 100 mg/ml in a 50-ml multidose vial. How many milligrams will the boar be administered each day?

_____

How many milliliters will the boar be administered each day? _____
How many bottles of medication does the owner need to purchase to treat the boar for 5 days?

_____

10. A cat weighing 8 lb who has a small laceration on its left hip is to be administered ketamine HCl for anesthesia. The veterinarian orders 15 mg/kg IM. The vial is labeled 100 mg/ml. How many milligrams will the cat be administered? _____
How many milliliters will be administered?

_____

11. The veterinarian orders 7 mEq of potassium chloride to be added into the IV fluids. The vial is labeled 20 mEq in 10 ml. How many milliliters will be added to the fluids? _____

12. The veterinarian orders 4 U of regular insulin to be administered to a diabetic cat. The regular insulin is labeled 40 U/ml. How many milliliters will be administered? _____

13. The veterinarian orders testosterone propionate for a 475-lb Landrace boar. The dose to be administered is 1 mg/10 lb. The label on the vial is 25 mg/ml. How many milligrams will be administered?

_____

How many milliliters will be administered?

_____

14. The veterinarian orders dexamethasone, 60 mg IV, to be given to a patient. The vial is labeled 2 mg/ml. How many milliliters will be administered?

_____

15. The veterinarian orders 15 mg of vitamin K_1. The vial is labeled 10 mg/ml. How many milliliters will be administered? _____

INJECTION PROBLEMS

Order	Stock	Give
1. 0.5 g IM	250 mg/ml	
2. 20 mEq IV	40 mEq/10 ml	
3. 0.75 mg IM	0.50 mg/ml	
4. 150 mg IM	0.2 g/5 ml	
5. 25 mg IM	100 mg/ml	
6. 0.5 mg IM	0.5 mg/2 ml	
7. 0.3 mg IV	0.4 mg/ml	
8. 300,000 U SC	40,000 U/ml	
9. 0.3 mg IM	0.5 mg/ml	
10. 55 mg SC	250 mg/ml	

PREPARING SOLUTIONS

1. Order: 100 ml of 10% formalin solution
On hand: Formaldehyde 37% (considered as 100% formalin) and water
Amount needed: _____

2. Order: 1000 ml 0.9% NaCl and 5% dextrose
On hand: 1000 ml 0.9% NaCl and 500 ml $D_{50}W$
Amount of each needed: _____

3. Order: 100 ml $D_{50}W$
On hand: 500 ml $D_{50}W$ and 250 ml sterile water for injection
Amount needed: _____

4. Order: 500 ml 0.45% NaCl and 5% dextrose
On hand: 500 ml 0.9% NaCl and 500 ml D_5W
Amount of each needed: _____

5. Order: 2000 ml lactated Ringer's solution and 2.5% dextrose
On hand: 2 containers of 1000 ml lactated Ringer's solution and 250 ml $D_{50}W$
Amount of each needed: _____

■ **Review Questions—cont'd**

6. Order: 50 ml D_5W
   On hand: 1000 ml sterile water for injection and 250 ml $D_{50}W$
   Amount of each needed: _____

7. Order: 500 ml 2.5% dextrose and 0.45% NaCl
   On hand: 1000 ml 0.45% NaCl and 500 ml $D_{50}W$
   Amount of each needed: _____

8. Order: 1000 ml of 10% glyceryl guaiacolate solution
   On hand: packets containing 50 g guaifenesin (GG) powder and 1000 ml sterile water for injection
   Amount of each needed: _____

9. Order: 8% thiamylal sodium solution
   On hand: One 5-g vial of powder and sterile water for injection
   Amount of sterile water needed:

   _____

10. Order: 5 ml of 2% cyclosporine ophthalmic solution
    On hand: 50 ml Sandimmune Oral Solution (cyclosporine) 100 mg/ml and 16 oz of extra virgin olive oil
    Amount of each needed: _____

11. Order: 50 ml of 2% formalin for Knott's heartworm test
    On hand: 37% formaldehyde and water
    Amount of each needed: _____

PROBLEMS CALCULATING IV DRIP RATES

1. What drip rate will you use to administer 500 ml of lactated Ringer's solution over a 3-hour period with a standard (15 gtt/ml) administration set?

2. What drip rate would you use to deliver 120 ml 0.9% NaCl over a 2-hour period using a microdrip (60 gtt/ml) administration set?

3. What drip rate would you use to deliver 1.2 L of Normosol over a 10-hour period using a standard (15 gtt/ml) administration set?

4. What drip rate would you use to deliver 8 mcg/kg/min of drug C (500 mg/250 ml) to a 83-lb dog using a microdrip (60 gtt/ml) administration set?

5. What drip rate would you use to deliver 10 mcg/kg/min of dopamine (0.2 mg/ml) to a 22-lb dog using the microdrip (60 gtt/ml) administration set?

Drugs Used in Nervous System Disorders

LEARNING OBJECTIVES

After studying this chapter, you should be able to:

1. Define terms related to the pharmacology of the nervous system
2. Develop a basic understanding of the anatomy and physiology of the nervous system
3. Describe the subdivisions, functions, and primary neurotransmitters of the autonomic nervous system (ANS)
4. Describe how drugs affect the ANS
5. List the different classes of ANS drugs
6. List the two major classification schemes of barbiturates
7. List indications and precautions for the use of the barbiturates
8. Describe dissociative anesthesia, and list three dissociative agents
9. List the opiate receptors and the basic function of each
10. List the indications for the use of the narcotics
11. List potential side effects of narcotic use or overdose
12. Describe how opioid antagonists exert their effect, and list three examples of this category of drug
13. Define neuroleptanalgesic and give an example
14. List examples of drugs used to control seizures
15. Describe the primary use of the central nervous system (CNS) stimulants
16. List drugs used in behavioral pharmacotherapy
17. Describe the characteristics of a good euthanasia agent

KEY TERMS

Acetylcholine A neurotransmitter that allows a nerve impulse to cross the synaptic junction (gap) between two nerve fibers or between a nerve fiber and an organ (e.g., muscle, gland).

Acetylcholinesterase An enzyme that brings about the breakdown of acetylcholine in the synaptic gap.

Adrenergic A term used to describe an action or a receptor that is activated by epinephrine or norepinephrine.

Analgesia Loss of pain sensation (other sensations may be present).

Anesthesia The loss of all sensations. May be described as local (affecting a small area), regional, or surgical (accompanied by unconsciousness).

Autonomic nervous system That portion of the nervous system that controls involuntary activities.

Catalepsy A state of involuntary muscle rigidity that is accompanied by immobility, amnesia, and variable amounts of analgesia. Some reflexes may be preserved.

Catecholamine The class of neurotransmitters that includes dopamine, epinephrine, and norepinephrine. When given therapeutically, catecholamines mimic the effect of stimulating the sympathetic nervous system.

Cholinergic A term used to describe an action or receptor that is activated by acetylcholine.

Effector A gland, organ, or tissue that responds to nerve stimulation with a specific action.

Ganglionic The site of the synapse between neuron one and neuron two of the autonomic nervous system.

Muscarinic Receptors activated by acetylcholine and muscarine that are found in glands, the heart, and smooth muscle. An acronym for remembering muscarinic effects is "SLUD." S = salivation; L = lacrimation; U = urination; D = defecation.

Nicotinic Receptors activated by acetylcholine and nicotine that are found at the neuromuscular junction of skeletal muscle and at ganglionic synapses.

Parasympathetic nervous system That portion of the autonomic nervous system that arises from the craniosacral portion of the spinal cord, is mediated by the neurotransmitter acetylcholine, and is primarily concerned with conserving and restoring a steady state in the body.

Parasympathomimetic A drug that mimics the effects of stimulating the parasympathetic nervous system.

Sympathetic nervous system That portion of the autonomic nervous system that arises from the thoracolumbar spinal cord, is mediated by catecholamines, and is concerned with the fight-or-flight response.

Sympathomimetic A drug that mimics the effects of stimulating the sympathetic nervous system.

INTRODUCTION

The nervous system is the body's primary communication and control center. It functions in harmony with the endocrine system to allow an animal to respond and adapt to its environment and to maintain a relatively constant internal environment (homeostasis) through control of the many internal organ systems. In broad terms, the nervous system serves three functions: (1) sensory, (2) integrative (analysis), and (3) motor (action). It senses changes within the environment and within the body, interprets the information, and responds to the interpretation by bringing about an appropriate action. The nervous system carries out this complex activity very rapidly by sending electric-like messages over a network of nerve fibers. The endocrine system works much more slowly by sending chemical messengers (hormones) through the bloodstream to target structures. The two systems are very closely interrelated functionally and anatomically.

The nervous system exerts control over the endocrine system through the influence of the hypothalamus (brain) on the pituitary gland.

ANATOMY AND PHYSIOLOGY

The nervous system has two main divisions, the CNS and the peripheral nervous system, and related subdivisions (Figure 4-1). The CNS is composed of the brain and spinal cord and serves as the control center of the entire nervous system. All sensory information must be relayed to the CNS before it can be interpreted and acted on. Most impulses that stimulate glands to act and muscles to contract originate in the CNS.

The nerve processes that connect the CNS with the various glands, muscles, and receptors in the body make up the peripheral nervous system. Functionally, the peripheral nervous system is divided into afferent and efferent portions. The afferent portion is composed of nerve cells that carry information from receptors in the periphery of the body to the CNS. The efferent system consists of nerve cells that carry impulses from the CNS to muscles and glands. Anatom-

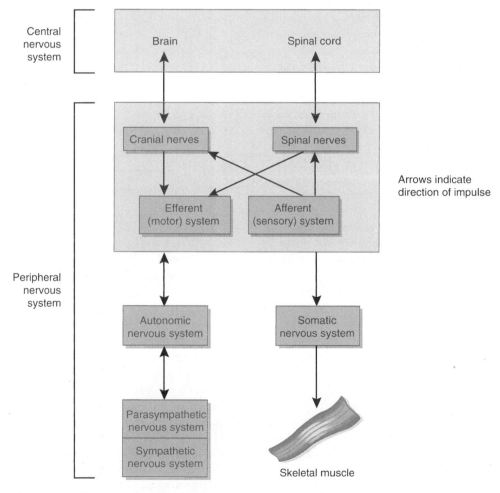

Figure 4-1

Organization of the nervous system.

ically, the peripheral nervous system is composed of cranial nerves and spinal nerves.

The peripheral nervous system is also subdivided into a somatic nervous system and an **autonomic nervous system.** The somatic nervous system consists of efferent nerves that carry impulses from the CNS to skeletal muscle tissue. It is under conscious control and is therefore called *voluntary.* The ANS consists of efferent nerve cells that carry information from the CNS to cardiac muscle, glands, and smooth muscle. It is under unconscious control and is called *involuntary.* The ANS has two subdivisions, the **sympathetic nervous system** and the **parasympathetic nervous system.** Most tissues innervated by the ANS receive both sympathetic and parasympathetic fibers. In general, one division stimulates an activity by a receptor and the other inhibits the activity to serve as a method of checks and balances.

The fundamental unit of all branches and divisions of the nervous system is the neuron (nerve cell). Neurons have the amazing ability to transmit information from point to point; the second point may be nearby or at a great distance. Like all cells in the body, neurons have a nucleus surrounded by cytoplasm. Unlike other cells, however, neurons have cellular extensions or processes called *axons* and *dendrites;* the axons carry electric-like messages away from the nerve cell, and the dendrites carry electric-like messages toward the nerve cell (Figure 4-2). Transmission of these messages along nerve fibers occurs through a wave of charge reversal moving down the fiber (Figure 4-3). The resting (polarized) fiber has positive charges lined up on the outside of its membrane and negative charges lined up on the inside of its membrane. When a stimulus of sufficient magnitude reaches the fiber, depolarization or charge reversal (positive in, negative out) occurs in a progressive wave down the fiber toward the synapse. Repolarization is the movement of the charges back to their original positions.

Axons may be short or long (up to 4 feet in humans), and they end, or terminate, in as many as 10,000 nerve endings called *telodendra* (Snyder, 1986). The large number of nerve endings allows for great variety in the number and type of connections made with other neurons. The synaptic end-bulbs of the telodendra pass nerve impulses to an adjacent

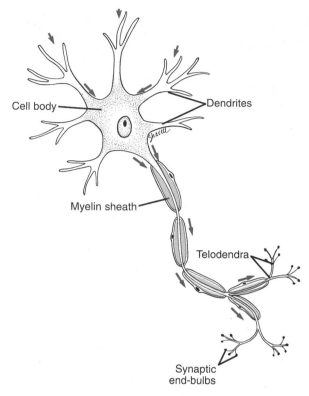

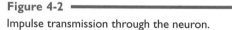

Figure 4-2

Impulse transmission through the neuron.

structure (another neuron, gland, or muscle) by emitting a chemical messenger called a *neurotransmitter* into the gap or junction (synapse) between the nerve ending and the adjacent structure (Figure 4-4). Neurotransmitters then combine with receptors on the dendritic side of the synapse and cause a stimulatory or inhibitory effect. Dendrites may respond to neurotransmitters by generating a nerve impulse, which is conducted via the axon to the adjacent structure (neuron, gland, or muscle). Neurotransmitters can be mimicked or blocked by the use of appropriate drugs (Figure 4-5).

Nerve fibers (nerves) may have a large diameter (A fibers), medium diameter (B fibers), or small diameter (C fibers) (Tortora and Anagnostakos, 1991). Fibers with large diameters conduct nerve impulses faster than those with small diameters. Fibers that are sur-

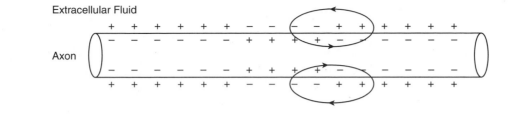

Figure 4-3

Electrical impulse transmission along a nerve fiber.

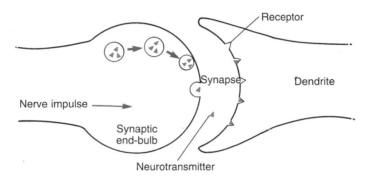

Figure 4-4

Neurotransmitter release.

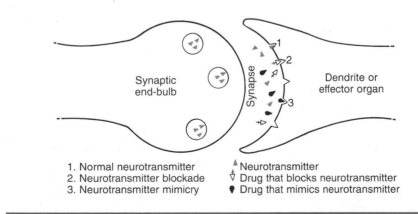

1. Normal neurotransmitter
2. Neurotransmitter blockade
3. Neurotransmitter mimicry

▲ Neurotransmitter
▽ Drug that blocks neurotransmitter
● Drug that mimics neurotransmitter

Figure 4-5

Neurotransmitter activity.

Spinal cord

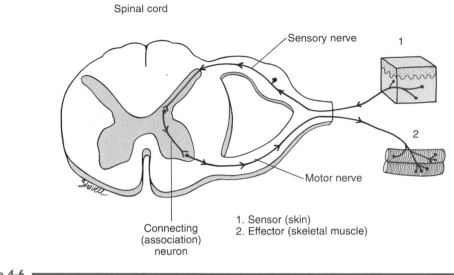

1. Sensor (skin)
2. Effector (skeletal muscle)

Figure 4-6

The reflex arc.

rounded by the insulating substance called *myelin* also transmit impulses faster than non-myelinated fibers. Type A and B fibers are generally myelinated.

The most basic impulse conduction system through the nervous system is the reflex arc (Figure 4-6). The reflex arc is composed of the following:

1. A receptor
2. A sensory neuron
3. A center in the CNS for a synapse
4. A motor neuron
5. An **effector**

The receptor of the reflex arc may be located in a peripheral site, such as the skin, or a central area, such as a muscle, tendon, or visceral organ. The sensory neuron carries the impulse from the receptor to the CNS. In the CNS, the sensory neuron synapses with interneurons in the spinal cord. These interneurons send the impulse to the brain for interpretation or send the impulse to a motor neuron. The motor neuron carries the message to an effector organ. If the impulse travels around the arc without going to the brain for analysis, the sequence of events is called a *spinal reflex* (see Figure 4-6). A spinal reflex can occur even if the spinal cord is completely severed; for example: a hemostat applied to the toe of a dog with a severed cord can cause the dog to withdraw its leg by means of the spinal reflex.

Areas of the brain that have importance to an understanding of the pharmacology of the CNS are illustrated in Figure 4-7. The cerebrum is responsible for higher functions of the brain, such as learning, memory, and interpretation of sensory input (vision, pain recognition, and so forth). The thalamus serves as a relay center for sensory impulses from the spinal cord, brain stem, and cerebellum to the cerebrum. The thalamus may also be involved in pain interpretation. The hypothalamus serves as the primary mediator between the nervous system and the endocrine system through its control of the pituitary gland. The hypothalamus also controls and regulates the ANS. The medulla carries both sensory and motor impulses between the spinal cord and the brain; it also contains centers that control vital physiologic activities such as breathing, heartbeat, blood pressure, vomiting, swallowing, coughing, body temperature, hunger, thirst, and others. The reticular formation is a network of nerve cells scattered through bundles of fibers that begin in the medulla and extend upward through the brain stem. The reticular activating system is a part of

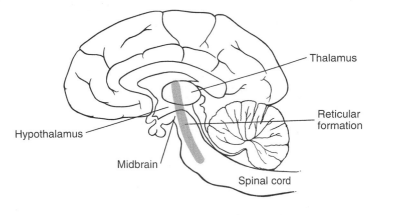

Figure 4-7 ━━

Pharmacologically important areas of the brain.

the reticular formation that functions to arouse the cerebral cortex and is responsible for consciousness, sleep, and wakefulness (DeLahunta, 1983).

In summary, nerve activity is usually described as the generation of nerve impulses occurring in a dendrite or cell body and then traveling down an axon by electric-like activity that is similar to the passage of an electric current down a wire. When this current reaches a synapse, a chemical "bridge" or neurotransmitter allows the message to be passed to one or as many as thousands of other neurons. Neurotransmitter substances include acetylcholine, norepinephrine, dopamine, serotonin, and gamma aminobutyric acid (GABA). These other neurons then carry the message to an interpretation center or a structure that takes appropriate action. CNS drugs act by mimicking or blocking the effect of neurotransmitters.

AUTONOMIC NERVOUS SYSTEM

The ANS is that portion of the nervous system that controls unconscious body activities. ANS fibers innervate smooth muscle, heart muscle, salivary glands, and other viscera. This system operates automatically and involuntarily to control visceral functions such as gastrointestinal (GI) motility, rate and force of the heartbeat, secretion by glands, size of the pupils, and

various other involuntary functions. Unlike the somatic nervous system, the ANS has two subdivisions: the parasympathetic (**cholinergic**) and the sympathetic (**adrenergic**). The sympathetic division regulates energy-expending activities (fight-or-flight responses), and the parasympathetic division regulates energy-conserving activities.

The ANS has two neurons carrying impulses to target structures (unlike the somatic nervous system, which has only one). The cell body of the first neuron arises in the CNS: the thoracolumbar cord for the sympathetic nervous system and craniosacral for the parasympathetic nervous system (Figure 4-8). The axon of the first neuron leaves the CNS and travels to a ganglion, where it synapses with dendrites of the second neuron. This second neuron then travels to the target structure (Figure 4-9). Axons of the first neuron are called *preganglionic,* and those of the second are called *postganglionic.*

Preganglionic fibers of the sympathetic nervous system are short; they end in ganglia adjacent to the spinal cord. The only exception is the preganglionic fiber to the adrenal medulla. The adrenal medulla itself is analogous to a postganglionic fiber because it releases epinephrine and norepinephrine directly into the bloodstream when stimulated by preganglionic fibers. Postganglionic sympathetic fibers are long.

Preganglionic fibers of the parasympathetic nervous system are generally long; they travel to ganglia

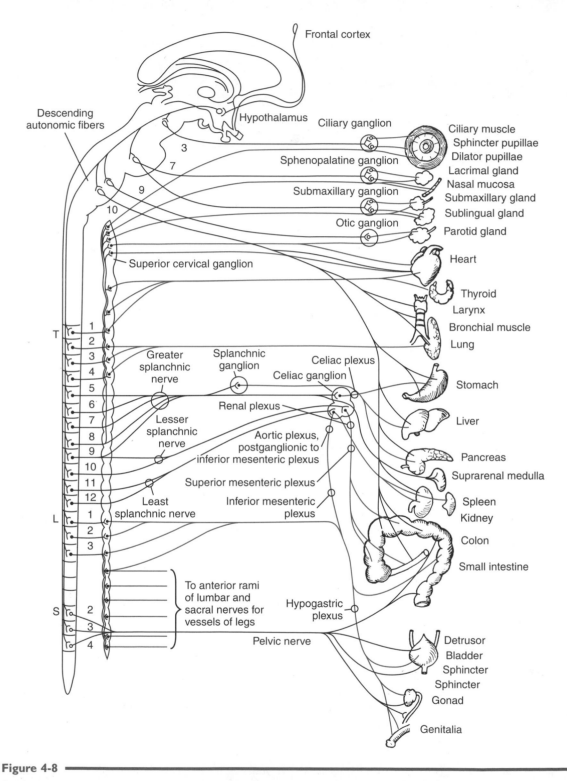

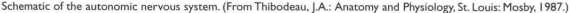

Figure 4-8

Schematic of the autonomic nervous system. (From Thibodeau, J.A.: Anatomy and Physiology, St. Louis: Mosby, 1987.)

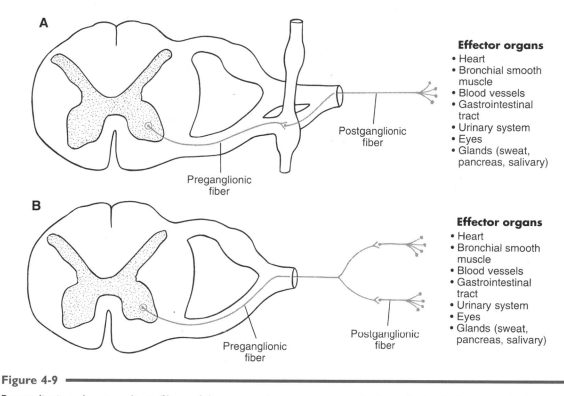

Figure 4-9

Preganglionic and postganglionic fibers of the autonomic nervous system. **A,** Sympathetic. **B,** Parasympathetic.

located in the wall of the target organ. Postganglionic fibers are consequently short.

Normally, target sites of the ANS have both sympathetic and parasympathetic innervation. The physiologic functions of the two systems usually oppose each other and thereby bring about a state of balance. When this balance is disrupted, drug therapy may be indicated to restore the balance. The adrenal medulla, sweat glands, and hair follicles have only sympathetic fibers.

Stimulation of the sympathetic nervous system causes an increase in heart rate and respiratory rate, a decrease in GI activity, dilation of the pupils, constriction of blood vessels in smooth muscle, dilation of blood vessels in skeletal muscle, dilation of bronchioles, and increase in blood glucose levels. These actions prepare an animal to fight or to flee. On the other hand, stimulation of the parasympathetic nervous system causes a decrease in heart rate and respiratory rate, an increase in GI activity, constriction of the pupils, and constriction of the bronchioles.

Receptors of the sympathetic (adrenergic) nervous system are subdivided as follows (Figure 4-10):

1. Alpha-1
2. Alpha-2
3. Beta-1
4. Beta-2
5. Dopaminergic

Generally, alpha receptors are stimulatory and beta receptors are inhibitory (Table 4-1). The parasympathetic (cholinergic) nervous system has **nicotinic** and **muscarinic** receptors. Effector organs have one or a combination of these receptors, and a drug's effect is determined by the number of receptors in the effector and the drug's specificity for the receptor (Williams and Baer, 1990).

The primary neurotransmitters for adrenergic sites are norepinephrine, epinephrine, and dopamine. Epinephrine stimulates both alpha and beta receptors equally and is therefore a potent stimulator of the

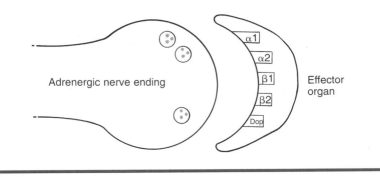

Figure 4-10

Adrenergic receptor types.

TABLE 4-1	Adrenergic Receptor Responses	
Receptor	**Target Organ**	**Response**
Alpha-1	Arterioles	Constriction
	Urethra	Increased tone
	Eye	Dilation of pupil
Alpha-2	Skeletal muscle	Constriction
Beta-1	Heart	Increased rate, conduction, and contractility
	Kidneys	Renin release
Beta-2	Skeletal blood vessels	Dilation
	Bronchioles	Dilation
Dopaminergic	Kidneys	Dilation of blood vessels
	Heart	Dilation of coronary vessels
	Mesenteric blood vessels	Dilation

heart and an equally powerful dilator of bronchioles. Acetylcholine is the neurotransmitter at sympathetic postganglionic fibers to sweat glands and the smooth muscle of blood vessels (**muscarinic** sites).

The neurotransmitter for cholinergic sites is **acetylcholine.** Acetylcholine combines with both nicotinic and muscarinic receptors.

Cholinergic sites are found in both the sympathetic and parasympathetic nervous systems. Nicotinic receptors are found in all autonomic ganglia, in the adrenal medulla, and at the neuromuscular junction of the somatic nervous system. Muscarinic receptors are found at the synapse of postganglionic fibers of the parasympathetic nervous system and at a few of the sympathetic postganglionic fibers.

HOW DRUGS AFFECT THE AUTONOMIC NERVOUS SYSTEM

Autonomic drugs bring about their effects by influencing the sequence of events involving neurotransmitters. Most autonomic drugs bring about this alteration of events by the following:

1. Mimicking neurotransmitters
2. Interfering with neurotransmitter release

3. Blocking the attachment of neurotransmitters to receptors
4. Interfering with the breakdown or reuptake of neurotransmitter at the synapse

CLASSES OF AUTONOMIC NERVOUS SYSTEM DRUGS

CHOLINERGIC AGENTS

Cholinergic agents are drugs that stimulate receptor sites mediated by acetylcholine. They achieve these effects by mimicking the action of acetylcholine (direct acting) or by inhibiting its breakdown (indirect acting). Cholinergic agents are also called **parasympathomimetic** because their effects resemble those produced by stimulating parasympathetic nerves.

Clinical Uses. Cholinergic agents do the following:

1. Aid in the diagnosis of myasthenia gravis
2. Reduce the intraocular pressure of glaucoma
3. Stimulate GI motility
4. Treat urinary retention
5. Control vomiting
6. Act as an antidote for neuromuscular blockers

Dosage Forms

Direct-Acting Cholinergics

1. Acetylcholine. Acetylcholine is seldom used clinically because it is broken down so rapidly by **acetylcholinesterase.**
2. Carbamylcholine. This product has been used to treat atony of the GI tract and to stimulate uterine contractions in swine.
3. Bethanechol (Urecholine). Bethanechol is used to treat GI and urinary tract atony.
4. Pilocarpine (Isopto Carpine, Akarpine, Pilocar). Pilocarpine reduces intraocular pressure associated with glaucoma.
5. Metoclopramide (Reglan). Metoclopramide is used to control vomiting and to promote gastric tract emptying.

Indirect-Acting Cholinergics (Anticholinesterase) Agents

1. Edrophonium (Tensilon). Edrophonium is used to diagnose myasthenia gravis.
2. Neostigmine (Prostigmine, Stiglyn). These products are used to treat urine retention and GI atony and as an antidote to neuromuscular blocking agents.
3. Physostigmine (Antilirium, Eserine). Uses of this product are similar to those of neostigmine.
4. Organophosphate compounds. These are commonly used as insecticide dips and may result in toxicity if used inappropriately; a drug called *2-PAM (Protopam)* can be used to reactivate cholinesterase that has been inactivated by organophosphates.
5. Demecarium (Humorsol). This drug is used in the preventive management of glaucoma.

Adverse Side Effects. Adverse side effects of the cholinergic drugs may include bradycardia, hypotension, heart block, lacrimation, diarrhea, vomiting, increased intestinal activity, intestinal rupture, and increased bronchial secretions.

CHOLINERGIC BLOCKING AGENTS (ANTICHOLINERGIC)

Cholinergic blocking agents are drugs that block the action of acetylcholine at muscarinic receptors of the parasympathetic nervous system.

Clinical Uses. Clinical uses of these drugs are as follows:

1. Treatment of diarrhea and vomiting by decreasing GI motility
2. As a preanesthetic to dry secretions and prevent bradycardia
3. To dilate the pupils for ophthalmic examination
4. To relieve ciliary spasm of the eye
5. To treat sinus bradycardia

The belladonna alkaloids of the deadly nightshade family of plants have been used as drugs for centuries and represent the prototype for this category of agents.

Dosage Forms

1. Atropine. Numerous generic and trade name products are available for parenteral or ophthalmic administration. Atropine is used as a preanesthetic to dry secretions and to prevent bradycardia, as an antidote to organophosphate poisoning, to dilate the pupils for ophthalmic examination, to control ciliary spasm of the eye, to treat sinus bradycardia, and to slow a hypermotile gut.
2. Scopolamine. Used in antidiarrheal medications.
3. Methscopolamine is an ingredient of Biosol-M. Methscopolamine is used to control diarrhea.
4. Glycopyrrolate (Robinul-V). Glycopyrrolate is a quaternary ammonium compound with actions similar to atropine; it provides longer action than atropine. It is used primarily as a preanesthetic.
5. Aminopentamide (Centrine). Aminopentamide is used to control vomiting and diarrhea in dogs and cats.
6. Propantheline (Pro-Banthine). Propantheline is used to treat diarrhea, urinary incontinence, and bradycardia and to reduce colonic peristalsis (horses) to allow rectal examination. Propantheline, like glycopyrrolate, is a quaternary ammonium compound.

Adverse Side Effects. Adverse side effects of the cholinergic blockers are dose-related. Overdose can cause drowsiness, disorientation, tachycardia, photophobia, constipation, anxiety, and burning at the injection site.

Technician's Notes

1. Atropine administered as a preanesthetic causes dilation of the pupils. It dries secretions and prevents bradycardia.
2. Atropine is packaged in small-animal and large-animal concentrations; care should be taken not to confuse the two preparations.

ADRENERGIC (SYMPATHOMIMETIC) AGENTS

Adrenergic (**sympathomimetic**) agents bring about action at receptors mediated by epinephrine or norepinephrine. Adrenergic agents may be classified as **catecholamines** or non-catecholamines, and either category can also be classified according to the specific receptor types (alpha-1, alpha-2, beta-1, beta-2) activated. In most cases, alpha receptor activity causes an excitatory response (except in the GI tract), and beta stimulation causes an inhibitory response (except in the heart). Adrenergic activity is a complex subject, and more advanced texts should be consulted for a thorough explanation.

Clinical Uses. Adrenergic agents are used for the following purposes:

1. To stimulate the heart to beat during cardiac arrest
2. To reverse the hypotension and bronchoconstriction of anaphylactic shock
3. To strengthen the heart during congestive heart failure
4. To correct hypotension through vasoconstriction
5. To reduce capillary bleeding through vasoconstriction
6. To treat urinary incontinence
7. To reduce mucous membrane congestion (vasoconstriction) in allergic conditions
8. To prolong the effects of local anesthetic agents by causing vasoconstriction of blood vessels at the injection site, thereby prolonging their absorption
9. To treat glaucoma (alpha stimulation increases the outflow of and beta stimulation decreases the production of aqueous humor)

Dosage Forms

1. Epinephrine (Adrenalin). Epinephrine stimulates all receptors to cause an increase in heart rate and cardiac output, constriction of the blood vessels in the skin, dilation of the blood vessels in muscle, dilation of the bronchioles, and an increase in metabolic rate.

2. Norepinephrine (Levophed, Noradrenalin). Norepinephrine is mostly an alpha stimulator with some beta stimulation; its primary effect is that of a vasopressor (to raise blood pressure).
3. Isoproterenol (Isuprel). Isoproterenol is a pure beta stimulator; its primary use is for bronchodilation.
4. Phenylephrine (Neo-Synephrine). Phenylephrine is an alpha stimulator that is used as a nasal vasoconstrictor.
5. Dopamine (Intropin). Dopamine is a precursor of epinephrine and norepinephrine. Its action is dose-dependent. It is used to treat shock and congestive heart failure and to increase renal perfusion.
6. Phenylpropanolamine (Ornade, Prolamine, Dexatrim). Phenylpropanolamine is used to treat urinary incontinence in dogs.
7. Dobutamine (Dobutrex). Dobutamine is a beta-1 agonist that is used for short-term treatment of heart failure.
8. Ephedrine (Vatronol), terbutaline (Brethine), and albuterol (Proventil). These products are beta agonists; their main use is bronchodilation.
9. Xylazine (Rompun, AnaSed). Xylazine is an alpha-2 agonist with analgesic and sedative properties.

Adverse Side Effects. These may include tachycardia, hypertension, nervousness, and cardiac arrhythmias. Hypertension, arrhythmias, and pulmonary edema may occur with overdoses.

Technician's Notes

Epinephrine is normally packaged as a 1:1000 dilution. Many clinicians prefer a 1:10,000 dilution for treating cardiac arrest. Mix 1 ml of the original dilution with 9 ml of sterile water to prepare a 1:10,000 dilution.

ADRENERGIC BLOCKING AGENTS

Adrenergic blocking agents are used to disrupt the activity of the sympathetic nervous system. They are classified according to the site of their action as alpha blocker, beta blocker, or ganglionic blocker. Drugs usually block only one category of receptor.

Alpha Blockers. Alpha blockers have had limited use in veterinary medicine. Phenoxybenzamine has been advocated by some clinicians for the treatment of laminitis in horses and urethral obstruction in cats. Yohimbine is used for xylazine antagonism.

Clinical Uses. See Dosage Forms, next.

Dosage Forms

1. Phenoxybenzamine (Dibenzyline). Phenoxybenzamine is a hypotensive (vasodilator) agent.
2. Tranquilizers (acepromazine, droperidol). These tranquilizers act as alpha blockers and cause vasodilation.
3. Prazosin (Minipress). Prazosin is a hypotensive agent.
4. Yohimbine (Yobine). Yohimbine is used as an antidote for xylazine toxicity.
5. Atipamezole (Antisedan) is a reversal agent for medetomidine.

Adverse Side Effects. Adverse side effects may include hypotension (phenoxybenzamine, tranquilizers, prazosin); tachycardia (phenoxybenzamine); muscle tremors (yohimbine); and seizures (acepromazine).

Beta Blockers. Beta blockers are used to treat glaucoma, arrhythmias, and hypertrophic cardiomyopathy.

Clinical Uses. See Dosage Forms, next.

Dosage Forms

1. Propranolol (Inderal). Propranolol is used to treat cardiac arrhythmias and hypertrophic cardiomyopathy.
2. Timolol (Timoptic). Timolol is an ophthalmic preparation used to treat glaucoma.

Adverse Side Effects. These include bradycardia, hypotension, worsening of heart failure, bronchoconstriction, heart block, and syncope.

Ganglionic Blockers. Ganglionic blockers are seldom used in veterinary medicine.

CENTRAL NERVOUS SYSTEM

CNS drugs have various uses in veterinary medicine. Depressant drugs are used to tranquilize or sedate animals to facilitate restraint or anesthetic procedures. They are also used to control pain, to induce **anesthesia,** and to prevent or control seizures. CNS drugs are also available to antagonize (reverse) the effects of some of the depressant drugs. Another group of CNS agents are used to stimulate the CNS to treat cardiac or respiratory depression or arrest. The euthanasia drugs allow veterinarians to provide a quick and painless end to hopeless medical situations.

Drugs affecting the CNS generally cause either depression or stimulation. They are thought to generate these changes by altering nerve impulse transmission between the spinal cord and the brain or within the brain itself. Altering impulse transmission within the thalamus could prevent messages concerning painful stimuli from reaching the interpretation centers within the cerebrum. Interfering with impulses within the reticular activating system could alter levels of consciousness or wakefulness (Upson, 1988). The changes that occur in the transmission of nerve impulses as a result of administration of CNS drugs are probably brought about by altered neurotransmitter activity.

The categories of CNS drugs that are covered in this chapter include the following:

1. Tranquilizers
2. Barbiturates
3. Dissociatives
4. Opioid/antagonists
5. Neuroleptanalgesics/antagonists
6. Drugs to prevent or control seizures
7. Miscellaneous CNS drugs
8. CNS stimulants
9. Euthanasia agents

TRANQUILIZERS

Phenothiazine Derivatives

The mechanism of action of the phenothiazine derivatives on the CNS is not well-understood; however, it has been proposed that they are dopamine blockers (Muir and Hubbell, 1989). The effects on the cardiovascular system are a result of alpha-adrenergic blockade.

The phenothiazine derivative tranquilizers produce sedation and allay fear and anxiety without producing significant **analgesia.** Sudden painful stimuli arouse the animal. Phenothiazine derivative tranquilizers produce an antiemetic effect by depressing the chemoreceptor trigger zone in the brain and have a mild antipruritic effect. These agents also reduce the tendency of epinephrine to induce cardiac arrhythmias.

Clinical Uses. Phenothiazine derivatives are used for prevention or treatment of vomiting, relief of mild pruritus, and sedation/tranquilization.

Dosage Forms

1. Acepromazine maleate (acepromazine, Promace)
2. Chlorpromazine hydrochloride (Thorazine)
3. Promazine HCl (Sparine)
4. Prochlorperazine/isopropamide (Darbazine, Compazine)

Adverse Side Effects. The phenothiazine derivative tranquilizers can cause hypotension and hypothermia because of their vasodilatory effect (alpha blockade). They also can induce seizures (by lowering the seizure threshold) in epileptic animals.

Technician's Notes

1. Phenothiazine derivatives should not be used within 1 month of worming with an organophosphate anthelmintic.
2. The tranquilizing effect may be reduced in an excited animal.

The phenothiazine derivative tranquilizers are approved for use in a wide variety of animals and for administration by almost any route. They generally are relatively safe drugs to use when administered appropriately; they should be given with care when used with other CNS depressants because of the additive effect. Most phenothiazine derivative tranquilizers are metabolized by the liver and excreted by the kidneys.

Benzodiazepine Derivatives

The mechanism of action of diazepam is through depression of the thalamic and hypothalamic areas of the brain. This drug produces sedation, muscle relaxation, appetite stimulation (especially in cats), and anticonvulsant activity. Diazepam also produces minimal depression of the cardiovascular and respiratory systems when compared with other CNS depressants. It is sometimes used in combination with ketamine for short-term anesthesia. Diazepam is very useful for treating seizures in progress.

Several potential drug interactions can occur when administering diazepam simultaneously with other drugs; appropriate references should be consulted.

Clinical Uses. Clinical uses include sedation, relief of anxiety and behavioral disorders, treatment of seizures, and appetite stimulation. Diazepam can be used as an injectable anesthetic.

Dosage Form

1. Diazepam (Valium, Vazepam)

Adverse Side Effects. These are limited when used as directed. Dogs can exhibit excitement. Overdose may cause excessive CNS depression.

Technician's Notes

1. Diazepam should be stored at room temperature and protected from light.
2. Diazepam should not be stored drawn up in plastic syringes or in solution bags because it can be absorbed into the plastic.
3. The manufacturers recommend that it not be mixed with other medications or solutions.
4. Diazepam is metabolized by the liver and eliminated by the kidneys.

Xylazine Hydrochloride

Xylazine is an alpha-2 agonist with sedative, analgesic, and muscle relaxant properties. It is approved for use in dogs, cats, horses, deer, and elk. This agent causes vomiting in a large percentage of cats and in some dogs. Xylazine is antagonized by yohimbine. It produces effective analgesia in horses and is often used for treating the pain associated with colic and for sedation for minor procedures. It is also used in combination with ketamine for short-term field procedures in horses, such as castration and suturing of extensive wounds, because this combination usually produces 15 to 20 minutes of recumbency. Extralabel use of xylazine for cesarean sections in cattle and other surgical procedures is common. Xylazine is used in cats and dogs as a tranquilizer and in combination with other injectable agents for surgical procedures.

Clinical Uses. Clinical uses include sedation, analgesia, short-term anesthesia (when combined with other agents), and induction of vomiting.

Dosage Forms

1. Rompun
2. AnaSed
3. Gemini
4. Sedazine

Adverse Side Effects. These include bradycardia, hypotension, respiratory depression, and increased sensitivity to epinephrine, resulting in cardiac arrhythmias. Overdose increases the potential for these effects.

Technician's Notes

1. Because of the potential of xylazine to cause bradycardia or heart block in dogs, atropine should be used as a premedicant in this species.
2. Xylazine is used in cattle at one-tenth of the equine dose.
3. Horses may appear heavily sedated with xylazine and still respond to painful stimuli by kicking.
4. Small-animal (20 mg/ml) and large-animal (100 mg/ml) concentrations are available. Care should be taken not to confuse them when dosing an animal.

Detomidine Hydrochloride

Detomidine, like xylazine, is an alpha-2 agonist. It is approved as a sedative/analgesic for horses, and clinicians often report excellent analgesic properties in their patients when using this product. It is used for procedures in horses when sedation and analgesia are needed and reportedly produces better analgesia of the rear limbs than does xylazine.

Clinical Uses. Detomidine is used for sedation and analgesia in horses.

Dosage Form

1. Dormosedan

Adverse Side Effects. These may include sweating, muscle tremors, penile prolapse, bradycardia, and heart block.

> **Technician's Notes**
>
> The manufacturer warns that detomidine should be used very carefully with other sedative drugs and that it should not be used with the potentiated sulfa drugs such as trimethoprim/sulfa.

Medetomidine

Medetomidine is an alpha-2–adrenergic agonist labeled for use as a sedative and analgesic in dogs more than 12 weeks of age. Atipamezole (Antisedan) is the reversal agent for this drug.

Clinical Uses. Uses include to facilitate clinical examination, minor surgical procedures, and minor dental procedures that do not require intubation.

Dosage Form

1. Domitor

Adverse Side Effects. Side effects include bradycardia, AV heart block, decreased respirations, hypothermia, urination, vomiting, hyperglycemia, and pain at the injection site.

> **Technician's Notes**
>
> 1. Treatment of medetomidine-induced bradycardia with anticholinergic drugs (atropine or glycopyrrolate) is not recommended because of the potential for more serious arrhythmias.
> 2. Antisedan is recommended for treatment of medetomidine-induced effects.
> 3. Before attempting the use of medetomidine in combination with other sedatives, references should be consulted for potential side effects and dosages.

BARBITURATES

The barbiturates are one of the oldest categories of CNS depressants used in veterinary medicine. They are derived from the parent compound barbituric acid and cause various responses ranging from sedation to death, depending on the dose and the circumstances of use. Barbiturates are used in veterinary medicine as sedatives, anticonvulsants, general anesthetics, and euthanasia agents. They are easy and cheap to administer but have much potential for complications because of their potent depressing effects on the cardiac and pulmonary systems (especially in cats) and because they are non-reversible and must be metabolized by the liver before elimination can occur. Individual patients with poor liver function, little body fat, or preexisting illnesses that cause acidosis may be at risk when receiving barbiturates. Because of their alkalinity, the ultrashort-acting barbiturates can cause necrosis of tissue if administered outside the vein in the subcutaneous space. The barbiturates are metabolized by the liver and are potent depressors of the respiratory system.

Barbiturates are classified according to their duration of action as long-acting, short-acting, and ultrashort-acting, or they are classified according to the chemical side chain on the barbituric acid molecule as an oxybarbiturate or a thiobarbiturate

TABLE 4-2	Barbiturate Classifications		
Generic Name	Proprietary Name	Classification	Duration of Action
Phenobarbital	Luminal	Long-acting oxybarbiturate	4-8 hours
Pentobarbital	Nembutal	Short-acting oxybarbiturate	$1/2$-2 hours
Thiopental	Pentothal	Ultrashort-acting thiobarbiturate	10-30 minutes

(Table 4-2). The long- and short-acting barbiturates have a side chain connected by oxygen and are therefore called *oxybarbiturates.* The thiobarbiturates have a side chain connected by a sulfur and are called *thiobarbiturates.* The thiobarbiturates are very soluble in fat and tend to move rapidly out of the CNS into the fat stores of the body, thus accounting for their ultrashort activity.

Clinical Uses. Clinical uses include the prevention and treatment of seizures, sedation, anesthesia, and euthanasia.

Dosage Forms

Long-Acting Barbiturates (Oxybarbiturates, 8 to 12 Hours)

1. Phenobarbital. Numerous proprietary and generic products exist. Phenobarbital is used primarily as an anticonvulsant to prevent epileptic seizures; it is administered by the oral route. Phenobarbital is a class IV controlled substance.

Short-Acting Barbiturates (Oxybarbiturates, 45 Minutes to 1.5 Hours)

1. Pentobarbital sodium (Nembutal and numerous generic products). Pentobarbital is given by intravenous injection (the intraperitoneal route may also be used) and provides 1 to 2 hours of general anesthesia. In the earlier days of veterinary anesthesia, it was the routine general anesthesia used in dogs. Today, pentobarbital is used primarily to control seizures

in progress and as a euthanasia agent. Intravenous administration of glucose or concurrent use of chloramphenicol may prolong the recovery period. Pentobarbital is a class II controlled substance.

Ultrashort-Acting Barbiturates (Thiobarbiturates, 5 to 30 Minutes)

The thiobarbiturates are very alkaline (especially at the higher concentrations) and must be given intravenously to avoid necrosis and subsequent sloughing of tissue. The thiobarbiturates are rapidly redistributed into the fat stores of the body within 5 to 30 minutes.

Extreme care should be taken when administering a thiobarbiturate to a thin animal because of the lack of fat stores. The thiobarbiturates are prepared as a sterile powder in vials for dilution up to the desired concentration; they are stable for long periods in the undiluted form. Sterile water for injection should be used as the diluent because solutions with electrolytes hasten precipitate formation. Solutions should not be administered if precipitates are present.

The thiobarbiturates can cause a period of apnea when they are rapidly administered intravenously. If spontaneous respirations do not resume in a short time, controlled respirations should be started. The barbiturates can also cause a period of CNS excitement when administered intravenously if they are given too slowly. It is often recommended to give one third to one half of the calculated dose rapidly to avoid the excitement phase. The remainder of the dose is administered to effect.

Dosage Forms

1. Thiopental (Pentothal). Thiopental is used as an intravenous agent to induce general anesthesia.
2. Methohexital (Brevane). Methohexital is an ultrashort-acting barbiturate that produces 5 to 10 minutes of anesthesia. It has been recommended for use in the sight hounds because of its rapid redistribution and metabolism by the liver.

Adverse Side Effects. These include excessive CNS depression, paradoxical CNS excitement, severe respiratory depression, and cardiovascular depression. Tissue irritation may occur when the barbiturates are injected perivascularly.

Technician's Notes

1. Recovery from pentobarbital is often prolonged, and dogs exhibit padding limb movements during this time.
2. Thiobarbiturates should not be used in sight hounds or in any very thin animal.
3. Giving additional doses of thiobarbiturates may prolong recovery.
4. The barbiturates are potent depressors of the respiratory system.

DISSOCIATIVE AGENTS

The dissociative agents belong to the cyclohexylamine family, which includes phencyclidine, ketamine, and tiletamine.

Dissociative anesthesia is characterized by involuntary muscle rigidity (**catalepsy**), amnesia, and analgesia; pharyngeal/laryngeal reflexes are maintained, and muscle tone is increased. Because deep abdominal pain is not eliminated (surgical stage III is not usually reached) with dissociative anesthesia, it is recommended only for restraint, diagnostic procedures, and minor surgery. Dissociative agents are often combined with other agents for abdominal surgery, however. Dissociative drugs produce minor cardiac stimulation, and

respiratory depression can occur at the higher doses. These agents act by altering neurotransmitter activity, causing depression of the thalamus and cerebral cortex and activation of the limbic system (Plumb, 1999).

Some species are often ataxic and hyperresponsive during induction and recovery with dissociatives agents (Muir and Hubbell, 1989). Tremors, spasticity, and convulsions can occur at the higher doses; hallucinations have been reported in humans and are suspected in cats.

Clinical Uses. Dissociative agents are used for sedation, restraint, and anesthesia.

Dosage Forms

1. Ketamine HCl (Ketaset, Vetalar, Ketalar). Ketamine is approved for use in humans, primates, and cats but has extralabel uses in various species including dogs, horses, birds, small ruminants, and reptiles. Tranquilizers such as acepromazine, xylazine, and diazepam are often used concurrently with ketamine to increase muscle relaxation and to deepen the level of anesthesia. Oral, ocular, and laryngeal reflexes are maintained when ketamine is used alone (except at the high doses). Occasional spastic jerking movements can occur in cats who are administered ketamine.

    Increased salivation may accompany administration of this drug and can be controlled or prevented with the use of atropine or glycopyrrolate. Because cats' eyes remain open after the administration of ketamine, an ophthalmic lubricant should be used. Ketamine is a class III controlled substance.
2. Tiletamine HCl (Telazol—tiletamine plus zolazepam HCl). Telazol is an injectable anesthetic that consists of a combination of tiletamine (chemically related to ketamine) and zolazepam (a tranquilizer). Telazol is approved for use in dogs and cats. The pharmacokinetics and pharmacotherapeutics of tiletamine are similar to those of ketamine. Because of the zolazepam in this product, additional agents are not needed for muscle relaxation. Ocular lubrication should be used in cats receiving Telazol. Telazol is a class III controlled substance.
3. Phencyclidine (Sernylan). This dissociative agent is no longer available. It was originally used as an im-

mobilizing agent for non-human primates. Its street name is "PCP" or "angel dust" (Upson, 1988).

Adverse Side Effects. These are usually associated with high doses and include spastic jerking movement, convulsions, respiratory depression, burning at the intramuscular injection site, and drying of the cornea.

Technician's Notes

1. Both ketamine and tiletamine may cause burning at the injection site. Adequate restraint should be used to ensure injection of all the medication.
2. The metabolites of the dissociative agents are excreted through the kidneys. These drugs may be contraindicated in animals with compromised kidney function.

OPIOID AGONISTS

An opioid is any compound derived from opium poppy alkaloids and the synthetic drugs with similar pharmacologic properties. These drugs produce analgesia and sedation (hypnosis) while reducing anxiety and fear. Morphine sulfate is the narcotic with which all others are compared. The effects of the narcotics are produced by combining with opiate receptors at the deep levels of the brain (e.g., thalamus, hypothalamus, limbic system). The opioid receptors are grouped into the following five classes (Plumb, 1999):

1. Mu—found in pain-regulating areas of the brain; contribute to analgesia, euphoria, respiratory depression, physical dependence, and hypothermic actions
2. Kappa—found in the cerebral cortex and spinal cord; contribute to analgesia, sedation, and miosis
3. Sigma—may be responsible for struggling, whining, hallucinations, and mydriatic effects
4. Delta—effects unknown
5. Epsilon—effects unknown

The opioids are used as preanesthetics or postanesthetics because of their sedative and analgesic proper-

ties. Sedation is more pronounced at the higher doses. They are sometimes used alone or in combination with tranquilizers as anesthetics for surgical procedures, for relief of colic pain in horses, and for restraint/capture of wild/zoo animals. At low doses, the opioids have antitussive (cough suppression) properties owing to depression of the cough center in the brain and antidiarrheal action because they cause a reduction in peristalsis or segmental contractions. Several potential adverse side effects are associated with the narcotics. Opioids are potent respiratory depressants. Because they affect the thermoregulatory centers in the brain (the body's thermostat), they may cause panting, defecation, flatulence, and vomiting; sound sensitivity may also occur. Excitement may occur in dogs if the narcotic is rapidly given intravenously. Cats and horses are reported to be sensitive to the opioids and may exhibit excitatory effects at high doses. Because opioids cross the placenta fairly slowly and their effects can be antagonized, they can be useful when performing cesarean sections. Opioids are metabolized by the liver, and the resulting metabolites are eliminated in the urine. Most of the opioid preparations are class II controlled substances, and they can be antagonized by the narcotic antagonists.

Clinical Uses. Opioid agonists are used for analgesia, sedation, restraint, anesthesia, treatment of coughing, and treatment of diarrhea.

Dosage Forms

Naturally Occurring Narcotics

1. Opium (laudanum—10% opium), paregoric. Opium is derived from the seed capsule of the opium poppy. Paregoric, also called *camphorated tincture of opium,* has been used for more than 100 years for the treatment of diarrhea. It has been used in veterinary medicine for treating diarrhea primarily in calves and foals.
2. Morphine sulfate (Duramorph). Morphine is an opium derivative used to treat severe pain; occasionally, it is used as a preanesthetic or anesthetic agent (e.g., cesarean section in dogs); and it is also used to relieve the anxiety associated with acute congestive heart failure. It exerts its effects primar-

ily on mu receptors. Morphine is a class II controlled substance that should be used under strict supervision because of its potential for abuse. It is the standard opioid with which all others are compared in terms of analgesic effect.

Synthetic Narcotics

1. Meperidine (Demerol). Meperidine is a mu agonist that is approximately one-eighth as potent an analgesic as morphine. It is used for relief of acute pain, such as that occurring after orthopedic procedures. It also may be combined with a tranquilizer for use as an anesthetic agent (neuroleptanalgesic). No meperidine products carry a veterinary label; however, the human products often have extralabel uses in animals. Naloxone is the preferred antagonist.

2. Oxymorphone (Numorphan). Oxymorphone is a semi-synthetic opioid that is a mu agonist; it is approximately 10 times more potent an analgesic than morphine. This drug is used primarily in dogs for restraint, for diagnostic procedures, and for minor surgical procedures. It may be combined with tranquilizers to produce neuroleptanalgesia; naloxone is the antagonist.

3. Butorphanol tartrate (Torbutrol; Torbugesic). Butorphanol is a synthetic, partial opioid agonist. Its narcotic activity is exerted on kappa and sigma receptors. It is a class IV controlled substance. Butorphanol has 2 to 5 times the analgesic properties of morphine and a much greater antitussive effect (4 times morphine and 100 times codeine) (Upson, 1988). Torbutrol is a product that is approved as an antitussive agent in dogs. It is also used in dogs and cats as an analgesic and preanesthetic. Torbugesic is approved for the treatment of the pain associated with colic in horses. It is also used in combination with other sedatives/tranquilizers in horses, dogs, and cats as a preanesthetic or for minor surgical procedures.

4. Fentanyl (Sublimaze). Fentanyl is an opioid agonist that is found in the neuroleptanalgesic Innovar-Vet. It has approximately 100 times the analgesic properties of morphine. Fentanyl is a class II controlled substance. Fentanyl transdermal patches are sometimes used in animals to control chronic pain (see Chapter 14).

5. Hydrocodone bitartrate (Hycodan; Tussigon). Hydrocodone is an opioid agonist that is used as an antitussive agent in dogs. It is a class III controlled substance.

6. Etorphine (M-99). Etorphine is an opioid that produces analgesic effects 1000 times those of morphine; it is restricted to use by veterinarians in zoo or exotic animal practice (Upson, 1988). It is lethal to people who accidentally inject themselves (it also can be absorbed through intact skin) if the antagonist (diprenorphine) is not administered immediately. Etorphine is a class II controlled substance.

7. Pentazocine (Talwin; Talwin-V). Pentazocine is a partial opioid agonist that is approved for pain relief in horses and dogs. It is a class IV controlled substance.

8. Diphenoxylate (Lomotil). Diphenoxylate is a synthetic opioid agonist that is combined with atropine for use as an antidiarrheal agent. This drug is a class V controlled substance.

9. Apomorphine—generic labeling. Apomorphine is an opioid with the principal effect of inducing vomiting by stimulating the chemoreceptor trigger zone in the brain. This drug is often administered by placing a portion of a tablet in the conjunctival sac for absorption (see Chapter 8).

10. Methadone (Dolophine). Methadone is a synthetic opioid that was developed as a treatment for morphine and heroin addiction in humans. Its primary use in veterinary medicine is in the treatment of colic pain in horses. Methadone is a class II controlled substance.

11. Codeine—generic labeling or in combination. Codeine is an opioid that is available in human-label products for use as an antitussive in dogs.

12. Carfentanil (Wildnil). Carfentanil is used for wildlife anesthesia. It has 10,000 times the potency of morphine.

Adverse Side Effects. These can include respiratory depression, excitement (cats and horses), nausea, vomiting, diarrhea, defecation, panting, and convulsions. Overdose causes profound respiratory depression.

OPIOID ANTAGONISTS

Opioid antagonists block the effects of opioids by binding with opiate receptors, displacing narcotic molecules already present, and preventing further narcotic binding at the sites. These antagonists are classified as pure antagonists or as partial antagonists. The partial antagonists may have some agonist activity (analgesic and respiratory depressant effects).

These drugs are usually administered by the intravenous route, and they exert their effects very rapidly (15 to 60 seconds).

Clinical Uses. Opioid antagonists are used to antagonize the effects of the opioid agonists.

Dosage Forms

1. Naloxone (naloxone HCl injection, Narcan). Naloxone is a pure opioid antagonist chemically similar to oxymorphone, with high affinity for mu receptors; it has no agonist activity.
2. Nalorphine (Nalline). Nalorphine is a partial antagonist that may produce untoward analgesic and respiratory depressant effects.

Adverse Side Effects. Nalorphine and levallorphan may induce respiratory depression. Naloxone usually has few adverse effects if dosed correctly.

NEUROLEPTANALGESICS

A neuroleptanalgesic agent consists of an opioid and a tranquilizer. Animals receiving neuroleptanalgesics may or may not remain conscious (Muir and Hubbell, 1989); they often defecate and are highly responsive to sound stimuli. The opioid effects of the neuroleptanalgesics can be antagonized with the opioid antagonists.

Clinical Uses. Neuroleptanalgesics are used for sedation, restraint, and anesthesia.

Dosage Forms

1. Fentanyl and droperidol (Innovar-Vet). Innovar-Vet is the only commercially available neuroleptanalgesic. It may be used for restraint, for diagnostic procedures, as a preanesthetic, and for minor surgical procedures.
2. Other neuroleptanalgesics may be prepared by a clinician and include the following:
   Acepromazine and morphine
   Acepromazine and oxymorphone
   Xylazine and butorphanol

Adverse Side Effects. These can include panting, flatulence, personality changes, increased sound sensitivity, and bradycardia. Overdose may cause severe depression of the CNS, respiratory system, and cardiovascular system.

DRUGS TO PREVENT OR CONTROL SEIZURES

Seizures occur in animals for various reasons, which include but are not limited to unknown (idiopathic), infectious (postdistemper), traumatic (head injury), toxicity (strychnine poisoning), and metabolic (heatstroke) factors. Prolonged seizures in progress require emergency action with intravenous therapy; periodic, recurring seizures require preventive oral medication. Oral preventive therapy often must be titrated to the individual patient and reviewed regularly for appropriate dose adjustment that controls the seizure activity.

Clinical Uses. These drugs are used to prevent seizures or to control seizures in progress.

Dosage Forms

1. Diazepam (Valium). Diazepam is a tranquilizer with potent antiseizure properties. It is administered intravenously and has a 3- to 4-hour duration of action.
2. Pentobarbital—generic products. Pentobarbital is a short-acting barbiturate that is effective for con-

trolling seizures. It is administered intravenously and has a 1- to 3-hour duration.

3. Phenobarbital (Luminal, Solfoton, generic formulations). Phenobarbital is an effective antiseizure drug that is available in oral and parenteral formulations. The oral route is the usual means of administering this drug to dogs and cats. The injectable form is used in horses (foals) by some clinicians. Drowsiness is a potential side effect of phenobarbital. Phenobarbital is a class IV controlled substance.

4. Primidone (Mylepsin). Primidone is similar chemically to phenobarbital, and a portion of the primidone dose is metabolized to phenobarbital by the liver. It is administered orally to dogs and cats, although its use in cats is controversial. Adverse side effects may include agitation, anxiety, polyuria, polydipsia, and dermatitis.

5. Phenytoin sodium (Dilantin). The use of phenytoin has declined considerably through the years because of its variable pharmacokinetics in dogs and cats (Plumb, 1999). It may occasionally be used in combination with other antiseizure medications.

6. Bromide is an old anticonvulsant that has sparked renewed interest, mainly as an adjunct to phenobarb or primidone therapy.

7. Clorazepate

8. Felbamate

Adverse Side Effects. These may include drowsiness, CNS depression, anxiety, agitation, polyuria, polydipsia, and hepatotoxicity (phenobarbital and primidone). Consult product inserts or appropriate references for specific effects.

Technician's Notes

1. Inadequate client compliance is a frequent cause of the failure of anticonvulsant therapy; clients should be advised about the importance of following medication instructions carefully.

2. Reserpine and phenothiazine drugs should not be given to epileptic animals.

MISCELLANEOUS CENTRAL NERVOUS SYSTEM DRUGS

Propofol

Propofol is a short-acting hypnotic unrelated to other general anesthetic agents; its mechanism of action is not well-understood. Chemically it is an alkylphenol derivative. The product that is commercially available is an emulsion that contains soybean oil, glycerol, and egg lecithin. Because of its white color, some clinicians have called this product "milk of amnesia." Propofol produces a rapid and smooth induction in dogs when given slowly IV. It produces sedation, restraint, or unconsciousness depending on the dose. A single bolus lasts 2 to 5 minutes, making it particularly useful when rapid recovery is important.

Clinical Uses. Propofol is useful for anesthetic induction before administration of an inhalant anesthetic, for outpatient procedures, as a substitute for barbiturates in sight hounds, and for patients with pre-existing cardiac arrhythmias.

Dosage Forms

1. Rapinovet
2. PropoFlo
3. Diprivan (human label)

Adverse Side Effects. Apnea may occur if propofol is given too rapidly IV. Occasional seizure-like signs may be seen. Prolonged recoveries and/or Heinz body production may be seen in cats with repeated use.

Technician's Notes

1. Propofol is an expensive agent that contains no preservatives. It is recommended that unused portions be discarded because bacteria may grow in the opened container.

Glyceryl Guaiacolate or Guaifenesin (Guailaxin, Gecolate)

Guaifenesin is a skeletal muscle relaxant that exerts it effects on the connecting neurons of the spinal cord and brain stem (Riebold, Goble, and Geiser, 1978). It is used primarily in equine medicine to induce general anesthesia or to extend the anesthetic activity of other injectable field anesthetics (i.e., ketamine and xylazine). It may be used as a 5% or 10% solution in 5% dextrose. Some clinicians add an ultrashort-acting barbiturate to the solution before administering it intravenously. Relatively large amounts are required to induce general anesthesia, and small increments are given to maintain or extend the anesthetic effects of other agents.

Clinical Uses. These include induction or prolongation of general anesthesia in large animals and occasional use as an expectorant.

Dosage Forms
1. Guailaxin
2. Gecolate

Adverse Side Effects. Adverse side effects are limited. Hemolysis has been reported when greater than 5% solutions are used.

Technician's Notes

1. Guaifenesin is packaged as a soluble powder; it may be difficult to dissolve when the diluent is added. Warming the 5% dextrose before mixing may aid solution preparation. It should be mixed only immediately before use because a precipitate forms if the solution is allowed to stand for several hours.
2. When administering increments of guaifenesin to maintain or extend anesthesia, communicate thoroughly with the veterinarian to understand the quantity of this drug to administer.

Chloral Hydrate/Magnesium Sulfate

This combination has been used as an intravenous agent for anesthesia in large animals. Because of the potential for severe irritation of tissue if administered outside of the vein and because of the advent of more efficacious agents, this combination is seldom used.

CENTRAL NERVOUS SYSTEM STIMULANTS

The primary medical use of the CNS stimulants is for treatment of respiratory depression or arrest. Many of the other uses of CNS stimulants are illegal or unethical (e.g., to enhance athletic performance).

Doxapram

Doxapram activates the respiratory system by stimulating respiratory centers in the medulla. It is labeled for use in dogs, cats, and horses. Its main indications are to stimulate respirations during or after general anesthesia, in newborns, and in cases of cardiopulmonary arrest. It is labeled for intravenous use but may administered under the tongue (1 to 2 drops) or into the umbilical vein of newborns.

Clinical Uses. These include stimulation of respiration in newborns and during or after anesthesia.

Dosage Forms
1. Dopram-V
2. Dopram. Approved for use in humans.

Adverse Side Effects. Adverse side effects are rare and usually associated with overdose. Hypertension, seizures, and hyperventilation may occur.

Technician's Notes

One to two drops of doxapram may be placed under the tongue or injected into the umbilical vein of newborns to stimulate respirations.

Pentyleneterazol (Metrazol)

Pentylenetetrazol is a generalized stimulant of the CNS that has been used to stimulate respirations and to hasten recovery from anesthesia. It has limited use in veterinary medicine.

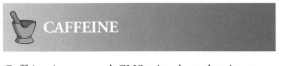

CAFFEINE

Caffeine is a general CNS stimulant that increases wakefulness.

AMPHETAMINES

Amphetamines, which are potent stimulants of the cerebral cortex, are similar chemically to epinephrine. They have no legitimate medical indications in veterinary medicine.

BEHAVIORAL PHARMACOTHERAPY

The use of drugs to treat behavioral problems in animals is a relatively new, but rapidly growing area of veterinary medicine. Behavior problems such as separation anxiety, fears and phobia, unruliness, hyperactivity, compulsive disorders, cognitive dysfunction in older dogs, and inappropriate elimination in cats are being diagnosed in increasing numbers. Many animals with behavioral disorders are taken in desperation to animal shelters, but a growing number of clients are willing to attempt to correct the conditions with environmental management, behavior modification, and/or pharmacotherapy.

Informed consent should be obtained from the client before these drugs are used (Shull, 1998) because many of the drugs used in behavioral pharmacotherapy are human psychiatric drugs that have not been approved for use in animals. The technician or veterinarian should explain to the animal owner the extralabel status of the drug, possible side effects or precautions, as well as the medical effects to be expected in the pet. Owners should also be aware that pharmacotherapy may not be a cure-all for problems of behavior and that the problems may return after therapy is discontinued.

All drugs used in psychotherapy are thought to produce their effects through altering neurotransmitter activity in the brain (Simpson, 1996a,b). The five neurotransmitters of clinical importance in behavioral pharmacotherapy are acetylcholine, dopamine, norepinephrine, serotonin, and gamma-aminobutyric acid (GABA).

Dopamine, norepinephrine, and serotonin are called *monoamine neurotransmitters* since they have similar chemical structures. Monoamines are found in large quantities in areas of the brain often associated with the expression and control of emotions. The primary method by which monamines are inactivated is by their reuptake from the synapse back into synaptic vesicles in nerve endings (see Figure 4-4). Drugs that block or inhibit their reuptake increase their activity. Acetylcholine is the most widely distributed neurotransmitter in the body. It is associated with a variety of behavioral effects and inactivated by cholinesterase at the synapse. Some of the most common side effects of drugs used in behavioral psychotherapy are related to their anti-cholinergic effects, such as dry mouth, increased heart rate, urine retention, and constipation. Gamma-aminobutyric acid is considered to be an inhibitory neurotransmitter and is widely distributed in the brain.

PHARMACOTHERAPEUTIC AGENTS

The most commonly used drugs in treating behavioral problems in veterinary medicine are the anti-anxiety medications, the antidepressants, and miscellaneous agents such as the synthetic progestins. All the drugs listed in the following carry a human label, except those otherwise indicated.

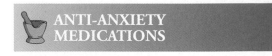

ANTI-ANXIETY MEDICATIONS

Benzodiazepines

The benzodiazepines most commonly used in veterinary medicine include diazepam, alprazolam, and lorazepam. All the benzodiazepines are similar in structure and mechanism of action. They are thought to bind with and promote GABA activity in both the cerebral cortex and in subcortical areas, such as the limbic system.

Clinical Uses. Behavioral uses of benzodiazepines include the treatment of fears and phobias, separation anxiety, fear, aggression, anxiety-induced stereotypes, urine marking in cats, and appetite stimulation.

Dosage Forms

1. Diazepam (Valium)
2. Alprazolam (Xanax)
3. Lorazepam (Ativan)

Adverse Side Effects. These may include lethargy, ataxia, polyuria and polydipsia (PUPD), hyperexcitability, and hepatic necrosis (cats).

Azapirones

Buspirone is the azapirone agent used in behavioral pharmacotherapy. Unlike the benzodiazepines, it possesses no muscle relaxant, anticonvulsant, or sedative effects. Its anti-anxiety effect is thought to be a result of blocking serotonin receptors.

Clinical Uses. Veterinary uses include the control of urine spraying/marking as well as the control of fearfulness and anxiety.

Dosage Form

1. Buspirone (BuSpar)

Adverse Side Effects. Few serious side effects appear to exist.

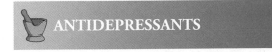 **ANTIDEPRESSANTS**

Tricyclics

The tricyclics used commonly in veterinary medicine include amitriptyline, imipramine, and clomipramine. These drugs are thought to exert their effects by preventing the reuptake of norepinephrine and serotonin. Clomipramine is apparently a selective inhibitor of serotonin reuptake. The tricyclic group is often used on a long-term basis and may take several weeks of use to become effective. Some of the tricyclics are available in the generic form and are relatively inexpensive to use.

Clinical Uses. Uses include the treatment of separation anxiety, obsessive disorders (e.g., lick granuloma, tail chasing), fearful aggression, hyperactivity, hypervocalization, and urine marking.

Dosage Forms

1. Amitriptyline (Elavil, generic forms)
2. Imipramine (Tofranil)
3. Clomipramine (Anafranil, Clomicalm [veterinary label])

Adverse Side Effects. Side effects may include sedation, tachycardia, heart block, mydriasis, dry mouth, reduced tear production, urine retention, and constipation.

Serotonin Reuptake Inhibitors

The serotonin reuptake inhibitors include fluoxetine, sertraline, paroxetine, and fluvoxamine. As their name indicates, these drugs increase the amount of serotonin in the synapse by inhibiting its reuptake back into the nerve terminal. The serotonin reuptake inhibitors have fewer potential side effects than the tricyclics but are usually more expensive.

Clinical Uses. Used for a variety of behavioral syndromes including obsessive disorders, phobias, aggression, and separation anxiety.

Dosage Forms

1. Fluoxetine (Prozac)
2. Sertraline (Zoloft)
3. Paroxetine (Paxil)
4. Fluvoxamine (Luvox)

Adverse Side Effects. Side effects are relatively few but include anorexia, nausea, lethargy, anxiety, and diarrhea.

Monoamine Oxidase-B Inhibitors

The neurotransmitter dopamine is broken down by the enzyme monoamine oxidase-B (MOA-B). Substances such as selegiline (a MOA-B inhibitor) block or inhibit MOA-B and allow dopamine levels to increase. Decreased dopamine levels may be associated with certain types of dementia seen in older dogs (canine cognitive dysfunction). Canine cognitive dysfunction is characterized by disorientation, decreased activity level, abnormal sleep-wake cycles, loss of house training, decreased or altered responsiveness, and decreased or altered greeting behavior.

Clinical Uses. Uses include treatment of old-dog dementia and treatment of canine Cushing's disease.

Dosage Form

1. Selegiline (Eldepryl, Atapryl, Anipryl [veterinary label])

Adverse Side Effects. Side effects include vomiting, diarrhea, anorexia, restlessness, lethargy, salivation, shaking, and deafness.

Synthetic Progestins

The synthetic progestins are sometimes used to treat behavioral problems through mechanisms associated with changing hormonal levels (reduced gonadotropins) or through some direct effect on the cerebral cortex.

Clinical Uses. Uses include the treatment of urine spraying/marking, intermale aggression, or dominance aggression.

Dosage Forms

1. Megestrol acetate (Megace, Ovaban [veterinary label])
2. Medroxy-progesterone (Depo-Provera)

Side Effects. Transient diabetes mellitus (cats), PUPD, increased weight gain, personality changes, endometritis, endometrial hyperplasia, mammary hypertrophy, mammary tumor, adrenal atrophy, and lactation.

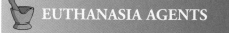 **EUTHANASIA AGENTS**

Euthanasia agents should have several properties to make them effective medically and esthetically for this emotion-laden procedure. These drugs should rapidly produce unconsciousness without struggling, vocaliza-

tions, or excessive involuntary movements. Death should follow quickly owing to the cessation of all vital functions, such as respiratory and cardiac functions.

The main component of most of the euthanasia agents is pentobarbital. Pentobarbital may also be combined with other agents such as propylene glycol and alcohol. Pentobarbital alone is a class II controlled substance, and pentobarbital combinations usually are class III controlled substances.

Clincial Uses. These agents are used to produce a rapid, humane death.

Dosage Forms

1. Pentobarbital sodium (Sleepaway, pentobarbital generic). These products are class II controlled substances for intravenous use.
2. Pentobarbital sodium (Beuthanasia-D). This drug is a class III controlled substance for intravenous use. This product is different from the pentobarbital sodium described above because it contains rhodamine B, a bluish-red dye to help distinguish it from other parenteral pentobarbital solutions, as well as phenytoin and preservatives.
3. Euthanasia-6. This product contains pentobarbital only.
4. T-61. T-61 is a non-narcotic, non-barbiturate agent that contains a general anesthetic, a local anesthetic, and a muscle paralyzer. It is not a controlled substance. It must be administered according to manufacturer instructions (first two-thirds slowly) to avoid apparent anxiety or pain.
5. Fatal-Plus. Contains pentobarbital sodium and is available as a sterile powder for dilution or as a prepared solution. The solution contains a stabilizer, a solvent, and a preservative.

Adverse Side Effects. These may include muscle twitching, and death may be delayed if the drug is injected outside the vein.

REFERENCES

DeLahunta, A.: Diencephalon. In DeLahunta, A. (ed.): Veterinary Neuroanatomy and Clinical Neurology. W.B. Saunders Company, Philadelphia, 1983.

Muir W.W., Hubbell, J.A.: Handbook of Veterinary Anesthesia. Mosby, St. Louis, 1989.

Plumb, D.C.: Veterinary Drug Handbook, ed. 3. Iowa State University Press, Ames, 1999.

Riebold, T.W., Goble, D.O., Geiser, D.R.: Principles and Techniques of Large Animal Anesthesia. Iowa State University Press, Ames, 1978.

Shull, E.A.: Psychopharmacology in Veterinary Behavioral Medicine. Annual Conference For Veterinarians and Technicians, UT-CVM, Knoxville, TN, 1998.

Simpson, B.S., Simpson, D.M.: Behavioral Pharmacotherapy. Part I. Antipsychotics and Antidepressants. Compend. Contin. Educ. Pract. Vet. 18(10):1067-1081, 1996.

Simpson, B.S., Simpson, D.M.: Behavioral Pharmacotherapy. Part II. Anxiolytics and Mood Stabilizers. Compend. Contin. Educ. Proc. Vet. 18(11): 1203-1210, 1996.

Snyder, S.: Mood modifiers. In Snyder, S. (ed.): Drugs and the Brain. Scientific American Library, New York, 1986.

Tortora, G.J., Anagnostakos, N.P.: The autonomic nervous system. In Tortora, G.J., Anagnostakos, N.P. (eds.): Principles of Anatomy and Physiology, 6th ed. Harper Collins Publishing Company, New York, 1991.

Upson, S.W.: Central nervous system. In Upson, S.W. (ed.): Handbook of Clinical Veterinary Pharmacology, 3rd ed. Dan Upson Enterprises, Manhattan, KS, 1988.

Williams, B.R., Baer, C.: Drugs affecting the autonomic nervous system. In Williams, B.R., Baer, C. (eds.): Essentials of Clinical Pharmacology in Nursing. Springhouse Corporation, Springhouse, PA, 1990.

■ Review Questions

1. Define the difference between an agonist and an opioid antagonist. _____

2. Define neurotransmitter. _____

3. The area of the brain that serves to relay information from the spinal cord and brain stem to the interpretation center in the cerebrum is the
   a. Cerebellum
   b. Thalamus
   c. Hypothalamus
   d. Hippocampus

4. Most CNS drugs act by _____ or _____ the effects of neurotransmitters.

5. What are the primary neurotransmitters for adrenergic receptors? _____

6. List the four primary ways in which drugs affect the ANS. _____

7. List five indications for the use of cholinergic agents. _____

8. Atropine, scopolamine, glycopyrrolate, and aminopentamide are examples of what specific drug class? _____

9. What category of drug is used to treat cardiac arrest and anaphylactic shock? _____

10. Propanolol is an example of what category of drug?
    a. Alpha agonist
    b. Beta agonist
    c. Alpha blocker
    d. Beta blocker

11. What are some adverse side effects of xylazine, and what drug may be used to antagonize its effects? _____

12. Why would you be concerned about using a thiobarbiturate to induce anesthesia in a very thin dog? _____

13. What are some of the characteristics of a cat anesthetized with ketamine? _____

14. List some of the signs of a narcotic overdose. _____

15. List two narcotic antagonists. _____

16. Why should glyceryl guaiacolate not be mixed until just before use? _____

17. You are assisting in the delivery of a litter of puppies and you deliver one that is not breathing adequately. What drug would the veterinarian instruct to give and by what route? _____

18. Why are euthanasia solutions containing only pentobarbital classified as class II controlled substances, whereas those containing pentobarbital and other substances are classified as class III controlled substances? _____

19. All psychotherapy drugs are thought to produce their effects by altering _____ activity in the brain.

20. Dissociative agents such as ketamine and tiletamine may cause _____ at the injection site.

21. A hypnotic (anesthetic) known for its very short duration and its white color is _____.

22. An inhibitory neurotransmitter widely distributed in the brain is _____

23. A benzodiazepine used as an anti-anxiety medication and as an appetite stimulant in cats is _____.

24. An example of a tricyclic antidepressant used in veterinary medicine for separation anxiety in dogs is _____

25. _____ is used to treat old-dog dementia.

Chapter 5

Drugs Used in Respiratory System Disorders

LEARNING OBJECTIVES

After studying this chapter, you should be able to:

1. Describe the basic anatomy and physiology of the respiratory system
2. List the protective mechanisms of the respiratory system
3. Describe the fundamental principles of treatment of the respiratory system
4. List the difference between the actions of the expectorants, antitussives, and mucolytics
5. Describe the action of the bronchodilators
6. Describe the use of antihistamines and decongestants in respiratory disease
7. List potential uses for respiratory stimulants

KEY TERMS

Antitussive A drug that inhibits or suppresses the cough reflex.

Bronchoconstriction Narrowing of the bronchi and bronchioles that results in increased airway resistance and decreased airflow.

Bronchodilation Widening lumen of bronchi and bronchioles, which results from relaxation of the smooth muscle in the walls of the bronchi and bronchioles. Airway resistance is decreased, and airflow is increased.

Decongestant A substance that reduces the swelling of mucous membranes.

Expectorant A drug that enhances the expulsion of secretions from the respiratory tract.

Humidification Addition of moisture to the air.

IgA The class of antibody produced on mucous membrane surfaces such as those of the respiratory tract.

Inspissated Thickened or dried out.

Mucolytic Having the ability to break down mucus.

Nebulization The process of converting liquid medications into a spray that can be carried into the respiratory system by inhaled air.

Non-productive cough A cough that does not result in coughing up of mucus, secretions, or debris (a dry cough).

Productive cough A cough that results in coughing up of mucus, secretions, or debris.

Reverse sneeze Aspiration reflex—short periods of noisy inspiratory effort in dogs.

Surfactant A mixture of phospholipids secreted by type II alveolar cells that reduces surface tension of pulmonary fluids.

Viscid Sticky.

INTRODUCTION

Veterinary references list a wide variety of diseases of the respiratory system. A partial listing of the general etiologies includes the following:

1. Allergy
2. Aspiration
3. Bacteria
4. Congenital defects
5. Fungi
6. Immunologic factors
7. Neoplasia
8. Neurologic conditions
9. Parasites
10. Trauma
11. Viruses

The respiratory system has a series of defense mechanisms for protecting itself from disease. These natural defenses can be damaged by management practices such as those that cause a buildup of ammonia in enclosed, poorly ventilated housing. They can also be suppressed by inappropriate therapy, such as the use of cough suppressants on a productive cough. Because it is essential that these defense mechanisms function optimally for prompt recovery from respiratory disease, it is very important that technicians have a basic understanding of respiratory anatomy and physiology, respiratory defense mechanisms, and respiratory therapeutics.

RESPIRATORY ANATOMY AND PHYSIOLOGY

The respiratory system consists of the lungs and the passageways that carry air into and out of the lungs (Figure 5-1). These passageways include the nostrils, nasal cavity, pharynx, larynx, trachea, bronchi, and bronchioles.

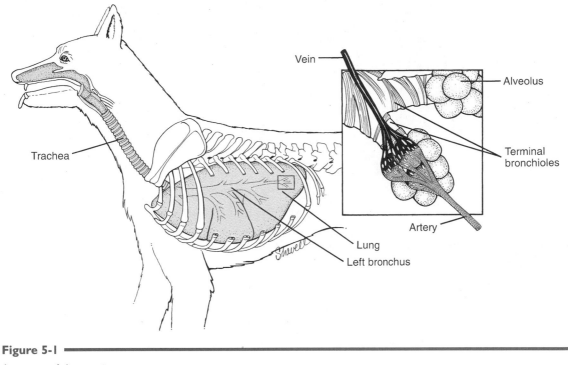

Figure 5-1

Anatomy of the respiratory system.

The passageways leading to the lungs are referred to as the *upper respiratory system.* The upper respiratory system begins with the nostrils, which open into the nasal cavity. The nasal cavity contains turbinates covered with mucous membranes. These turbinates increase the surface area of the nasal cavity to allow for **humidification** and warming of inspired air. Air passing out of the nasal cavity moves in turn through the pharynx and the larynx into the trachea. The trachea bifurcates into a right and left bronchus, which lead to the right and left lung. Each bronchus then divides into a series of passageways of decreasing size, called *bronchioles.* Smooth muscle fibers are found in the walls of the bronchioles. Contraction of the smooth muscle fibers decreases the diameter of the bronchioles, and relaxation of the fibers allows the diameter to return to normal size (Figure 5-2).

The upper respiratory tract is lined with ciliated, pseudostratified columnar epithelial cells. Interspersed

between the epithelial cells are goblet cells capable of secreting mucus. Mucus is secreted onto the surface of the epithelial cells and is moved toward the pharynx by the movement of the cilia (mucociliary apparatus).

Sympathetic stimulation results in decreased mucus production by the goblet cells and relaxation of the smooth muscle in the walls of the bronchioles, leading to **bronchodilation**.

Parasympathetic stimulation causes increased secretion of mucus and constriction of smooth muscle **(bronchoconstriction)** (Figure 5-3).

The bronchioles terminate in small, saclike structures called *alveoli.* The alveoli are arranged in grapelike clusters and are lined with a chemical substance called **surfactant,** which reduces the surface tension of the alveoli and helps to keep them from collapsing. The alveoli are surrounded by capillaries, thus making it possible for the blood to unload its carbon dioxide into the alveoli and pick up oxygen from the alveoli.

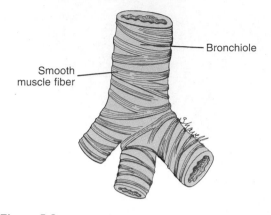

Figure 5-2

Smooth muscle fibers in the walls of the bronchioles relax to allow bronchodilation and contract to cause bronchoconstriction.

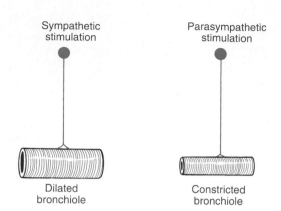

Figure 5-3

Effects of autonomic stimulation on bronchioles.

The functions that the respiratory system serves include the following:

1. Oxygen-carbon dioxide exchange
2. Regulation of acid-base balance
3. Body temperature regulation
4. Voice production

The work of the respiratory system can also be divided into the following four parts:

1. Ventilation—the movement of air into and out of the lungs. The inspiratory portion of ventilation is usually an active process, whereas expiration is usually a passive process. Forced inspiration may be associated with upper airway obstruction, and active expiration may be related to intrathoracic airway obstruction (McKiernan, 1988).
2. Distribution—the distributing of the inspired gases throughout the lungs.
3. Diffusion—the movement of gases across the alveolar membrane.
4. Perfusion—the supply of blood to the alveoli. The ratio of perfusion to ventilation of the alveoli is normally 1.

RESPIRATORY DEFENSE MECHANISMS

The respiratory system has several effective methods of defense against disease processes, including the following:

1. Nasal cavity: The turbinates of the nasal cavity provide a large surface area for warming and humidifying inspired air. Hair in the nasal passages also may help to filter out larger particulate matter.
2. Protective reflexes: The cough, sneeze, and perhaps the **reverse sneeze** respond to stimulation of receptors on the surface of the air passageways to expel foreign material forcefully. Laryngospasm and bronchospasm also help to prevent introduction of materials into the lung tissue.
3. Mucociliary clearance: The layer of mucus secreted onto the surface of the epithelial lining of the respiratory tract helps to trap foreign debris that enters the respiratory passages. The wavelike action of the cilia then move the debris up the passages ("escalator" action) to the pharynx, where it can be swallowed or expelled. Macrophages and immunoglobulins (**IgA**) also contribute to the defensive qualities of the mucociliary apparatus by immobilizing or phagocytizing foreign material.

PRINCIPLES OF RESPIRATORY THERAPEUTICS

It is important that a specific diagnosis be made through radiology, cytology, or appropriate culture before beginning treatment of respiratory disease, because the correct treatment for one type of disease may be contraindicated for another. Once the diagnosis has been made, the treatment of respiratory disease is divided into the following three general goals (McKiernan, 1988):

1. Control of secretions: Secretions may be reduced by decreasing their production or increasing their elimination. Removing the cause of the secretions through antibiotic, antifungal, antiparasitic, or other appropriate therapy is of vital concern. Methods are also aimed at making the secretions less **viscid** through the use of expectorants or through **nebulization** of **mucolytics** (aerosol therapy).
2. Control of reflexes: Coughing may be suppressed through the use of antitussives or bronchodilators if the cough is **non-productive.** Sneezing is controlled by removing the offending agent or through the use of vasoconstrictors. Bronchospasms may be controlled with bronchodilators and corticosteroids.
3. Maintaining normal airflow to the alveoli: Airflow to the alveoli may be maintained by reversing bronchoconstriction, by removing edema or mucus from alveoli and air passages, and by providing oxygen therapy. Intermittent positive-pressure ventilation and other ventilation strategies are often used in humans and may have application in selected animal cases.

CATEGORIES OF RESPIRATORY DRUGS

 EXPECTORANTS

Expectorants are drugs that liquefy and dilute viscid secretions of the respiratory tract and thereby help in evacuating those secretions. Most expectorants are administered orally, although a few are given by inhalation or parenterally. Expectorants are thought to act directly on the mucus-secreting glands or by reducing the adhesiveness of the mucus. Expectorants are indicated when a **productive cough** is present and are often combined with other substances such as ammonium chloride, antihistamines, or dextromethorphan.

Guaifenesin (Glyceryl Guaiacolate)

Guaifenesin is found in a few veterinary label products as well as many human label over-the-counter cough preparations. Guaifenesin is more commonly used in equine practice to induce or maintain general anesthesia.

Clinical Uses. These include relief of cough symptoms related to upper respiratory tract conditions.

Dosage Forms. These are primarily liquid (syrup) and tablet preparations.

1. Antitussive syrup
2. Cough syrup
3. Cough tablets
4. Robitussin-AC
5. Triaminic Expectorant

Adverse Side Effects. Adverse side effects of guaifenesin are rare, although mild drowsiness or nausea may occur.

MUCOLYTICS: ACETYLCYSTEINE

Mucolytics such as acetylcysteine decrease the viscosity of respiratory secretions by altering the chemical composition of the mucus through the breakdown of chemical (disulfide) bonds. Acetylcysteine is the only mucolytic of clinical significance in veterinary medicine. It is administered by nebulization for pulmonary uses. This drug is also administered orally as an antidote for acetaminophen toxicity.

Clinical Uses. Acetylcysteine is used to break down thick or **inspissated** respiratory mucus or to treat acetaminophen toxicity.

Dosage Forms. Dosage forms (human label) include a 10% solution and a 20% solution in 4-ml, 10-ml, and 30-ml vials.

1. Mucomyst
2. Mucosil-10
3. Mucosil-20

Adverse Side Effects. Adverse side effects are few when acetylcysteine is nebulized; however, the drug may cause nausea or vomiting when administered orally.

ANTITUSSIVES: CENTRALLY ACTING AGENTS

Antitussives are drugs that inhibit or suppress coughing. Antitussives are classified as centrally acting or peripherally acting (Figure 5-4). Centrally acting agents suppress coughing by depressing the cough center in the brain, whereas peripherally acting agents depress cough receptors in the airways. The peripherally acting antitussives are seldom used in veterinary medicine because they are usually prepared as cough drops or lozenges, which are not practical to administer to animal patients.

Butorphanol Tartrate

Butorphanol is a synthetic opiate partial agonist with significant antitussive activity. It is a C-IV controlled substance. It is also used as a preanesthetic and as an analgesic.

Clinical Uses. Butorphanol tartrate is used for the relief of chronic non-productive cough in dogs and for analgesia and preanesthesia in dogs and cats.

Dosage Forms. Dosage forms include injectable and tablet forms.

1. Butorphanol (Torbutrol) injection (0.5 mg/ml, 10-ml vial). This dosage is approved for use in dogs

2. Butorphanol (Torbugesic) injection (10 mg/ml, 50 ml). Approved for use in horses
3. Butorphanol (Torbutrol) tablets (1 mg, 5 mg, and 10 mg; 100/bottle)

Adverse Side Effects. Adverse side effects may include sedation and ataxia.

Hydrocodone Bitartrate

Hydrocodone is a schedule III opiate agonist used for the treatment of non-productive coughs in dogs.

Clinical Uses. Hydrocodone is primarily used as an antitussive for harsh, non-productive coughs.

Dosage Forms. Dosage forms include several human label combination products in syrup and tablet form.

1. Hycodan (hydrocodone and homatropine) tablets
2. Tussigon (hydrocodone and homatropine) tablets
3. Hycodan (hydrocodone and homatropine) syrup
4. Hydropane (hydrocodone and homatropine) syrup
5. Codan syrup (hydrocodone and homatropine)
6. Generic hydrocodone syrup

Adverse Side Effects. These include potential sedation, constipation, and gastrointestinal upset.

Codeine

Codeine is a schedule V opiate agonist that is used as an antitusive in human label combination products.

Clinical Uses. The clinical uses of codeine are similar to those of hydrocodone.

Dosage Forms. These include combination human label products primarily in the syrup form.

1. Codeine phosphate oral tablets, 30 mg and 60 mg
2. Codeine sulfate oral tablets, 15 mg, 30 mg, and 60 mg
3. Codeine phosphate with aspirin (Empirin with codeine)

Adverse Side Effects. Adverse side effects include sedation and constipation.

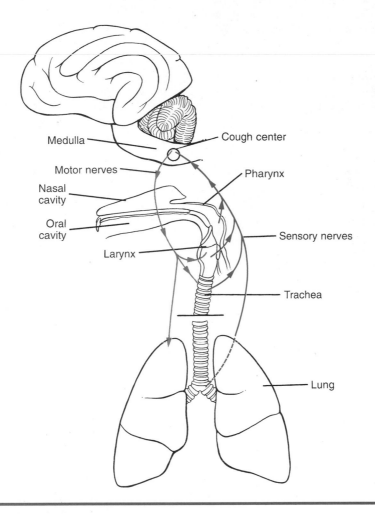

Figure 5-4

Antitussives act peripherally on sensory nerve endings or centrally on cough centers.

Dextromethorphan

Dextromethorphan is a non-narcotic antitussive that is chemically similar to codeine. It has no analgesic or addictive properties. It acts centrally and elevates the cough threshold. Like the two drugs previously mentioned, it is available primarily in human label combination products.

Clinical Uses. Dextromethorphan is used to suppress non-productive cough.

Dosage Forms. The primary dosage form is the syrup product.

1. Phenergan with dextromethorphan
2. Dimetapp DM (dextromethorphan, phenylpropanolamine, and bromepheniramine)

3. Robitussin DM (dextromethorphan and guaifensin)

Adverse Side Effects. Adverse side effects are rare when this drug is dosed correctly but can include drowsiness or gastrointestinal upset.

Technician's Notes

Technicians administering combination products to cats should take special precautions to ensure that the product does not contain acetaminophen.

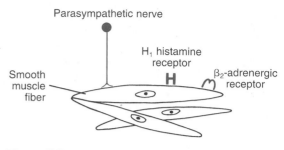

Figure 5-5

Bronchoconstriction may result from *(1)* acetylcholine release at parasympathetic nerve endings, *(2)* stimulation of H₁ histamine receptors, *(3)* blockade of beta-2–adrenergic receptors.

Temaril-P

Temaril-P is a combination product that contains a centrally acting antitussive (trimeprazine tartrate) and a corticosteroid (prednisolone).

Clinical Uses. Temaril-P is used as an antitussive and as an antipruritic.

Dosage Forms. Dosage forms include tablets.

1. Temaril-P tablets (5 mg trimeprazine tartrate, 2 mg prednisolone)

Adverse Side Effects. These include sedation, depression, hypotension, and minor central nervous system signs.

BRONCHODILATORS

Contraction of the smooth muscle fibers surrounding the bronchioles results in bronchoconstriction and often a corresponding dyspnea. Contraction of these smooth muscle fibers can result from the following three basic mechanisms (Bill, 1993) (Figure 5-5):

1. Release of acetylcholine at parasympathetic nerve endings or inhibition of acetylcholinesterase. In-

creased acetylcholine levels also tend to increase the secretions of the respiratory tract, thus reducing airflow and adding to the level of dyspnea.

2. Release of histamine through allergic or inflammatory mechanisms. Histamine combines with H₁ receptors on the smooth muscle fibers to cause bronchoconstriction. Histamine also increases the inflammatory response in the airways, further leading to increased levels of secretions and viscosity.

3. Blockade of beta-2–adrenergic receptors by drugs such as propranolol results in bronchoconstriction. Stimulation of beta-2–adrenergic receptors, however, produces bronchodilation.

Drugs that cause bronchodilation are of four basic categories. Those categories include the cholinergic blockers, the antihistamines, the beta-2 adrenergics, and the methylxanthines (Upson, 1988).

Cholinergic Blockers

The cholinergic blockers produce bronchodilation by combining with acetylcholine receptors on the smooth muscle fibers and preventing the bronchoconstricting effects of acetylcholine. Cholinergic blockers such as atropine, aminopentamide (Centrine), and glycopyrrolate (Robinul-V) have limited use in treating bronchoconstriction except in cases of organophosphate or carbamate toxicity.

Antihistamines

The antihistamines are addressed later in this chapter.

Beta-2–Adrenergic Agonists

Beta-2–adrenergic agonists combine with appropriate receptors on the smooth muscle fibers and effect relaxation of those fibers. They also stabilize mast cells and reduce the amount of histamine released (Bill, 1993). It is desirable that these drugs have limited beta-1 activity because beta-1 stimulation can produce tachycardia.

Clinical Uses. Beta-2–adrenergic agonists are used as a bronchodilator.

Dosage Forms

1. Epinephrine. This drug is a potent bronchodilator used only in life-threatening situations (e.g., anaphylactic shock) because it also produces significant tachycardia.
2. Isoproteronol (Isuprel). Also causes beta-1 stimulation and has limited use as a bronchodilator in veterinary medicine.
3. Albuterol (Ventolin, Proventil), clenbuterol (Ventipulmin syrup and clenbuterol HCl oral syrup), terbutaline (Brethine), and metaproterenol (Alupent) are beta-2 agonists that have little stimulatory effect on the heart. Clenbuterol is veterinary approved for horses not intended for food. None of the other products carry a veterinary label.

Adverse Side Effects. These include tachycardia and hypertension.

Methylxanthines

The methylxanthine derivatives that are used therapeutically include aminophylline and theophylline. These two products are very similar in their chemistry and pharmacologic effects. Both inhibit an enzyme in smooth muscle cells called phosphodiesterase. When beta-2 receptors are stimulated, a chemical messenger called *cyclic adenosine monophosphate (cyclic AMP)* released in the smooth muscle cell completes the relaxation response to allow dilation. Phosphodiesterease inhibits cyclic AMP in the cell and thereby tends to promote bronchoconstriction. By inhibiting the inhibitor (phosphodiesterase) and allowing cyclic AMP to accumulate, the methylxanthines tend to promote bronchodilation.

The methylxanthines also cause mild stimulation of the heart and respiratory muscles and minor diuresis.

Caffeine and theobromine (found in chocolate) are methylxanthines.

Aminophylline is an ethylenediamine salt of theophylline. It is available in various human label products. One hundred milligrams of aminophylline contain approximately 80 mg of theophylline (Plumb, 1999). Injectable forms are available, as well as immediate- and sustained-release oral forms.

Clinical Uses. Methylxanthines are used for bronchodilation in respiratory and cardiac conditions and for mild heart stimulation (positive ionotropic effect).

Dosage Forms

1. Theo-Dur
2. Slo-bid
3. Choledyl SA
4. Aminophylline (generic)

Adverse Side Effects. These may include gastrointestinal upset, central nervous system stimulation, tachycardia, ataxia, or arrhythmias.

Technician's Notes

Because theophylline may interact adversely with many drugs, including phenobarbital, cimetidine, erythromycin, thiabendazole, clindamycin, and lincomycin, appropriate precautions should be taken before administering this drug.

DECONGESTANTS

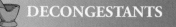

Decongestants are drugs that reduce the congestion of nasal membranes by reducing the associated swelling. Decongestants may be administered as a spray or as nose drops or may be given orally as a liquid or tablet. These drugs act directly or indirectly (Williams and Baer, 1990) to reduce congestion through vasoconstriction of nasal blood vessels. These products have limited use in veterinary medicine but may be used to treat selected feline upper respiratory tract disease.

Many human label decongestants are available. Those that are given orally and act systemically include ephedrine (Primatene), pseudoephedrine (Sudafed), and phenylpropanolamine (Ornade). Topically applied decongestants include oxymetazoline (Afrin) and phenylephrine (Neo-Synephrine).

ANTIHISTAMINES

Antihistamines are substances that are used to block the effects of histamine. Histamine is released from mast cells in the allergic response and combines with H_1 receptors on bronchiole smooth muscle to cause bronchoconstriction. Antihistamines may be useful in treating respiratory disease because they prevent mast cell degranulation and they block H_1 receptors on smooth muscle. Antihistamines are thought to be more effective when used preventively because they apparently do not replace histamine that has already combined with receptors (Bill, 1993).

Respiratory conditions that may be treated using antihistamines include "heaves" in horses, pneumonias in cattle, feline asthma, and insect bites.

Generic names for antihistamines are often easily recognized because most end in the suffix -*amine* (e.g., pyrilamine, diphenhydramine, chlorpheniramine).

Veterinary label antihistamines for treating respiratory conditions are available in injectable and oral preparations.

Clinical Uses. Antihistamines are used in the treatment of allergic and respiratory conditions. They may also be used for their antiemetic effect.

Dosage Forms
1. Pyrilamine (Histavet-P)
2. Tripelennamine (Re-Covr)
3. Probahist Syrup
4. Antihistamine Injection
5. Diphenhydramine (Benadryl). Human approved
6. Doxylamine (A-H, inhection or tablets)
7. Hydroxyzine (Atarax)
8. Terfenadine (Seldane). Human approved
9. Clemastine (Tavist)

Adverse Side Effects. These include sedation and, occasionally, gastrointestinal effects.

MISCELLANEOUS RESPIRATORY DRUGS

Many other drugs are used to treat respiratory disorders. These include antimicrobials, corticosteroids, and diuretics. Antimicrobials are used in cases of bacterial infections of the respiratory tract and may be administered parenterally or by nebulization. Corticosteroids are used in respiratory conditions to reduce the inflammatory component of the disease. They should be used with care in infectious disease because they also suppress the immune response. Diuretics are used to treat respiratory disease in which pulmonary edema is a major problem.

Respiratory Stimulants
Doxapram Hydrochloride

Doxapram is a general central nervous system stimulant that is used primarily as a stimulant of the respiratory system.

Clinical Uses. Doxapram is used for stimulation of respiration during and after anesthesia and to speed awakening and restoration of reflexes after anesthesia. In neonatal animals, doxapram is used to stimulate respiration after dystocia or cesarean section.

Dosage Form

1. An injectable form is Dopram-V for injection (20 mg/ml, 20-ml vial)

Adverse Side Effects. These include hypertension, arrhythmias, hyperventilation, central nervous system excitation, and seizures. These effects are most likely at high doses (Plumb, 1999). The safety of doxapram in pregnant animals has not been established.

Naloxone

Naloxone is used to stimulate respirations in narcotic overdose.

Yobine

Yobine is used to stimulate respirations in xylazine overdose.

REFERENCES

Bill, R.: Drugs affecting the respiratory system. In Bill, R. (ed.): Pharmacology for Veterinary Technicians. American Veterinary Publications, Goleta, CA, 1993.

McKiernan, B.: Respiratory therapeutics. In Proceedings of the 17th Seminar for Veterinary Technicians, The Western Veterinary Conference, Las Vegas, 1988.

Plumb, D.C.: Veterinary Drug Handbook. Iowa State University Press, Ames, 1999.

Upson, D.W.: Respiratory system. In Upson, D.W.: Handbook of Clinical Veterinary Pharmacology, 3rd ed. Dan Upson Enterprises, Manhattan, KS, 1988.

Williams, B.R., Baer, C.: Essentials of Clinical Pharmacology in Nursing. Springhouse Publishing Corporation, Springhouse, PA, 1990.

■ Review Questions

1. What structures would a molecule of oxygen pass over or through as it travels from the environment to the alveoli? _____

2. What are the four primary functions of the respiratory system? _____

3. Describe the function of the three basic defense mechanisms of the respiratory system.
_____

4. What are three important principles of respiratory therapeutics? _____

5. Expectorants are indicated when what type of cough is present? _____

6. Mucolytics decrease the viscosity of respiratory mucus by what mechanism?
_____

7. Acetylcysteine is administered by what method for pulmonary uses? _____

8. What is the mechanism of action of most antitussives used in veterinary medicine?
_____

9. Codeine is classified in what category of controlled substances? _____

10. List three mechanisms that can cause smooth muscle contraction in the bronchioles.
_____

11. List two bronchodilators that are beta-2–adrenergic agonists. _____

12. The methylxanthines bring about bronchodilation by inhibiting what cellular enzyme?
_____

13. List two potential uses for antihistamines in veterinary medicine. _____

14. What suffix is found at the end of many antihistamine names? _____

15. List two potential uses for dopram.
_____

16. Use your textbook and formulary to complete the following questions.

    Maxi Jones is being treated for canine infectious tracheobronchitis. Dr. Ladd has instructed you to dispense Hycodan tablets at 0.22 mg/kg b.i.d. for 7 days. Maxi weighs 50 lb.

    What dose of Hycodan does Maxi require?
    _____

    How many tablets will you dispense?
    _____

    Create a label for this prescription.
    _____

Drugs Used in Renal and Urinary Tract Disorders

LEARNING OBJECTIVES

After studying this chapter, you should be able to:

1. Identify the anatomic features of the urinary system
2. Discuss the formation of urine through glomerular filtration, tubular reabsorption, and tubular secretion
3. Compare the different classes of drugs and understand the indications for each class
4. Understand how renal dysfunction can affect the metabolization and excretion of many drugs and their metabolites

Agonist A drug that competes for the same receptor site as another drug or natural substance and enhances or stimulates the receptor's functional properties.

Antagonist A drug that competes for the same receptor site as another drug or natural substance but does not produce a physiologic effect itself.

Atony The absence or lack of normal tone or strength.

Catecholamine A group of sympathomimetic amines including dopamine, norepinephrine, and epinephrine.

Detrusor The smooth muscle of the urinary bladder that is mainly responsible for emptying the bladder during urination.

Detrusor areflexia The absence of detrusor contractions.

Enuresis Involuntary discharge of urine while sleeping.

Hypertension Persistently high blood pressure.

Hypertonus The state characterized by an increased tonicity or tension.

Hypokalemia Abnormally low potassium concentration in the blood.

Hypotonus The state characterized by a decreased tonicity or tension.

Lower motor neurons Peripheral neurons whose cell bodies lie in the central gray columns of the spinal cord and whose terminations are in skeletal muscles. A sufficient number of lesions of lower motor neurons causes muscles supplied by the nerve to atrophy, resulting in weak reflexes and flaccid paralysis.

Micturition Urination.

Nocturia Excessive urination at night.

Polydipsia Excessive thirst.

Polyuria Excessive urination.

Upper motor neurons Neurons in the cerebral cortex that conduct impulses from the motor cortex to the motor nuclei of the cerebral nerves or to the ventral gray columns of the spinal column. A sufficient number of lesions of upper motor neurons interrupts the inhibitory effect that upper motor neurons have on lower motor neurons, resulting in exaggerated or hyperactive reflexes.

Uremia Abnormally high concentrations of urea, creatinine, and other nitrogenous end products of protein and amino acid metabolism in the blood.

Urinary incontinence Lack of voluntary control over the normal excretion of urine.

Urinary tract infection Infection of the urinary tract. The infection may be localized or may affect the entire urinary tract.

INTRODUCTION

The urinary system is composed of the kidneys, ureters, bladder, and urethra (Figures 6-1 to 6-4). The urinary system regulates several functions, including water balance, acid-base balance, osmotic pressure, electrolyte levels, and concentration of many plasma substances. This system is also active in the elimination of many drugs and toxins from the body. Homeostasis may be interrupted by changes in plasma composition, cardiovascular changes (e.g., arterial blood pressure), hormones, the autonomic nervous system, and certain drugs and toxins.

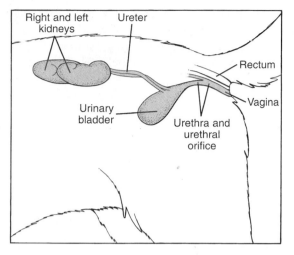

Figure 6-1
Side view of the urogenital system of a female dog.

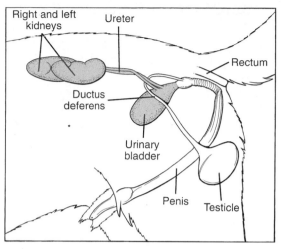

Figure 6-2
Side view of the urogenital system of a male dog.

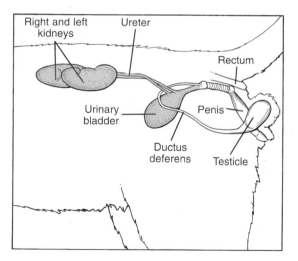

Figure 6-3
Side view of the urogenital system of a male cat.

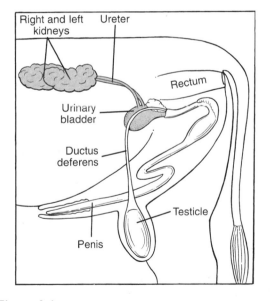

Figure 6-4
Side view of the urogenital system of a bull.

PHYSIOLOGIC PRINCIPLES

The formation of urine is a rather complex process that involves glomerular filtration, tubular reabsorption, and tubular secretion (Figure 6-5). The glomerular filtrate is composed of water and dissolved substances, which pass from the plasma into the glomerular capsule. The formation of glomerular filtrate is controlled by the effective filtration pressure [EFP = arterial blood pressure − (plasma osmotic pressure + capsule pressure)]. The amount of glomerular filtrate is directly proportional to the effective filtration pressure (Figure 6-6). Any changes in blood flow through the glomerulus, glomerular blood pressure, plasma osmotic pressure, or capsule pressure affect glomerular filtration. The kidney tubules are responsible for the reabsorption, or the secretion, of certain substances. Substances needed by the body are reabsorbed from the filtrate, pass through the tubular cell wall, and re-enter the plasma. This process filters needed substances and returns them to the body. Reabsorbed materials include water, glucose, amino acids, urea, and ions such as Na^+, K^+, Ca^{2+}, Cl^-, $HCO3^-$, and HPO_4^{2-}. Any excess of these substances, as well as substances that are not useful, remains in the filtrate and is excreted in the urine. Tubular secretion occurs when substances are carried to the tubular lumen. This includes the active transport of certain endogenous substances and many exogenous substances. These secreted substances include potassium and hy-

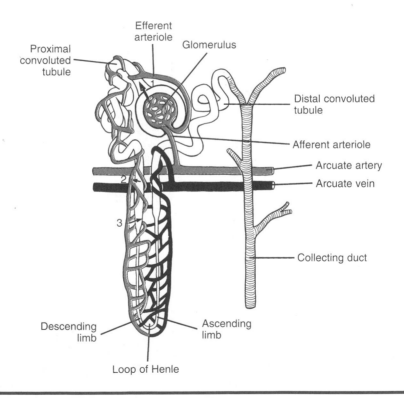

Figure 6-5

Shown are the direction and location of glomerular filtration: *1,* tubular reabsorption; *2,* tubular secretion; *3,* as they would occur in the glomerulus and proximal tubule.

drogen ions, ammonia, creatinine, and some drugs. The main effects of tubular secretion are to rid the body of certain materials and help control blood pH (Figure 6-7). Because the kidneys are active in the metabolization and excretion of many drugs and their metabolites, it is very important to remember that these actions may be inhibited in cases of renal failure or dysfunction. Drug therapy in animals with renal dysfunction has increased risks. Renal failure can impair a drug's absorption from an administration site or affect a drug's distribution in the body. **Uremia** can increase the sensitivity of some tissues to certain drugs. For example, sensitivity to central nervous system depressants is increased, and therefore, the dose of opiates, barbiturates, and tranquilizers should be reduced in uremic patients. Xylazine (Rompun) and ketamine

hydrochloride (Ketaset) are contraindicated in uremic patients. Impaired renal excretion or biotransformation causes delayed elimination of many drugs and increases their toxicity and duration of action. Box 6-1 lists common drugs that may require dosage modification in renal insufficiency. Modification can be made by measuring the plasma concentration of drugs and adjusting the dose accordingly. Because this is usually impractical in most clinical settings, a veterinarian may use the normal dose but lengthen the time intervals at which it is administered or give a smaller dose at the normal time intervals. Because many technicians are responsible for administering anesthesia, it is important to remember that patients with renal failure are a greater anesthetic risk and require even closer monitoring than patients with normal renal function.

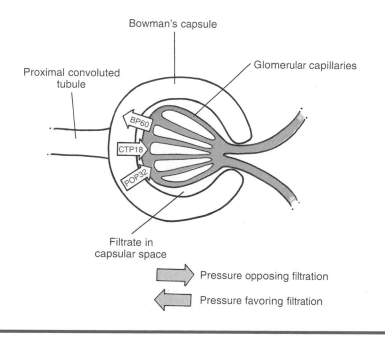

Figure 6-6

Filtration occurs through the glomerular membrane within Bowman's capsule. The amount of filtrate produced is determined by the difference between the pressures favoring filtration and those opposing filtration. This diagram shows that filtration occurs because 60 − (32 + 18) = 10 mm Hg. Values greater than or less than 10 mm Hg would correlate with more or less filtration, respectively. Pressure values (60, 32, 18) are measured in mm Hg. *BP,* blood pressure; *CTP,* capsular tissue pressure; *POP,* plasma osmotic pressure.

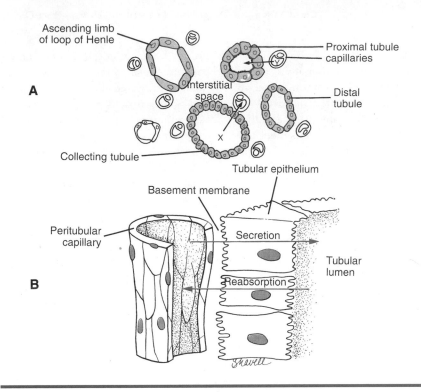

Figure 6-7

Tubular reabsorption and secretion. **A,** Cross-section of nephron tubules and peritubular capillaries. Interstitial fluid occupies the interstitial space. Reabsorption is represented by substance X going from tubule to capillary, and secretion is represented by substance Y going from capillary to tubule. **B,** Longitudinal section of nephron tubule. Shown is the relationship among the tubular lumen, epithelial cell, and capillary. (From Reece, W.O.: Physiology of Domestic Animals. Lea & Febiger, Philadelphia, 1991.)

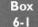 **Box 6-1**   Dosage Modification in Renal Insufficiency

Drugs That Require Dosage Modification or That Are Contraindicated in Renal Insufficiency

Acetazolamide	Colistin and polymyxin	Mannitol	Procainamide
Antimonials	Decamethonium	Mercurials	Spironolactone
Aspirin	Digoxin	Methenamine	Streptomycin
Atropine	Erythromycin	Methotrexate	Sulfonamides
Barbital	Furosemide	Neomycin	Tetracyclines
Bendroflumethiazide	(increased dose)	Neostigmine	Tetraethyl-ammonium
Cephalothins	Gentamicin	Nitrofurantoin	Tubocurarine, gallamine
Chelating agents	Iodide	Ouabain	Vancomycin
Chlorothiazide	Kanamycin	Penicillins	
Clindamycin	Lincomycin	Phenazopyridine	

Drugs That Do Not Require Dosage Modification or That Are Contraindicated in Renal Insufficiency

Acetaminophen	Narcotic analgesics	Phenobarbital	Procaine
Chloramphenicol	Novobiocin	Phenothiazines	Propranolol
Diazepam	Pentobarbital	Phenytoin	

From Kirk, R.W.: Current Veterinary Therapy VII: Small Animal Practice. W.B. Saunders Company, Philadelphia, 1980.

RENAL FAILURE

Renal failure is among the major causes of non-accidental death in dogs and cats. Although the disease is most common in older animals, it may be diagnosed in younger animals. Renal damage may stem from many causes, including infectious diseases, toxins, neoplasia, congenital disorders, immunologic problems, and amyloidosis. Diets with excessive protein, phosphorus, and sodium are also factors that may cause renal damage. Renal damage may be categorized as prerenal, renal, and postrenal. Renal failure may be differentiated as acute or chronic according to certain parameters common to each condition.

COMMON DRUGS FOR THE TREATMENT OF RENAL DYSFUNCTION AND ASSOCIATED HYPERTENSION

 DIURETIC DRUGS

Diuretics are used to remove excess extracellular fluid by increasing urine flow and sodium excretion and reducing **hypertension.** A number of conditions may indicate the need for a diuretic drug. The classifications of commonly used diuretics are loop diuretics, osmotic diuretics, thiazide and thiazide-like diuretics, potassium-sparing diuretics, and carbonic anhydrase inhibitors.

Loop Diuretics

Loop diuretics are highly potent diuretics that inhibit the tubular reabsorption of sodium. Their actions are generally rapid once they are administered. Loop diuretics also increase the excretion of chloride, potassium, and water.

Dosage Forms

1. Furosemide (Lasix, Disal, Diuride)
2. Ethacrynic acid (Edecrin—human label)

Adverse Side Effects. These include **hypokalemia** because of the increased excretion of potassium.

> **Technician's Notes**
>
> To prevent hypokalemia, a potassium supplement is commonly given to patients who are receiving long-term diuretic therapy.

Osmotic Diuretics

Osmotic diuretics can be administered intravenously to promote diuresis by exerting high osmotic pressure in the kidney tubules and limiting tubular reabsorption. Water is drawn into the glomerular filtrate, reducing the reabsorption and increasing the excretion of water. These drugs may be used to treat oliguric acute renal failure and to reduce intracranial pressure.

Dosage Forms

1. Mannitol 20%
2. Glucose

Adverse Side Effects. These are uncommon.

> **Technician's Notes**
>
> These drugs are administered over a 10- to 15-minute period.

Thiazide Diuretics

Thiazide diuretics reduce edema by inhibiting reabsorption of sodium, chloride, and water. Their duration of action is longer than that of loop diuretics.

Dosage Forms

1. Chlorothiazide (Diuril—human label)
2. Hydrochlorothiazide (HydroDIURIL—human label)

Adverse Side Effects. These include hypokalemia if therapy is prolonged.

Technician's Notes

1. Like loop diuretics, thiazide diuretics cause an increase in potassium excretion, and a potassium supplement may be necessary to prevent hypokalemia.
2. These drugs will cross the placental border.

Potassium-Sparing Diuretics

Potassium-sparing diuretics have weaker diuretic and antihypertensive effects than other diuretics, but they have the ability to conserve potassium. These agents are also referred to as *aldosterone antagonists*. They work by antagonizing aldosterone, an adrenal mineralocorticoid. This action increases the excretion of sodium and water and reduces the excretion of potassium. Aldosterone secretion may be a factor in edema associated with heart failure.

Dosage Forms

1. Spironolactone (Aldactone—human label)
2. Triamterene (Diazide, Dyrenium—human label)

Adverse Side Effects. These are uncommon, but hyperkalemia may result if these drugs are administered concurrently with potassium supplements or angiotensin-converting enzyme (ACE) inhibitors such as captopril or enalapril.

Technician's Notes

These drugs may be used alone or with other diuretic agents.

Carbonic Anhydrase Inhibitors

Carbonic anhydrase inhibitors block the enzyme carbonic anhydrase, thereby producing a bicarbonate diuresis and promoting the excretion of sodium, potassium, and water (Giovanoni, 1983). These drugs also reduce intraocular pressure by reducing the production of aqueous humor and may be used in the treatment of glaucoma.

Dosage Forms

1. Acetazolamide (Diamox—human label)
2. Dichlorphenamide (Daranide—human label)

Adverse Side Effects. These include the ability to cause hypokalemia.

Technician's Notes

Carbonic anhydrase inhibitors have the least efficacy when compared with the other tubular inhibitors and are not commonly used to treat edema.

CHOLINERGIC AGONISTS

Cholinergic agents act directly or indirectly to promote the function of acetylcholine. The cholinergic agents may also be referred to as *parasympathomimetic agents* because their effects mimic the stimulation of the parasympathetic nervous system. Cholinergic **agonists** mimic the action of natural acetylcholine by directly stimulating cholinergic receptors. Once the cholinergic agonist binds with the receptors on the cell membrane of smooth muscles, the permeability of the cell membrane changes, permitting calcium and sodium to enter into the cells. Depolarization of the cell membrane occurs, and muscle contraction is achieved.

Clinical Uses. Cholinergic agents are used to promote voiding of the urinary bladder. Their action increases the tone of the detrusor muscle of the bladder and decreases bladder capacity.

Dosage Form

1. Bethanechol (Urecholine—human label)

Adverse Side Effects. These include the potential for cholinergic toxicity.

ANTICHOLINERGIC DRUGS

The action of anticholinergic drugs is the opposite of the cholinergic agents. They block the action of acetylcholine at receptor sites in the parasympathetic nervous system. These drugs may also be described as parasympatholytic because of their ability to block the passage of impulses through the parasympathetic nerves. Their action produces muscle relaxation.

Clinical Uses. Anticholinergic drugs can be used for treating urge incontinence by promoting the retention of urine in the urinary bladder.

Dosage Forms

1. Propantheline (Pro-Banthine—human label)
2. Butyl hyoscine (Buscopan)

Adverse Side Effects. These include decreased gastric motility and delayed gastric emptying, which may decrease the absorption of other medications.

 ## ADRENERGIC ANTAGONISTS

Adrenergic blocking agents disrupt the sympathetic nervous system by blocking impulse transmission at adrenergic neurons, adrenergic receptor sites, or adrenergic ganglia. These agents may also be described as sympatholytic because of their ability to block sympathetic nervous system stimulation. The classification of adrenergic **antagonists** is based on their site of action (i.e., alpha blockers, beta blockers, or autonomic ganglionic blockers).

Alpha-Adrenergic Antagonists

Alpha-adrenergic antagonists relax vascular smooth muscle, increase peripheral vasodilation, and decrease blood pressure by interrupting the actions of sympathomimetic agents at alpha-adrenergic receptor sites.

Clinical Uses. In the urinary system, these drugs reduce internal sphincter tone when the urethral sphincter is in **hypertonus**. This action is useful in the treatment of urinary retention because of **detrusor areflexia** or functional urethral obstruction. Prazosin is effective in controlling moderate to severe hypertension, which may be a complicating factor in chronic renal failure.

Dosage Forms

1. Phenoxybenzamine (Dibenzyline—human label)
2. Nicergoline (Sermion)
3. Moxisylyte (Carlytene)
4. Prazosin (Minipress—human label)

Adverse Side Effects. These include rapid decrease of blood pressure, resulting in weakness or syncope after the first dose of prazosin. This is usually self-limiting.

Beta-Adrenergic Antagonists

Beta-adrenergic antagonists inhibit the action of **catecholamines** and other sympathomimetic agents at beta-adrenergic receptor sites and thereby inhibit stimulation of the sympathetic nervous system.

Clinical Uses. These include control of mild to moderate hypertension associated with chronic renal failure.

Dosage Form

1. Propranolol (Inderal—human label)

Adverse Side Effects. These include decreased cardiac output and the promotion of bronchospasm; therefore, caution should be exercised with their use in patients with cardiac or pulmonary disease (Cowgill, 1991).

Technician's Notes

Combination with a diuretic is common because of beta-adrenergic antagonists' tendency to cause salt and fluid retention.

ANGIOTENSIN-CONVERTING ENZYME INHIBITORS

ACE inhibitors block the conversion of angiotensin I to angiotensin II, decrease aldosterone secretion, decrease peripheral arterial resistance, and alleviate vasoconstriction.

Clinical Uses. ACE inhibitors are used to treat non-responding hypertension or moderate to severe hypertension.

Dosage Forms

1. Captopril (Capoten—human label)
2. Enalapril (Enacard)

Adverse Side Effects. These include complications in patients with renal insufficiency because of excretion by the kidneys.

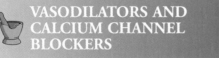

VASODILATORS AND CALCIUM CHANNEL BLOCKERS

A vasodilator or calcium channel blocker may be substituted for or used in combination with other medications if previous drug therapy to control hypertension fails.

Clinical Uses. These drugs are used to treat non-responding hypertension. Dopamine may be used to promote diuresis in patients unresponsive to loop or osmotic diuretics.

Dosage Forms

1. Vasodilators
   a. Hydralazine (Apresoline—human label)
   b. Dopamine (Intropin—human label)
2. Calcium channel blockers
   a. Diltiazem (Cardizem—human label)
   b. Verapamil (Isoptin—human label)

Adverse Side Effects. These include hypotension, edema, conduction disturbances, heart failure, and bradycardia (Cowgill, 1991). Hydralazine is excreted by the kidneys and requires dosage modification when used to treat hypertension in patients with renal failure.

ANTIDIURETIC HORMONE

Antidiuretic hormone (ADH) is normally secreted by the posterior pituitary gland. This secretion regulates fluid balance in the body. In some conditions such as pituitary diabetes insipidus, this hormone fails to be synthesized or excreted properly and **polyuria** and **polydipsia** occur.

Clinical Uses. ADH is used to treat diabetes insipidus.

Dosage Form

1. Vasopressin (Pitressin—human label)

Adverse Side Effects. These are uncommon.

Technician's Notes

Chlorpropamide (Diabinese, Glucamide) is a human product used to control type II diabetes mellitus. It potentiates the action of ADH and may be used to treat mild diabetes insipidus.

URINARY ACIDIFIERS

Urinary acidifiers are used to produce acid urine, which assists in dissolving and preventing formation of struvite uroliths. Since the introduction of urinary acidifying diets, urinary acidifiers have not been routinely prescribed.

Dosage Forms

1. Methionine (Methigel, Methio-tabs)
2. Ammonium chloride (Uroeze)

Adverse Side Effects. These include gastro-intestinal disturbance. These products should not be administered to patients with severe liver, kidney, or pancreatic diseases or to those exhibiting acidosis.

Technician's Notes

It is very important to inform clients who may change from using an acidifier to one of the available acidifying diets that while administering the diet, no acidifiers, salt, vitamin or mineral supplements, or any other food items than what is allowed on the diet should be given to the patient.

XANTHINE OXIDASE INHIBITORS

Xanthine oxidase inhibitors decrease the production of uric acid and are used in combination with a urate calculolytic diet for the dissolution of ammonium acid urate uroliths. Once dissolution occurs, a urine-alkalizing, low-protein, low-purine, low-oxalate diet is usually prescribed to prevent recurrence of the uroliths.

Dosage Form

1. Allopurinol (Zyloprim—human label)

Adverse Side Effects. These are uncommon, but because excretion occurs via the kidneys, the dosage may be altered in patients with renal insufficiency.

Technician's Notes

In case of recurrence, allopurinol may once again be prescribed.

URINARY ALKALIZERS

Urinary alkalizers may be used in the management of ammonium acid urate, calcium oxalate, and cystine urolithiasis.

Dosage Forms

1. Potassium citrate (Uracit-K—human label)
2. Sodium bicarbonate, administered orally
3. Tiopronin tablets (Thiola—human label)

Adverse Side Effects. These include possible fluid and electrolyte imbalance with the use of sodium bicarbonate.

PHARMACOTHERAPY OF RENAL FAILURE COMPLICATIONS

Because the renal cortex produces erythropoietin, chronic renal failure can cause an absolute or relative deficiency in its production. The resulting complication is normocytic, normochromic anemia. Parenteral androgens such as nandrolone (Durabolin) and testosterone enanthate are capable of stimulating the production of red blood cell precursors and may increase the level of erythropoietin. Recombinant human erythropoietin (Epogen) has been shown to correct anemia associated with chronic renal failure (Ettinger, 1993). Vitamin D supplementation may be used in the control of renal secondary hyperparathyroidism. Rocaltrol and dihydrotachysterol (Hytakerol) may be used for this purpose. Serum calcium, creatinine, and phosphate levels should be monitored in patients receiving this therapy because hypercalcemia, hyperphosphatemia, or deteriorating renal function can occur (Ettinger, 1993).

PHARMACOTHERAPY OF URINARY INCONTINENCE

Ettinger (1993) states that "pharmacologic agents are selected for management of **urinary incontinence** when **urinary tract infection,** morphologic abnormalities, and mechanical types of excessive outlet resistance have been excluded as possible causes of the problem." Urinary incontinence may be described as a neurogenic disorder or a non-neurogenic disorder. A neurogenic disorder is evidenced by a neurologic lesion that affects either the **upper motor neuron** seg-

ments or the **lower motor neuron** segments. When the upper motor neuron segments are affected, the result is a spastic neuropathic bladder. The **detrusor** muscle contractions are normal but the bladder and urethral functions are abnormal. Therefore, as the bladder fills with urine, contractions will occur more frequently (hypercontractility), and the bladder capacity is decreased. Also the contraction of the detrusor muscle and the relaxation of the urethral sphincter are often not coordinated. This results in interrupted, incomplete, and involuntary urination. Functional urinary obstruction and urinary retention may also be present. When the lower motor neuron segments are affected, the result is an **atonic** neuropathic bladder. With this disorder the detrusor muscle contractions are abnormal and there is an absence of sensation of fullness when the bladder fills (hypocontractility). This causes the bladder to become distended, and eventually bladder capacity is increased. The bladder distention may

TABLE 6-1 Pharmacotherapy of Urinary Incontinence

Drug	Action	Examples of Indications
Bethanechol (Urecholine)	Cholinergic agonist	Bladder hypocontractility
Propantheline (Pro-Banthine)	Anticholinergic agent	Urge incontinence, bladder hypercontractility
Butyl hyoscine (Buscopan)	Anticholingeric agent	Urge incontinence, bladder hypercontractility
Phenoxybenzamine (Dibenzyline)	Alpha-adrenergic antagonist	Urethral hyperreflexia
Nicergoine (Sermion)	Alpha-adrenergic antagonist	Urethral hyperreflexia
Moxisylyte (Carlytene)	Alpha-adrenergic antagonist	Urethral hyperreflexia
Aminopropazine (Jenotone)	Smooth muscle relaxant	Urge incontinence, bladder hypercontractility
Dantrolene (Dantrium)	Skeletal muscle relaxant	Urethral hyperreflexia
Diazepam (Valium)	Tranquilizer/skeletal muscle relaxant	Urethral hyperreflexia
Phenylpropanolamine (Propagest)	Alpha-adrenergic agonist	Urethral incompentence
Diethylstilbestrol (DES)	Estrogene hormone	Hormone-responsive urethral incompetence
Testosterone cypionate	Hormone	Hormone-responsive urethral incompetence
Testosterone propionate	Hormone	Hormone-responsive urethral incompetence

also cause damage to the tight junctions between the smooth muscle fibers. Urination eventually occurs when the pressure inside the bladder exceeds the urethral outlet resistance. Non-neurogenic disorders occur as a result of some type of anatomic anomaly of the lower urinary tract. In the young dog this is usually a congenital anomaly. A congenital anomaly seen in young female dogs is ectopic ureter, which causes constant dribbling of urine. This occurs when the ureters end in abnormal places rather than at the normal sphincters. In the older dog, acquired anatomic anomalies are usually responsible for non-neurogenic disorders. The conditions that commonly cause such problems include chronic cystitis, chronic urethritis, neoplasia, urolithiasis, and postsurgical adhesions. Other non-neurogenic disorders include functional abnormalities such as urethral incompetence and partial urethral obstruction. One type of non-neurogenic urethral incompetence is often seen in spayed female dogs and is usually responsive to hormonal therapy. Once the cause of the urinary incontinence is identified, medical or surgical management will begin. If there is a morphologic abnormality that is causing urinary incontinence, surgical correction of the problem will be necessary. Medical management will include treatment of infection, if present, and treatment for the cause of the urinary incontinence (e.g., urethral incompetence or bladder hypercontractility or hypocontractility). The drugs used in the medical management of urinary incontinence include the previously mentioned cholinergic agonists, anticholinergics, alpha-adrenergic antagonists, smooth muscle relaxants, skeletal muscle relaxants, tranquilizers, alpha-adrenergic agonists, and hormones such as estrogen and testosterone. Table 6-1 outlines these drugs for easy reference.

TECHNICIAN'S ROLE

Veterinary technicians have a vital role in the care of patients with problems affecting the urinary system. This role includes providing client support and education, carrying out patient nursing care, performing necessary laboratory or radiologic examinations, giving surgical assistance, and understanding the various drugs and diets available for the treatment of renal diseases.

REFERENCES

Cowgill, L.D.: Clinical significance, diagnosis, and management of systemic hypertension in dogs and cats. In Cowgill, L.D.: Managing Renal Disease and Hypertension. Harmon-Smith, 1991.

Ettinger, S.J.: Textbook of Veterinary Internal Medicine, vol. I and II. W.B. Saunders Company, Philadelphia, 1993.

Giovanoni, R., Warren, R.G.: Principles of Pharmacology. Mosby, St. Louis, 1983.

■ Review Questions

1. What organs compose the urinary system?
   _____

2. What are the functions of the urinary system?
   _____

3. Distinguish the difference between tubular reabsorption and tubular secretion.
   _____

4. Explain why caution should be exercised when drug therapy is used in patients with renal dysfunction.
   _____

5. How are renal damage and renal failure categorized or differentiated?_____

6. Define diuretic._____

7. Describe the classifications of diuretics and give examples of each._____

8. Describe the differences in the actions of cholinergic and anticholinergic drugs. Give examples of each.
   _____

9. What important factors should be remembered when educating clients who use prescription diets in the prevention and treatment of struvite urolithiasis?
   _____

10. List the most common uroliths and indicate whether acidifying or alkalizing agents are used in the management of each._____

Drugs Used in Cardiovascular System Disorders

LEARNING OBJECTIVES

After studying this chapter, you should be able to:

1. Describe the basic anatomy and physiology of the cardiovascular system
2. List four compensatory mechanisms of the cardiovascular system
3. List five basic objectives of the treatment of cardiovascular disease
4. Differentiate between an inotropic and a chronotropic drug
5. List and describe the indications, physiologic effects, and toxic side effects of the cardiac glycosides
6. List the four categories of antiarrhythmic drugs and an example in each category
7. List potential adverse side effects of the antiarrhythmic drugs
8. Describe the actions and potential side effects of the vasodilator drugs
9. Describe the actions and potential side effects of the angiotensin-converting enzyme (ACE) inhibitors
10. Describe the actions and potential side effects of the diuretics used to treat cardiovascular disease
11. Describe the purpose of dietary sodium restriction in the therapy of cardiovascular disease
12. List ancillary drugs or procedures that may be used in the treatment of cardiovascular disease

KEY TERMS

Afterload The resistance (pressure) in arteries that must be overcome to empty blood from the ventricle.

Arrhythmia (Dysrhythmia) A variation from the normal rhythm.

Automaticity The ability of cardiac muscle to generate impulses.

Bradyarrhythmia Bradycardia associated with an irregularity of heart rhythm.

Bradycardia A slower-than-normal heart rate.

Chronotropic Affecting the heart rate.

Depolarization Neutralizing of the polarity of a cardiac cell by an inflow of sodium ions. Depolarization results in contraction of the cardiac cell and renders it incapable of further contraction until repolarization occurs.

Inotropic Affecting the force of cardiac muscle contraction.

Preload The volume of blood in the ventricles at the end of diastole.

Premature ventricular contraction (PVC) Contraction of the ventricles without a corresponding contraction of the atria. PVCs arise from an irritable focus or foci in the ventricles.

Repolarization The return of the cell membrane to its resting polarity after depolarization.

Stroke volume The amount of blood ejected by the left ventricle with each beat.

Tachyarrhythmia Tachycardia associated with an irregularity of normal heart rhythm.

Tachycardia A faster-than-normal heart rate.

INTRODUCTION

Heart disease has a relatively high incidence in veterinary medicine. Studies have found that approximately 11% of all dogs presented to veterinary clinics exhibited some degree of heart disease (Lewis et al, 1987). Heart disease may be congenital or acquired; however, the acquired form accounts for most of the cases. The incidence and cause may vary from location to location. Heartworm disease accounts for a large percentage of heart disease in some parts of the country, whereas acquired disease of the atrioventricular valves or myocardium has a more uniform distribution. Acquired disease is encountered more often in older animals, and congenital disease is more prevalent in younger ones.

Whatever the cause, treatment of heart disease is often individualized to the particular patient according to the cause, degree of progression, and owner cooperation. The response to treatment must be carefully monitored and adjusted as the disease progresses and causes poor liver or kidney function or as toxic side effects develop. Many cardiovascular drugs have a narrow margin of safety (that is, they are potentially toxic at low doses), and failing liver and kidney function may reduce the body's ability to metabolize or eliminate the drugs.

Because veterinary technicians are often the persons monitoring the progress of hospitalized patients, they must be aware of the signs of cardiovascular disease and of the normal and abnormal responses to the drugs used to treat this disease.

ANATOMY AND PHYSIOLOGY OF THE HEART

The heart is a four-chambered pump that is responsible for moving blood through the vascular system. The two dorsal chambers are called *atria,* and the two ventral chambers are called *ventricles* (Figure 7-1). Each of the chambers is composed primarily of strong muscle tissue called *myocardium,* which contracts to eject the blood. Even though the heart is considered one organ, it is functionally two pumps (Spinelli and

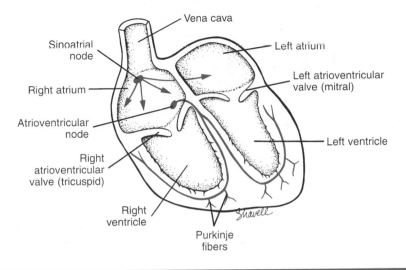

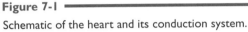

Figure 7-1

Schematic of the heart and its conduction system.

Enos, 1978). The right atrium and ventricle consti-tute the "right-side pump," and the left atrium and ventricle make up the "left-side pump." Blood from the general circulation returns by way of the vena cava to the right atrium, enters the right ventricle through the right atrioventricular valve (tricuspid valve), and is pumped through the pulmonary artery to the lungs. In the lungs, the blood gives up carbon dioxide and picks up oxygen. The oxygenated blood returns to the heart via the pulmonary veins, where it fills the left atrium, passes through the left atrioventricular valve (mitral valve), and enters the left ventricle. The mitral and tricuspid valves swing open when the atria con-tract and snap shut when the ventricles contract; the closing of the valves as the ventricles contract prevents blood from flowing back into the atria. The left ven-tricle then contracts and ejects the oxygenated blood through the aorta out into the branching arteries. These arteries divide into arterioles and end in the thin-walled capillaries throughout the body where car-bon dioxide is loaded to the blood and oxygen is un-loaded to the tissues. Because the left ventricle must work harder to pump blood throughout the body than the right ventricle must work to pump blood to the lungs, the left ventricular wall is thicker than the right ventricular wall.

The pumping action of the heart is divided into two phases, systole and diastole. Systole is the period of contraction of the chambers, and diastole represents the relaxation phase when the chambers are filling with blood. Because each cell in the heart is capable of contracting spontaneously, the interaction of these two phases must be carefully coordinated to create an efficient pumping action. Diastolic time must be ad-equate to allow the atria to fill completely, and atrial systole must occur shortly before ventricular systole to allow the ventricles to fill maximally. Coordination of these two phases is achieved primarily by a wave of electric activity that arises in a specialized group of cells in the right atrium and is then conducted throughout the myocardium by a special conduction system.

The structures that make up the cardiac conduc-tion system (see Figure 7-1) include the sinoatrial node, the atrioventricular node, the bundle of His and its branches, and the Purkinje system. Under abnor-mal conditions, parts of the myocardium as well as the parts of the conduction system are capable of sponta-neous discharge. Normally, however, the sinoatrial node discharges most rapidly and spreads a wave of depolarization over the remaining areas of the heart before they can depolarize spontaneously. The rate of

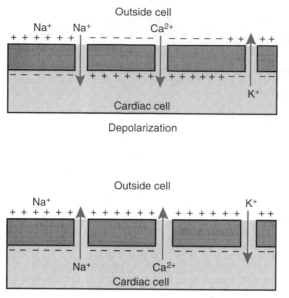

Figure 7-2

Depolarization and repolarization of a cardiac cell. Repolarization: The $Na^+ = K^+ = ATPase$ pump restores the electrolytes to their resting sites.

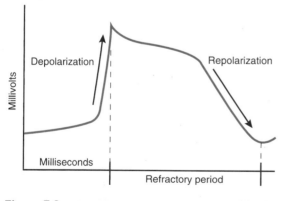

Figure 7-3

Schematic of the refractory period of a cardiac cell. After depolarization (contraction), cardiac muscle cells are unable to contract again until they have undergone repolarization. The time while they are unable to contract is the refractory period.

discharge of this node therefore controls the heart rate and is called the *cardiac pacemaker*. The impulses generated by the sinoatrial node travel over the atria to the atrioventricular node, face a brief delay (about 0.1 second) in the atrioventricular node, travel down the bundle of His to its left and right branches, and pass into the ventricular muscle via the Purkinje fibers. Myocardial cells are joined together by structures called *intercalated disks* and by fusing of cell membranes into an interconnected mass of cells called a *syncytium*. The syncytium of cells in the atria is separate from the syncytium in the ventricles (Giovanoni and Warren, 1983). An electric stimulus from the sinoatrial node is transmitted over the entire atrial mass by the syncytial arrangement of cells. The impulse is not, however, transmitted directly into the ventricular syncytium. The impulse first must be picked up and transmitted by the atrioventricular node through its conduction system to the ventricular syncytium. Stimulation of a single atrial or ventricular muscle fiber causes the entire atrial or ventricular muscle mass to contract as a unit. When situations cause spontaneous depolarization of cardiac muscle or abnormalities of the conduction system, **arrhythmias** may occur.

When a cardiac cell is stimulated by electric activity arising in the sinoatrial node, it undergoes depolarization and contracts. **Depolarization** is characterized by the rapid influx of sodium ions into the cell through channels or "gates," the slower influx of calcium ions, and the outflow of potassium ions (Figure 7-2). Until the sodium, potassium, and calcium ions have returned to the positions they had before depolarization, the cell is in a refractory period (Figure 7-3). A cell in an absolute refractory state cannot normally depolarize. In a relative refractory period, however, a cardiac cell can depolarize again but the stimulus must be stronger than normal (Bill, 1993). A refractory period is essential for a cardiac cell to prevent it from remaining in a constant state of contraction resulting from stimulation by recycling impulses. The return of the ions to their original positions is brought about in part by the sodium-potassium pump and is an essential part of the **repolarization** process. The summed electric activity arising from the con-

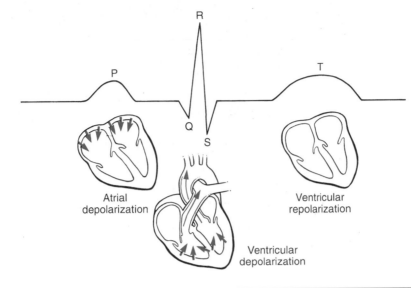

Figure 7-4

Cardiac events as depicted on an electrocardiogram tracing.

traction of all the heart cells represents the electrocardiogram (Figure 7-4), with each of its waves signifying activity in a particular area (Ganong, 1993).

Even though the heart establishes its own inherent rate of beating, this rate is also subject to outside influences through the autonomic nervous system. The sympathetic portion of the autonomic nervous system through beta-1 receptors produces positive **chronotropic** and **inotropic** effects on the heart. The parasympathetic branch of the autonomic nervous system causes negative chronotropic effects through cholinergic receptors.

The heart pumps blood through a series of arteries (arterial tree) to deliver it to the tissues. The larger of these arteries have elastic properties that allow them to stretch and recover when blood is pumped into them, thereby serving as a second pump (Upson, 1988). The smaller arteries are capable of changing their diameter (constricting or dilating) through the action of smooth muscle in their walls to increase or decrease the resistance that the heart must pump against. Stimulation of alpha-1 receptors causes vessels to constrict, and stimulation of beta-2 receptors causes vessels to dilate.

The amount of blood that the heart is capable of pumping per minute is called *cardiac output,* which is calculated by multiplying the heart rate by the stroke volume. The **stroke volume** is determined in part by the amount of blood that fills the ventricle during diastole, called the **preload,** and the arterial resistance that the ventricle must pump against, called the **afterload.**

COMPENSATORY MECHANISMS OF THE CARDIOVASCULAR SYSTEM

The cardiovascular system has a built-in reserve capacity that allows it to increase its output during times of need (e.g., athletic performance) and to compensate for cardiac disease. The four basic factors of cardiac reserve or compensation are described in the following (Upson, 1988):

1. Increasing heart rate. Increasing the rate of contraction increases cardiac output up to the point at which the rate is so fast that there is inadequate time for ventricular filling.

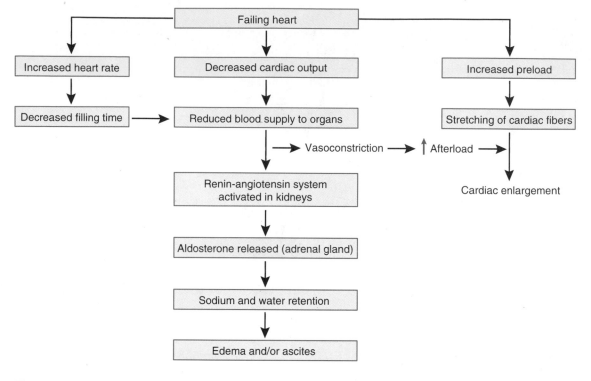

Figure 7-5

Pathophysiology of congestive heart failure.

TABLE 7-1 Stages and Treatment of Cardiac Disease

Stage	Signs	Treatment
I	None/murmur	None
II	Cough	Restricted sodium diet
		Diuretic
		Bronchodilator
III	Cough	Exercise restriction
	Reduced exercise tolerance	Sodium restriction
		Digitalis
		Diuretic
		Vasodilators
IV	Dyspnea at rest	Oxygen
		Diuretics
		Sedatives
		Vasodilators
		Others

2. Increasing the stroke volume. Up to a point, an increased force of contraction results in an increased amount of blood being pumped.
3. Increasing the efficiency of the heart muscle.
4. Physiologic heart enlargement. The heart is composed of muscle that responds to work by increasing its size and becoming stronger.

Many disorders can result in cardiac disease; however, most that respond to pharmacologic therapy fall into one of the following categories:

1. Valvular disease. Valvular insufficiency, a backflow or leakage of blood backward through the valve, is a relatively common acquired heart disorder of dogs. If the tricuspid valve is affected, ascites may occur. If the mitral valve is involved, pulmonary edema may result. Valvular disease may be a result of progressive bacterial endocarditis.
2. Cardiac arrhythmias. If a focus of cardiac tissue depolarizes more rapidly than the sinoatrial node, an arrhythmia may result. Various types of arrhythmias may occur, including **tachyarrhythmias** (arrhythmias with a rapid rate) and **bradyarrhythmias** (arrhythmias with a slow rate). Arrhythmias may occur in the atria (supraventricular) or in the ventricles (ventricular). Several categories of drugs predispose the heart to arrhythmias (catecholamines, thiobarbiturates, xylazine, digoxin, and others).
3. Myocardial disease. Cardiomyopathy, a disease of the myocardium, primarily affects dogs and cats. It may be classified as congestive (the myocardium becomes thin and ineffective in its pumping action) or hypertrophic (the myocardium becomes thickened and restricts ventricular filling). Each type is often accompanied by various arrhythmias.
4. Other potential causes of cardiac disease include congenital defects and abnormalities of cardiac innervation or the blood vessels.

Congestive heart failure (CHF) (Figure 7-5) results when the pumping ability of the heart is impaired to the extent that sodium and water are retained in an effort to compensate for inadequate cardiac output. It is associated with exercise intolerance, pulmonary edema, and ascites. The heart usually becomes enlarged in this condition.

Cardiac disease has been divided into four phases according to the degree of severity. Table 7-1 lists the phases with corresponding clinical signs and treatments.

BASIC OBJECTIVES IN THE TREATMENT OF CARDIOVASCULAR DISEASE

The basic objectives of the treatment of cardiovascular disease include the following (Ettinger, 1989; Upson, 1988):

1. Control rhythm disturbances
2. Maintain or increase cardiac output
   a. Increase the strength of contraction
   b. Decrease the afterload
      (1) Arteriolar dilator
   c. Decrease the preload
      (1) Venodilator
3. Relieve fluid accumulations
   a. Diuretics
   b. Dietary salt restriction
4. Increase the oxygenation of the blood
   a. Bronchodilation
5. Ancillary treatment
   a. Narcotics/sedatives
   b. Oxygen

CATEGORIES OF CARDIOVASCULAR DRUGS

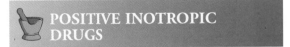

POSITIVE INOTROPIC DRUGS

The general principle of the use of the drugs that improve the strength of contraction is that the heart, even in the presence of disease, has reserve capacity for contraction that can be called on to improve car-

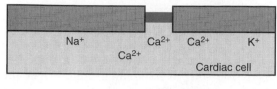

Figure 7-6

Effect of digitalis on the $Na^+ = K^+ = ATPase$ pump. Digitalis compounds block the $Na^+ = K^+ = ATPase$ enzyme, reduce the amount of Ca^2 pumped out of the cell during repolarization, and increase the amount of Ca^2 available for depolarization.

diac output. Some clinicians advise cautious use of positive inotropic drugs because these can increase the oxygen demand of cardiac muscle, can potentially damage the contractile apparatus, and can increase the tendency for arrhythmias. Despite the academic questions that are raised over their use, these agents often bring about improvement in the clinical signs associated with heart disease, thus accounting for their widespread use (Ettinger, 1989).

Cardiac Glycosides (Digitalis)

The digitalis compounds (digoxin and digitoxin) are obtained from the dried leaves of the plant *Digitalis purpurea*. The beneficial effects of these compounds have been known for hundreds of years and include (1) improved cardiac contractility, (2) a decrease in heart rate, (3) antiarrhythmic effect, and (4) decreased signs of dyspnea.

Digitalis increases the strength of contraction by increasing the level of calcium ions available in the contractile filaments within the cardiac muscle cells. This action occurs as a result of inhibition of sodium-potassium-adenosine triphosphatase (Figure 7-6). The heart rate is slowed by prolonging the atrioventricular conduction time and by increasing parasympathetic, autonomic stimulation (Ettinger, 1989). The primary actions of the digitalis drugs are to (1) increase force of contraction, (2) decrease rate of contraction, (3) increase excitability of cardiac muscle, and (4) increase automaticity (Upson, 1988).

Digitalis use is indicated in patients with cardiac disease that results from impaired cardiac contraction

or atrial arrhythmias as suggested by clinical signs such as exercise intolerance, weak peripheral pulses, pulmonary edema, and coughing or by electrocardiographic diagnosis.

Clinical Uses. Clinical uses of the digitalis compounds include the treatment of CHF, atrial fibrillation, and supraventricular tachycardia.

Dosage Forms. Dosage forms include tablets and elixirs. Veterinary and human label products are available for both digoxin and digitoxin.

1. Veterinary approved
   a. Digoxin elixir (Cardoxin LS, 0.05 mg/ml; Cardoxin, 0.15 mg/ml)
   b. Digitoxin—none available
2. Human approved
   a. Digoxin for injection (Lanoxin, 0.25 mg/ml or 0.1 mg/ml in ampules and vials)
   b. Digoxin tablets (Lanoxin, 0.125, 0.25, and 0.5 mg)
   c. Digoxin capsules (Lanoxicaps, 0.05, 0.1, and 0.2 mg)
   d. Digoxin elixir (Lanoxin, 0.05 mg/ml, 60-ml bottle)

Adverse Side Effects. Adverse side effects from the use of the digitalis compounds are often associated with high or toxic serum levels of the drugs and can include anorexia, vomiting, diarrhea, and various arrhythmias. Cats are relatively more sensitive than dogs to toxic effects (Plumb, 1999). Digitalis compounds are adversely affected when given concurrently with many drugs (cimetidine, metoclopramide, diazepam, anticholinergics, and others); consult appropriate references for suitability.

Technician's Notes

1. The bioavailability of digoxin varies from 60% in tablet form to 75% in the elixir form, and adjustments are probably needed if the dosage form is changed.
2. Clients should be advised to monitor their pets carefully for signs of toxicity and to advise the veterinarian if any arise.

Catecholamines

The catecholamines include a group of sympathomimetic (adrenergic) compounds that (1) increase the force and rate of muscular contraction of the heart (increase cardiac output), (2) constrict peripheral blood vessels (increase blood pressure), and (3) elevate blood glucose levels. Catecholamines increase cardiac contractility primarily by stimulating beta-1 receptors. Because of their short serum half-lives, catecholamines are used mainly for short-term management of severe heart failure.

Epinephrine

Epinephrine is the preferred drug for providing stimulation for contraction of the heart and for supporting the circulatory system after cardiac arrest. It may be administered by the intracardiac, intratracheal, or intravenous route, and a 1:10,000 solution is preferred. Most products provide a 1:1000 solution. Because epinephrine greatly increases the workload of the heart and increases the tendency for arrhythmias, it is not used for therapy of chronic heart failure.

Clinical Uses. Epinephrine is used in veterinary medicine for cardiac resuscitation and for the treatment of anaphylaxis.

Dosage Forms. Human label forms of epinephrine are used.

1. Epinephrine HCl for injection, 0.1 mg/ml (1:10,000) in 10-ml syringes
2. Epinephrine HCl for injection (Adrenalin Chloride, 1 mg/ml [1:1,000] in ampules and vials)

Adverse Side Effects. These include hypertension, arrhythmias, anxiety, and excitability.

> **Technician's Notes**
>
> A 1:10,000 solution can be prepared from a 1:1000 solution by mixing 1 ml of the drug with 9 ml of sterile water for injection. Alternatively, 0.5 ml of drug can be mixed with 4.5 ml of sterile water for injection.

Isoproterenol

Isoproterenol is seldom used in the treatment of cardiac disease. It is indicated in atropine-resistant **bradycardia.**

Dopamine

Dopamine is a biosynthetic precursor of norepinephrine. It stimulates dopaminergic receptors in coronary, mesenteric, renal, and cerebral vascular beds. It also is capable of stimulating alpha- and beta-adrenergic receptors to increase heart contractility, heart rate, and blood pressure. Dopamine use in cardiac cases is mainly limited to heart failure associated with anesthetic emergencies or after cardiac resuscitation.

Clinical Uses. Dopamine is used for adjunctive treatment of acute heart failure and oliguric renal failure and for the supportive treatment of shock.

Dosage Forms

1. Inotropin
2. Dopamine HCl
3. Dopamine HCl in 5% dextrose

Adverse Side Effects. These include vomiting, tachycardia, dyspnea, and blood pressure variations (hypotension or hypertension).

Dobutamine

Dobutamine is a synthetic inotropic agent related structurally to dopamine. It causes increased cardiac contractility, as does dopamine, but does not produce its dilation of selected vascular beds. Dobutamine is a direct beta-1–adrenergic agent. It produces increased cardiac output with little tendency to cause arrhythmias or increased heart rate. It is available only as a human label product (Dobutrex solution) and is administered in a diluted form by intravenous infusion. Consult the *Veterinary Drug Handbook* (Plumb, 1999) for directions on preparation of the solution for infusion.

Bipyridine Derivatives

Amrinone and milrinone are representatives of a new class of positive inotropic drugs that appear to work by inhibiting enzymes that ultimately lead to an increase in cellular calcium. Amrinone (Inocor) is given intravenously and is limited to short-term inpatient use, whereas milrinone is given orally and has potential for long-term use.

ANTIARRHYTHMIC DRUGS

An arrhythmia is a variation from the normal rhythm of the heart. Such a variation may result from an abnormality of impulse generation (increased **automaticity**) or from abnormalities of impulse conduction. Many arrhythmias arise when a localized group of cells begin to depolarize faster than the sinoatrial node (pacemaker), causing disruption of the normal depolarization pattern of the heart. The location of this group of cells is called an *ectopic focus* (foci if more than one location is involved). Arrhythmias usually result in reduced cardiac output resulting from poorly coordinated pumping activity. Some arrhythmias may be auscultated by an experienced ear, but arrhythmias more often are diagnosed through their production of abnormal waveforms seen on an electrocardiogram tracing.

Factors that may cause or predispose the heart to arrhythmias include the following:

1. Conditions that cause hypoxia
2. Electrolyte imbalances
3. Increased levels of or increased sensitivity to catecholamines
4. Drugs such as digitalis compounds, thiobarbiturates, inhalant anesthetics (halothane), xylazine, and others
5. Cardiac trauma or disease resulting in altered cardiac cells

Arrhythmias are classified in relation to the heart rate as either tachyarrhythmias or bradyarrhythmias. Tachyarrhythmias are further classified into ventricular or atrial, depending on their location, and can lead to rapid contraction rates (200 units) of the corresponding chambers. At these rapid rates, pumping efficiency is greatly reduced because of decreased filling time. Rapid, incoordinated activity called *flutter* or *fibrillation* may also result.

Pharmacologists classify antiarrhythmic drugs into the following four basic categories (Williams and Baer, 1990):

1. Class IA includes quinidine, procainamide, and others.

2. Class IB includes lidocaine, tocainide, and mexiletine.
3. Class IC includes flecainide and encainide.
4. Class II includes the beta-adrenergic blockers (propranolol).
5. Class III includes bretylium and amiodarone.
6. Class IV includes the calcium channel blockers (verapamil, nifedipine, and diltiazem).

Class IA

Drugs in class IA depress myocardial excitability, prolong the refractory period, decrease automaticity, and increase conduction times. Class IA drugs are used to treat both atrial and ventricular arrhythmias and may be given orally on a long-term basis.

Quinidine

Quinidine is an alkaloid obtained from cinchona plants or is prepared from quinine (Plumb, 1999).

Clinical Uses. Quinidine is used to treat ventricular arrhythmias, ventricular tachycardia, and atrial fibrillation (drug of choice).

Dosage Forms. Human label forms are used.

1. Quinidine sulfate
   a. Tablets, 200 and 300 mg (Quinora)
   b. Sustained-release tablets, 300 mg (Quinidex Extentabs)
2. Quinidine gluconate
   a. Sustained-release tablets (Quinaglute Dura-Tabs [324 mg])
   b. Injection, 80 mg/ml
3. Quinidine polygalacturonate
   a. Tablets, 275 mg (Cardioquin)

Adverse Side Effects. These include anorexia, vomiting, diarrhea, weakness, and laminitis (horses).

Technician's Notes
Quinidine doses must be reduced in animals being concurrently treated with digoxin.

Procainamide

Procainamide is an antiarrhythmic that is chemically related to procaine.

Clinical Uses. Procainamide is used to treat **premature ventricular contractions (PVC),** ventricular tachycardia, and some forms of atrial tachycardia.

Dosage Forms. Human label procainamide hydrochloride is used.

1. Injection, 100 mg/ml in 10-ml vials and 500 mg/ml in 2-ml vials (Pronestyl)
2. Tablets or capsules, 250, 375, and 500 mg (Pronestyl)

Adverse Side Effects. These include anorexia, vomiting, diarrhea, hypotension, and others; however, these effects are generally dose-related.

Class IB

Drugs in this category exert their effect by stabilizing myocardial cell membranes. By blocking the influx of sodium into the cell, these drugs prevent depolarization and decrease cell automaticity (Figure 7-7). They are used to treat ventricular arrhythmias, but they are not approved by the Food and Drug Administration (FDA) for this use.

Lidocaine

Lidocaine is a local anesthetic and antiarrhythmic that is prepared only in the injectable form and is administered intravenously. It is frequently used in emergency medicine and acute care.

Clinical Uses. Lidocaine is primarily used for the control of PVCs and for the treatment of ventricular tachycardia.

Dosage Forms. Various veterinary brand name forms are available in 1% and 2% solutions.

Adverse Side Effects. These are rare but may include drowsiness, depression, ataxia, and muscle tremors. Cats are potentially sensitive to the central nervous system effects of lidocaine; they should be monitored carefully when receiving this drug.

Technician's Notes

When administering lidocaine for an arrhythmia, make certain that it is lidocaine without epinephrine. Epinephrine (a catecholamine) predisposes the heart to arrhythmia.

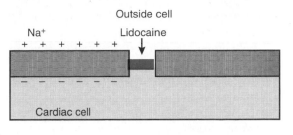

Figure 7-7

Effect of lidocaine on sodium channels. Lidocaine blocks sodium channels and reduces the automaticity of the cardiac cells.

Tocainide and Mexiletine

Tocainide and mexiletine are other class IB agents that may be given orally, but they have had limited use in veterinary medicine at this time.

Class IC

Class IC agents are seldom used in veterinary medicine.

Class II

Class II antiarrhythmics are the beta-adrenergic blockers. Propranolol and acebutolol are FDA-approved agents in this category, but acebutolol has little use in veterinary medicine. These drugs may be used for atrial or ventricular arrhythmias.

Propranolol

Propranolol reduces automaticity of cardiac conduction cells by blocking beta-1 and beta-2 receptor sites. Myocardial oxygen demand is reduced by propranolol. Reducing the myocardial oxygen demand reduces the tendency for ischemia, in turn reducing automaticity (Williams and Baer, 1990). Propranolol reduces the heart rate, cardiac output, and blood pressure.

Clinical Uses. In veterinary medicine, propranolol is used to treat hypertrophic cardiomyopathy and various atrial and ventricular arrhythmias.

Dosage Forms

1. Propranolol HCl tablets, 10, 20, 40, 60, 80, and 90 mg (Inderal)

2. Propranolol HCl extended-release capsules, 60, 80, 120, and 160 mg (Inderal LA)
3. Propranolol for injection, 1 mg/ml in 1-ml ampules or vials (Inderal)
4. Propranolol oral solution, 4, 8, and 80 mg/ml concentrate (Intensol)

Adverse Side Effects. These include bradycardia, hypotension, worsening of heart failure, lethargy, and depression.

Technician's Notes

1. Propranolol is contraindicated in patients with overt heart failure, greater than first-degree heart block, and sinus bradycardia (Plumb, 1999).
2. Do not discontinue therapy abruptly, because tachycardia or hypertension may occur.

Class III

The class III antiarrhythmics bretylium (Bretylol) and amiodarone (Cordarone) are not in common use in veterinary medicine. Some clinicians have reported that Bretylol has promise for treating ventricular fibrillation in the absence of a defibrillation unit. These drugs are used in human medicine to treat ventricular arrhythmias.

Class IV

Class IV antiarrhythmic drugs work by blocking the channels that permit entry of calcium ions through the cardiac cell membrane. This effect causes depression of the contractile mechanism in myocardial and smooth muscle cells and depresses automaticity and impulse transmission (Williams and Baer, 1990).

Verapamil Hydrochloride

Verapamil is a channel blocking agent that is available in oral and injectable forms. It has had limited use in veterinary medicine.

   Clinical Uses. Verapamil is used to treat supraventricular tachycardia, atrial flutter, or atrial fibrillation.

   Dosage Forms. Human label products are used.

1. Verapamil HCl tablets, 40, 80 and 120 mg (Calan, Isoptin)
2. Verapamil HCl sustained-release tablets, 120, 180, 240, and 360 mg (Calan SR, Isoptin SR)
3. Verapamil HCl for injection, 5 mg/2 ml in ampules, vials, and syringes (Isoptin)

Adverse Side Effects. These include hypotension, bradycardia, tachycardia, pulmonary edema, and worsening of CHF.

Other Class IV Antiarrhythnics

Other channel blockers used in human medicine include nifedipine (Adalat) and diltiazem (Cardizem).

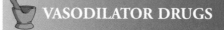

VASODILATOR DRUGS

When heart failure occurs, cardiac output is reduced, resulting in hypotension and poor perfusion of tissues. As a reaction to this poor perfusion of tissues, the body activates compensatory mechanisms to increase the blood pressure and to improve blood supply to tissues. The first compensatory activity is stimulation of the sympathetic nervous system to increase the heart rate and to cause constriction of small arteries, which in turn raises the blood pressure. Next, the renin-angiotensin system is activated by the release of renin from the poorly perfused kidneys (Figure 7-8). Renin causes angiotensinogen to be converted to angiotensin I. Angiotensin I is then converted by ACE to angiotensin II. Angiotensin II causes further vasoconstriction and stimulates the adrenal glands to release aldosterone. Aldosterone acts on the kidney tubules to cause reabsorption of sodium ions and osmotic retention of water. The water that is retained helps to expand the circulating blood volume to improve tissue perfusion.

   In the short term, these compensatory mechanisms are beneficial. In the long term, however, they become harmful because the heart must work harder to pump blood through vessels constricted by sympathetic nervous stimulation and by the effects of angiotensin II

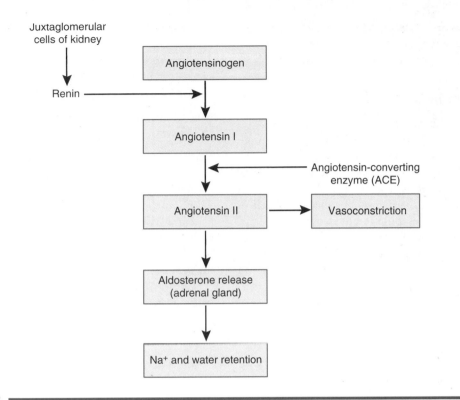

Figure 7-8

The renin-angiotensin scheme.

(increased afterload). The ever-increasing blood volume (increased preload) caused by aldosterone release and water retention also necessitates more strenuous activity by the heart, whose weakened state initiated the preceding chain of events.

Vasodilator drugs act by dilating arteries (arteriolar dilator), veins (venodilator), or both (combined vasodilator). Dilatory activity may be brought about by direct action on vessel smooth muscle, through blockage of sympathetic stimulation, or by preventing conversion of angiotensin I to angiotensin II. Dilation of constricted arteries tends to decrease the afterload and improve cardiac output. Preload is also reduced because of pooling of blood in dilated veins.

Many forms of CHF are improved by the use of vasodilators, which can be used in conjunction with other heart medications such as digitalis and diuretics and a reduced-salt diet (Lewis et al, 1987).

Hydralazine

Hydralazine is primarily an arteriolar dilator. It acts directly on smooth muscle in the arterial wall by interfering with calcium movements and inhibiting the contractile state (Plumb, 1999). The net result is that peripheral resistance is reduced and cardiac output is often greatly improved in animals with CHF. Some clinicians recommend that hydralazine be used with a diuretic because it may activate the renin-angiotensin system and cause water retention (Bill, 1993).

Clinical Uses. Hydralazine is used for afterload reduction associated with CHF, especially that caused by mitral valve insufficiency.

Dosage Forms. Human forms are used.

1. Hydralazine HCl tablets, 10, 25, 50, and 100 mg (Apresoline)
2. Hydralazine for injection, 20 mg/ml in ampules or vials (Apresoline)

Adverse Side Effects. Adverse side effects in small animals include hypotension, vomiting, diarrhea, sodium and water retention, and tachycardia.

Nitroglycerin Ointment

Nitroglycerin is primarily a venodilator that reduces preload resulting from the pooling of blood in peripheral vessels and decreased venous return to the heart. Some arteriolar dilation may occur at the higher doses. Nitroglycerin is applied topically in hairless areas of small animal patients. The medical vehicle of nitroglycerin causes it not to be explosive.

Clinical Uses. In small-animal medicine, nitroglycerin is used as a vasodilator to improve cardiac output and reduce associated pulmonary edema. In equine medicine nitroglycerin is used as a leg sweat to reduce swelling and to treat laminitis.

Dosage Forms. Human forms are used, such as nitroglycerin topical ointment, 2% in 20-, 30-, and 60-g tubes (Nitro-Bid, Nitrol).

Adverse Side Effects. Adverse side effects are minimal and may include rashes at the application site and hypotension.

Technician's Notes
1. Gloves should be worn when applying nitroglycerin.
2. Rotate application sites.
3. Do not pet animals at application sites.
4. The dose is measured in inches by application of a strip of ointment to measuring paper supplied with the product.
5. The veterinarian should be contacted if a rash appears at the application site.

Prazosin

Prazosin is a combined vasodilator. It reduces blood pressure and peripheral vasoconstriction by blocking alpha-1–adrenergic receptor sites. Prazosin apparently does not activate the renin-angiotensin system.

Clinical Uses. Prazosin is used for adjunctive treatment of CHF, dilated cardiomyopathy in dogs, systemic hypertension, and pulmonary hypertension.

Dosage Forms. Human forms are used: prazosin capsules, 1, 2, and 5 mg (Minipress).

Adverse Side Effects. These include hypotension, syncope, vomiting, and diarrhea.

Angiotensin-Converting Enzyme Inhibitors

Captopril and enalapril are combined vasodilators that exert their effects on blood vessels by preventing formation of the potent vasoconstrictor angiotensin II. They prevent the conversion of angiotensin I to angiotensin II by inhibiting ACE. Drugs in this category are sometimes called *ACE inhibitors.* Both products may be administered with cardiac glycosides and furosemide.

Clinical Uses. ACE inhibitors act as vasodilators in the treatment of class II, III, and IV heart failure.

Dosage Forms
1. Veterinary approved: enalapril tablets, 1 mg, 2.5 mg, 5 mg, 10 mg, 20 mg (Enacard)
2. Human approved: captopril tablets, 12.5, 25, 50, and 100 mg (Capoten)
3. Human approved: Vasotec tablets, 2.5, 5, 10, and 20 mg
4. Human approved: Vasotec injection for IV use, 1.25 mg/ml

Adverse Side Effects. These include hypotension, azotemia, vomiting, diarrhea, hyperkalemia, and others. The safety of enalapril in breeding dogs has not been established.

Technician's Notes
1. Care should be taken when administering captopril or enalapril with other vasodilators and certain diuretics because of potential hypotension.
2. Concurrent use of non-steroidal anti-inflammatory drugs may reduce the effectiveness of captopril.
3. Captopril may cause a false-positive urine acetone finding.

DIURETICS

Diuretics have been some of the most commonly used drugs in the treatment of heart failure because of their ability to promote the reduction of preload through diuresis. The diuretics reduce the harmful effects of CHF (pulmonary edema, ascites, and increased cardiac work) by reducing the plasma volume through various mechanisms.

Many different diuretics are available, and most work by inhibiting reabsorption of sodium and water in the loop of Henle or the distal tubules. If sodium ions remain in the tubules, they exert an increased osmotic "pull" on water molecules to cause them to remain in the tubules and be excreted as urine. The diuretics used most in veterinary medicine include furosemide, the thiazides, and spironolactone.

Furosemide

Furosemide is very powerful and is the diuretic of choice for treating CHF in dogs and cats (Lewis et al, 1987). Furosemide may be administered intravenously, intramuscularly, subcutaneously, or orally and works rapidly to reduce pulmonary edema and other signs of CHF. It causes diuresis by reducing reabsorption of sodium and other electrolytes in the kidney tubules. Because much of the reabsorption occurs in the loop of Henle, furosemide is sometimes called a *loop diuretic.*

Clinical Uses. Furosemide is used for diuretic therapy (in CHF and other conditions) in all species.

Dosage Forms. Injectable and oral (solution, tablet, and bolus) human label products are used.

1. Lasix
   a. Tablets, 12.5 and 50 mg
   b. Bolus, 2 g
   c. Oral solution, 10 mg/ml
   d. Injection, 5% (50 mg/ml)
2. Furosemide injection, generic 5%
3. Furosemide tablets, generic, 12.5 and 50 mg

Adverse Side Effects. These include low blood potassium (hypokalemia), dehydration, low blood sodium (hyponatremia), ototoxicity (cats), weakness, and shock.

> **Technician's Notes**
> 1. Furosemide should be administered carefully to animals that are dehydrated or in shock.
> 2. Furosemide can cause hypokalemia that can increase the chances of digitalis toxicity (anorexia increases the chances of hypokalemia).
> 3. Animals who are receiving diuretics such as furosemide should always have free access to water.
> 4. Dose at convenient times for the client because urination follows within 20 to 30 minutes.

Thiazides

Thiazide diuretics such as (chlorothiazide) Diuril acts on the loops of Henle and distal tubules to inhibit reabsorption of sodium. The thiazides are seldom used in veterinary medicine.

Spironolactone

Spironolactone is a potassium-sparing diuretic (it does not normally cause hypokalemia) that is an antagonist of aldosterone. By inhibiting aldosterone, it reduces the amount of sodium reabsorbed from the kidney tubules. Spironolactone (Aldactone) is usually not used alone but is combined with a loop diuretic or a thiazide (Plumb, 1999). Like the thiazides, it has limited use in veterinary medicine.

DIETARY MANAGEMENT OF HEART DISEASE

Dietary management is an important part of the overall treatment of patients with heart disease. Dietary measures are often instituted early in the pathogenesis of heart disease, before clinical signs are observed or drug therapy is begun. The two primary goals of dietary management of heart disease are (1) sodium restriction and (2) control of debilitation and weight loss (cardiac cachexia) (Ettinger, 1989).

Sodium restriction has long been recognized as an important part of the management of CHF. As previously mentioned, increased sodium levels in the body lead to water retention, increased plasma volume, and exacerbation of the clinical signs of heart failure. The primary source of sodium is food; however, water and treats must also be considered when limiting dietary intake. Prescription diets (Hill's and Purina) provide sodium-restricted nutrition for dogs and cats.

Diets fed to animals with heart failure should not only be sodium restricted but also should be balanced with adequate (but not excessive) levels of high-biologic–value protein, simple sugars, and emulsified fats (Lewis et al, 1987). Protein of high biologic value (1) reduces the amount of deamination required by the liver, (2) reduces the amount of nitrogenous waste to be excreted by the kidneys, and (3) increases the absorption of amino acids from the gastrointestinal tract. Simple sugars and emulsified fats provide good energy sources for tissues. All these factors tend to reduce the tendency for weight loss, a condition noted in CHF.

> **Technician's Notes**
>
> Clients should be instructed not to supplement their pet's diet with treats, human foods, or vitamin-mineral supplements when the animal is receiving a prescription sodium-restricted diet.

ANCILLARY TREATMENT OF HEART FAILURE

Various ancillary drugs and procedures are used in the treatment of heart failure. The following section provides a partial list of these therapies.

BRONCHODILATORS

Bronchodilators such as aminophylline and theophylline are sometimes used in the treatment of heart failure. These agents increase the size of lung passageways to allow more efficient oxygenation of blood, exert a mild positive ionotropic effect on heart muscle, and provide a mild diuretic effect.

OXYGEN THERAPY

Oxygen therapy can be crucial in treating animals in the advanced stages of CHF. Animals with pulmonary edema benefit greatly from the administration of 40% to 50% oxygen via cage, mask, or nasal cannula.

SEDATION

Animals with pulmonary edema resulting from heart failure often experience a great deal of anxiety because of the dyspnea that they encounter. This anxiety often leads to hyperventilation and even more oxygen demand and anxiety. To break the cycle and calm the animal, sedative drugs are often administered. The clinician may chose morphine, meperidine, diazepam, or other drugs.

ASPIRIN

Aspirin is known for its ability to reduce pain and inflammation, fever, and platelet aggregation. It is sometimes used in heart disease when clot formation may be a potential problem. It is used by some veterinarians to reduce the tendency for clot formation in heartworm treatment and for the same purpose in congestive cardiomyopathy in cats.

THORACOCENTESIS AND ABDOMINOCENTESIS

When heart failure is accompanied by excessive fluid (effusion) in the thoracic cavity, drawing the fluid from the cavity may be lifesaving. Removal of ascitic fluid is controversial but may relieve pressure on the diaphragm and improve ventilation.

REFERENCES

Bill, R.: Drugs affecting the cardiovascular system. In Bill, R. (ed.): Pharmacology for Veterinary Technicians. American Veterinary Publications, Goleta, CA, 1993.

Ettinger, S.: Therapy of heart failure. In Ettinger, S. (ed.): Textbook of Veterinary Internal Medicine. W.B. Saunders Company, Philadelphia, 1989.

Ganong, W.: Origin of the heartbeat and the electrical activity of the heart. In Ganong, W. (ed.): Review of Medical Physiology. Appleton and Lange, Norwalk, CT, 1993.

Giovanoni, R., Warren, R.C.: Cardiovascular drugs. In Giovanoni, R., Warren, R.C. (eds.): Principles of Pharmacology. Mosby, St. Louis, 1983.

Lewis, L.D., Ross, J.N., Morris, M.L., et al.: Heart failure. In Lewis, L.D., Ross, J.N., Morris, M.L., et al. (eds.): Small Animal Clinical Nutrition. Mark Morris Associates, Topeka, KS, 1987.

Plumb, D.C.: Veterinary Drug Handbook. Iowa State University Press, Ames, 1999.

Spinelli, J.S., Enos, L.R.: Drugs for treatment of cardiovascular disorders. In Spinelli, J.S., Enos, L.R. (eds.): Drugs in Veterinary Practice. Mosby, St. Louis, 1978.

Upson, D.W.: Cardiovascular system. In Upson, D.W. (ed.): Handbook of Clinical Veterinary Pharmacology, 3rd ed. Dan Upson Enterprises, Manhattan, KS, 1988.

Williams, B.R., Baer, C.: Antiarrythmic agents. In Williams, B.R., Baer, C. (eds.): Essentials of Clinical Pharmacology in Nursing. Springhouse Publishing Company, Springhouse, PA, 1990.

■ Review Questions

1. Why is the heart considered to be two pumps functionally? _____

2. Cardiac cells are connected by intercalated disks and a fusion of cell membranes to form a
_____.

3. Depolarization of cardiac cells is characterized by a rapid influx of _____ ions,
a slower influx of _____ ions, and the outflow of
_____ ions.

4. A relatively long _____ is important to cardiac cells to prevent a constant state of contraction from recycling impulses.

5. Define chronotropic and inotropic effects in relation to the heart. _____

6. Define preload and afterload in relation to the pumping mechanism of the heart.

_____

7. List the four basic compensatory mechanisms of the cardiovascular system.

_____

8. List five objectives of the treatment of heart failure.

_____

9. List four beneficial effects and one potential toxic effect of the use of the cardiac glycosides.

_____

10. Catecholamines such as epinephrine are used in veterinary cardiology primarily for

_____.

11. List five factors that may predispose the heart to arrhythmias. _____

12. List six categories of antiarrhythmic drugs and an example of each. _____

13. List four vasodilator drugs and classify each as arteriodilator, venodilator, or mixed.

_____

14. Why is Lasix sometimes called a loop diuretic?

_____

15. The use of many diuretics can lead to a dangerous loss of what electrolyte? _____

16. What are the two primary objectives of dietary management of cardiovascular disease?

_____

17. List five ancillary methods of the treatment of cardiovascular disease. _____

Chapter 8

Drugs Used in Gastrointestinal System Disorders

LEARNING OBJECTIVES

After studying this chapter, you should be able to:

1. Develop a basic understanding of the anatomy and physiology of the gastrointestinal (GI) system
2. Become familiar with the various mechanisms of control of the GI system
3. Understand the difference between vomiting and diarrhea
4. Develop a working knowledge of drugs that induce vomiting and those that inhibit it
5. Become familiar with antiulcer medications used in veterinary medicine
6. Develop a knowledge of the pathophysiology of diarrhea and the medications used to control this condition
7. List the different categories of laxatives and their respective mechanisms of action
8. List the two basic categories of GI prokinetics and stimulants
9. Understand the reasons for using digestive enzymes
10. Become acquainted with the use of antibiotics and anti-inflammatory agents in GI disease
11. List the categories of oral products and an example of each category

137

Adsorbent A drug that inhibits GI absorption of drugs, toxins, or chemicals by attracting and holding them to its surface.

Anticholinergic Blocking nerve impulse transmission through the parasympathetic nervous system; also called parasympatholytic. Anticholinergic drugs may be used for the treatment of diarrhea or vomiting.

Chemoreceptor trigger zone (CRTZ) An area found in the brain that, when stimulated by certain toxic substances in the blood, activates the vomiting center.

Cholinergic Activated by or transmitted through acetylcholine; also called parasympathomimetic. Cholinergic drugs increase activity in the GI tract.

Dentifrice A preparation for cleansing teeth, as a powder, paste, or liquid.

Emesis The act of vomiting.

Hematemesis Vomiting of blood (the character of the vomitus often resembles coffee grounds).

Melena Dark or black stools resulting from blood staining. The bleeding has occurred in the anterior part of the GI tract.

Motilin A hormone secreted by cells in the duodenal mucosa that causes contraction of intestinal smooth muscle.

Parietal cell A cell located in the gastric mucosa that secretes hydrochloric acid.

Peristalsis A wave of smooth muscle contraction passing along a tubular structure (GI or other) that moves the contents of that structure forward.

Regurgitation Casting up of undigested or semi-digested (ruminant) foodstuff from the esophagus or rumen.

Segmentation Periodic constrictions of segments of intestine without movement backward or forward; a mixing rather than a propulsive movement.

Vomiting center An area found in the medulla that may be stimulated by the CRTZ, the cerebrum, or peripheral receptors to induce vomiting.

INTRODUCTION

Problems of the GI system are common reasons for visits to a veterinary practice. These problems include **regurgitation,** vomiting, diarrhea, weight loss, colic, bloat, flatulence, abnormal stools, and constipation. Because veterinary technicians are expected to answer clients' questions about the GI tract, administer therapeutic GI medications, and monitor the response to GI medications, they must be knowledgeable about this system. They should have a basic knowledge of GI anatomy, physiology, pathophysiology, therapeutic principles, and medications.

ANATOMY AND PHYSIOLOGY

The anatomic and physiologic differences between the GI systems of different animal species are greater than for any other organ system (Bill, 1993). Despite these differences, the functions are basically the same in each species: (1) taking food and fluid into the body, (2) absorption of nutrients and fluid, and (3) excretion of waste products. A discussion of the anatomy and physiology of the GI tract with an emphasis on the similarities and differences between the species follows.

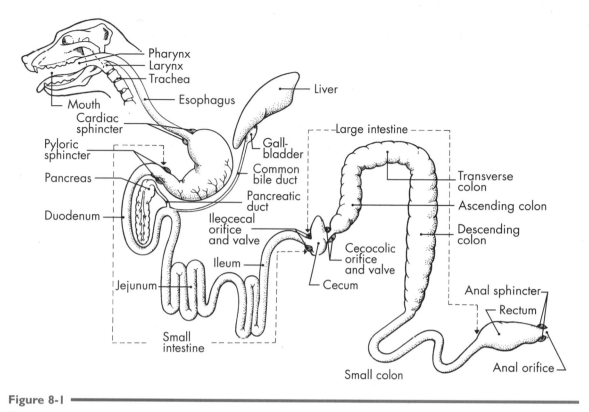

Figure 8-1

The monogastric gastrointestinal system.

The basic structures of the GI tract include (depending on the species) the mouth, teeth, tongue, salivary glands, esophagus, outpocketings of the esophagus (crop, reticulum, rumen, and omasum), stomach, liver, pancreas, duodenum, jejunum, ileum, cecum, colon, rectum, and anus.

Carnivorous or omnivorous species (cats, dogs, and primates) are often described as monogastric or simple-stomach animals because they have no outpocketings or forestomachs arising from the basic configuration (Figure 8-1). The function of the stomach in these monogastric animals is primarily to store ingested material and to begin some enzymatic breakdown of protein. The salivary glands begin enzymatic digestion by producing enzymes that break down starch into simpler carbohydrates. Pancreatic enzymes delivered to the duodenum break down fats, carbohydrates, and

proteins, and sodium bicarbonate from the pancreas neutralizes hydrochloric acid from the stomach. Bile salts produced in the liver and delivered to the duodenum aid in digestion by emulsifying fats. Bile is stored in the gallbladder except in animals in which it is absent (horses and rats). Digestion and its control mechanisms are complex, and students should consult an appropriate text for further information.

Ruminant animals are herbivorous and have a GI system characterized by three forestomachs, the reticulum, rumen, omasum, and a "true" stomach—the abomasum (Figure 8-2). The reticulum receives ingested material and passes it on to the rumen, where it is mixed and acted on by microorganisms to digest cellulose and other coarse plant material (roughage). Some refer to the rumen as a "fermentation vat," where microorganisms break down coarse feeds into

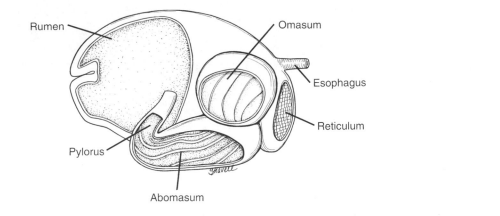

Figure 8-2

Compartments of the ruminant forestomach.

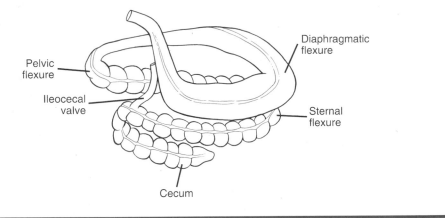

Figure 8-3

The large intestine of a horse.

forms that can be used by the simple stomach portion of the GI system in ruminants. Partially digested material (cud) in the rumen is regurgitated and remasticated to further facilitate digestion. In an immature ruminant, an esophageal groove allows milk to bypass the rumen and flow directly into the abomasum, and the rumen gains full function only after several months.

Equines, rabbits, and some rodents are chiefly herbivorous animals that have a monogastric GI configuration. They possess, however, a large cecum that is capable of limited roughage digestion (Figure 8-3).

Birds have an outpocketing of the esophagus called the *crop*, which is used for food storage. They also have a *ventriculus*, or *gizzard*, which serves to grind coarse food material (Figure 8-4).

The small intestine comprises three sections: the duodenum, which forms a sharp turn in which the pancreas is located; the long and highly coiled jejunum; and the short ileum, which connects to the large intestine. In the small intestine, contents passing from the stomach are mixed with intestinal secretions, pancreatic juice, and bile. The digestive process that began in the mouth and stomach is com-

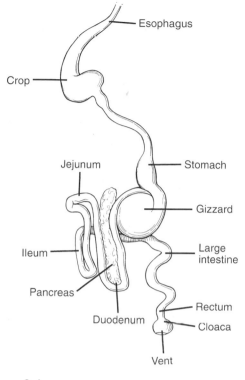

Figure 8-4

The digestive system of a bird.

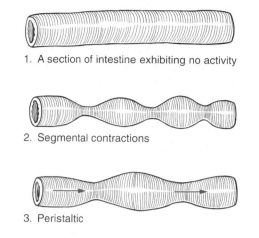

1. A section of intestine exhibiting no activity

2. Segmental contractions

3. Peristaltic

Figure 8-5

Peristalsis and segmentation.

pleted in the small intestine, in which the products of this process are absorbed together with most of the vitamins and a great deal of fluid. Villi and microvilli protrude from the mucosal surface into the lumen of the small intestine and greatly enhance the absorptive process.

The movements of the small intestine mix the intestinal contents, called *chyme,* and move them toward the large intestine. Normal intestinal motility includes two different patterns—**peristalsis** and **segmentation** (Figure 8-5). Peristalsis is a wave of contraction that propels contents along the digestive tract. Segmentation is a periodic, repeating pattern of intestinal constrictions that serve to mix and churn the contents.

The colon has a considerably larger diameter than the small intestine. The colon is connected to both the ileum and the cecum through the ileocecocolic valve. The surface of the colon may exhibit one or more lon-

gitudinal bands (depending on the species) called *teniae.* The wall of the colon may also form outpocketings called *haustra.* The colon of monogastric animals has an ascending portion, a transverse portion, and a descending portion leading into the rectum. The functions of the colon include the absorption of water, the synthesis of certain vitamins, and the storage of waste material.

The movements of the colon include peristalsis and segmentation (like the small intestine) and a third type called *mass action contraction* (Ganong, 1993). Mass action contraction is a result of simultaneous contraction of smooth muscle over a large area and serves to move fecal material from one portion of the colon to another and from the colon into the rectum.

REGULATION OF THE GASTROINTESTINAL SYSTEM

Regulation of GI system activity is complex but can be said to be under the influence of the following three basic control systems:

1. The autonomic nervous system (ANS).
   a. Stimulation of the parasympathetic portion of the ANS increases intestinal motility and

tone, increases intestinal secretions, and stimulates relaxation of sphincters. Drugs that mimic parasympathetic stimulation (**cholinergic,** or parasympathomimetic) cause similar results. **Anticholinergic,** or parasympatholytic, drugs inhibit these ANS actions.

b. Stimulation of the sympathetic branch of the ANS decreases intestinal motility and tone, decreases intestinal secretions, and inhibits sphincters.

c. Stimulation of various intrinsic receptors in the GI tract, such as the myenteric plexus (stretch receptor), also may increase peristaltic activity. Some physiologists consider the intrinsic receptors (myenteric plexus and Meissner's plexus) to be a third portion of the ANS called the *enteric nervous system* (Ganong, 1993).

2. GI hormones such as gastrin, secretin, and cholecystokinin released from intestinal cells exert control over many functions, such as gastric secretions, emptying of the gallbladder, and gastric emptying.

3. Substances such as histamine, serotonin, and prostaglandin are released from specialized cells of the GI tract. Histamine attaches to H_2 receptors in gastric parietal cells to cause the increased release of hydrochloric acid in the stomach. The influence of serotonin and prostaglandin is less well-defined.

Another factor that can have a major influence on GI activity is the presence of bacterial endotoxins. Endotoxins are components of the bacterial cell wall of certain bacteria (often gram-negative bacteria) that may increase the permeability of intestinal blood vessels and cause increased fluid loss as well as fever.

VOMITING

Vomiting is forceful ejection of the contents of the stomach, and sometimes those of the proximal small intestine, through the mouth. Vomiting is initiated by activation of the **vomiting** (emetic) **center** in the

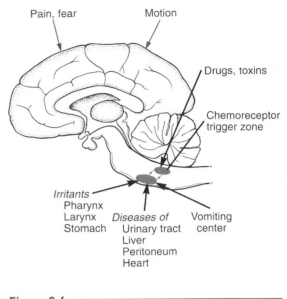

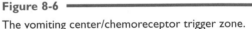

Figure 8-6

The vomiting center/chemoreceptor trigger zone.

medulla of the brain. The vomiting center is connected by nerve pathways to the **chemoreceptor trigger zone (CRTZ);** the cerebral cortex; and peripheral receptors in the pharynx, GI tract, urinary system, and heart. Impulses from any of these areas activate the vomiting reflex, which requires a coordinated effort of the GI, musculoskeletal, respiratory, and nervous systems (Figure 8-6). Impulses may be generated by (1) pain, excitement, or fear (cortex); (2) disturbances of the inner ear (CRTZ); (3) drugs such as apomorphine and digoxin (CRTZ); (4) metabolic conditions such as uremia, ketonemia, or endotoxemia (CRTZ); and (5) irritation of peripheral receptors (Dimski, 1989).

Occasional vomiting by a dog or cat is considered normal; however, persistent vomiting is not normal. Horses and rats do not normally vomit. Persistent vomiting can cause serious problems because of resulting dehydration, electrolyte disturbances, and acid-base imbalances. Sizable amounts of sodium, potassium, and chloride are lost in vomitus; however, potassium loss is usually the most significant abnormality.

EMETICS

Emetics are drugs that induce vomiting. Emetics are administered to animals that have ingested toxins, but they must be used carefully to avoid serious complications. Emetics should *not* be used in animals that (1) are comatose or having a seizure; (2) have depressed pharyngeal reflexes; (3) are in shock or dyspneic; or (4) have ingested strong acids, alkali, or other caustic substances. Obviously, emetics should not be given to animals that do not normally vomit, such as rabbits, some rodents, and horses. Emetics usually remove about 80% of the stomach contents; therefore, the animal should still be closely monitored for signs of toxicity after induced vomiting (Plumb, 1999).

Emetics are classified according to the site of their action. Those acting on the CRTZ are called *centrally acting*, and those that act on peripheral receptors are called *locally acting*.

Centrally Acting Emetics

Apomorphine

Apomorphine is a morphine derivative that stimulates dopamine receptors in the CRTZ, which then activates the vomiting center. This drug is poorly absorbed after oral administration and is therefore usually administered topically in the conjunctival sac or parenterally. Vomiting follows rapidly after intravenous administration, 5 to 10 minutes after intramuscular injection, and variably (10 to 20 minutes) after conjunctival administration.

Clinical Uses. Apomorphine is primarily used for induction of vomiting in dogs. It is considered by many to be the emetic of choice for dogs. Its use in cats is controversial and possibly contraindicated. Xylazine, which is safer than apomorphine, is effective as an emetic in most cats.

Dosage Form

1. Apomorphine HCl soluble tablets, 6 mg (human label), are commonly used. Apomorphine is a class II controlled substance.

Adverse Side Effects. These include protracted vomiting, restlessness, and depression.

> **Technician's Notes**
> 1. Whole or divided apomorphine tablets may be placed in the conjunctival sac of the eye. The tablets or portions can also be crushed, dissolved in saline, and placed in the conjunctiva. Once vomiting has occurred, the remaining apomorphine should be rinsed out of the conjunctiva to prevent protracted vomiting.
> 2. Naloxone may be used to treat overdosage or toxicity.

Xylazine

Although xylazine is not classified as an emetic, the label indicates that it induces vomiting in 3 to 5 minutes in cats and occasionally in dogs. Some clinicians consider xylazine to be the agent of choice to induce vomiting in cats. Normal precautions should be followed for the administration of this product.

Locally Acting Emetics

Syrup of ipecac is the primary agent. Other locally acting emetics that have been used with various degrees of effectiveness include mustard and water, hydrogen peroxide, and salt water (warmed).

Syrup of Ipecac

Ipecac is obtained from plant roots and contains alkaloids that irritate the gastric mucosa and induce vomiting within 10 to 30 minutes. Some stimulation of the CRTZ is thought to occur also. This agent may be used in dogs and cats. Some veterinarians question the efficacy of this emetic.

Clinical Uses. Ipecac is used to induce **emesis** in dogs and cats.

Dosage Form

1. Ipecac oral syrup in 15-ml, 30-ml, pint, and gallon bottles (generic) is an over-the-counter product.

Adverse Side Effects. These include cardiotoxicity (high doses), lacrimation, and salivation.

> ### Technician's Notes
>
> 1. Ipecac should be administered with caution to animals with an existing heart condition. It is cardiotoxic at high doses.
> 2. Extract of ipecac should never be substituted for syrup of ipecac because it is several times more potent than the syrup.

ANTIEMETICS

Antiemetics are drugs used to prevent or control vomiting. The use of antiemetics is a form of symptomatic treatment because the underlying cause of the vomiting is not necessarily corrected by these drugs. Many cases of vomiting in small-animal patients are self-limiting or can be controlled by withholding food and water for 24 to 48 hours. Other cases are more difficult to control and require the use of antiemetic agents and careful attention to determining the underlying cause. Antiemetics are usually given parenterally because vomiting precludes use of the oral route.

Phenothiazine Derivatives

Phenothiazine derivative antiemetics act centrally by blocking dopamine receptors in the CRTZ and possibly by direct inhibition of the vomiting center. These agents are in widespread use. They are very useful in preventing motion sickness in dogs and cats but may be less effective against irritant emetics (Upson, 1988). Common side effects include hypotension and sedation.

Chlorpromazine

Chlorpromazine is a phenothiazine derivative tranquilizer that has little popularity as a tranquilizer in veterinary medicine but is more often used as an antiemetic.

Clinical Uses. Chlorpromazine is used as an antiemetic in dogs and cats. It is more effective in dogs than in cats.

Dosage Forms

1. Chlorpromazine tablets (Thorazine), various sizes
2. Chlorpromazine extended-release capsules (Thorazine Spansule), various sizes
3. Chlorpromazine oral solution (Thorazine), 2 mg/ml, 30 mg/ml, and 100 mg/ml
4. Rectal suppositories (Thorazine), 25 and 100 mg
5. Chlorpromazine injection (Thorazine), 25 mg/ml in ampules and vials

Adverse Side Effects. These are primarily limited to sedation, ataxia, or hypotension.

> ### Technician's Notes
>
> 1. Chlorpromazine is incompatible when mixed with several other injectable agents. Check the label before administering.
> 2. Chlorpromazine may interact adversely when given concurrently with several other drugs. Read the label before administering to determine whether the combination is compatible.

Prochlorperazine

Prochlorperazine is a phenothiazine derivative agent that has moderate sedative effects and strong antiemetic effects. The approved form of this drug is a combination product that contains an anticholinergic agent (Darbazine). Prochlorperazine is available singly as Compazine (human label).

Clinical Uses. These include control of vomiting (prochlorperazine alone) in dogs and cats and treatment of vomiting, gastroenteritis, diarrhea, spastic colitis, and motion sickness (combination product).

Dosage Forms

1. Prochlorperazine. Injection, oral syrup, sustained-release capsules, and suppositories (Compazine)
2. Prochlorperazine/isopropamide. Injectable and capsule (Darbazine)

Adverse Side Effects. These are similar to those of chlorpromazine but may also include dry mucous membranes, dilated pupils, and urinary retention because of the effects of the anticholinergic in the combination product.

Procainamide Derivatives: Metoclopramide

Metoclopramide is a derivative of procainamide that has both central and peripheral antiemetic activities. Centrally it blocks the dopamine receptors in the CRTZ, whereas peripherally it increases gastric contraction, speeds gastric emptying, and strengthens cardiac sphincter tone. Metoclopramide has limited effect on GI secretions. This drug has a short half-life and may have to be administered often or in a continuous drip in severe cases of vomiting (Dimski, 1989).

Clinical Uses

1. As an antiemetic (especially for parvoviral enteritis, uremic vomiting, and vomiting associated with chemotherapy)
2. For the treatment of gastric motility disorders

Dosage Forms

1. Metoclopramide HCl tablets (Reglan), 5 and 10 mg
2. Metoclopramide HCl oral solution (Reglan), 1 mg/ml in containers of various sizes
3. Metoclopramide HCl injection (Reglan), 5 mg/ml

Adverse Side Effects. The most common side effects in horses, dogs, and cats are behavioral or other disorders associated with the central nervous system (CNS). Constipation may also occur.

Technician's Notes

1. Reglan is contraindicated if GI obstruction is suspected.
2. Atropine and the opioid analgesics may antagonize the action of metoclopramide.

Antihistamines

Antihistamines are most effective as antiemetics in dogs and cats when the vomiting is a result of motion sickness or inner ear abnormalities. Antihistamines block vomiting at the level of the CRTZ. All antihistamines may cause sedation.

Dosage Forms

1. Trimethobenzamide HCl (Tigan). Trimethobenzamide is an antiemetic for use in dogs only.
2. Dimenhydrinate (Dramamine). Dimenhydrinate is an antihistamine labeled for treatment of motion sickness in dogs and cats; it is available in tablet, liquid, and injectable forms.
3. Diphenhydramine (Benadryl). Diphenhydramine is used in veterinary medicine as an antiemetic and for the treatment of motion sickness, pruritus, and allergic reactions; it is available in tablet, capsule, oral elixir, and injectable forms.
4. Meclizine (Antivert)
5. Promethazine (Phenergan)

Anticholinergics

Anticholinergic or parasympatholytic drugs block the effects of acetylcholine at parasympathetic nerve endings. The result is reduction of GI spasms, intestinal motility, and intestinal secretions. These drugs act peripherally, except for atropine sulfate and aminopentamide, which have some capacity to cross the blood-brain barrier and block the CRTZ. Many clinicians believe that these drugs have a limited ability to reduce vomiting. Gastric emptying is slowed by anticholinergics, which may actually increase the tendency for vomiting.

Aminopentamide Hydrogen Sulfate

Aminopentamide is an anticholinergic, antispasmodic agent for use in dogs and cats.

Clinical Uses. These include the treatment of acute abdominal spasm and associated nausea, vomiting, and diarrhea.

Dosage Forms

1. Aminopentamide hydrogen sulfate tablets (Centrine), 0.2 mg
2. Aminopentamide hydrogen sulfate injection (Centrine), 0.5 mg/ml, 10-ml vials

Adverse Side Effects. These include dry mucous membranes and urinary retention.

Propantheline

Propantheline is a quaternary ammonium compound with anticholinergic activity similar to that of atropine.

Clinical Uses. The antispasmodic and antisecretory activity of propantheline is useful in the treatment of vomiting and diarrhea.

Dosage Form

1. Propantheline bromide tablets, 7.5 and 15 mg (Pro-Banthine)

Adverse Side Effects. These are similar to those of atropine and include dry mucous membranes, tachycardia, urinary retention, and constipation.

Butyrophenones

The butyrophenones are a group of tranquilizers that are capable of blocking both the CRTZ and the vomiting center. These drugs are relatively effective antiemetics but are seldom used for this purpose in veterinary medicine. Domperidone has been used in Europe but has seldom been used as an antiemetic in the United States.

Dosage Forms

1. Droperidol/fentanyl (Innovar-Vet)
2. Haloperidol (Haldol)
3. Pimozide (Orap)

Opioids

Opioids are not usually used as antiemetics. They may penetrate the vomiting center and cause a strong blockade of the vomiting reflex (Willard, 1998). Some opioids may penetrate the CRTZ and cause vomiting first before they block further vomiting.

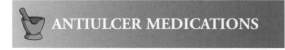

ANTIULCER MEDICATIONS

Gastric ulcers may occur in animals for various reasons including stress, metabolic disease, gastric hyperacidity, and drug therapy (corticosteroids or non-

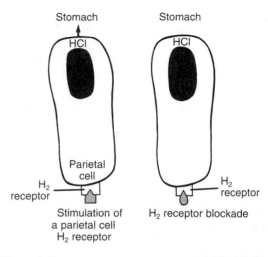

Figure 8-7

H_2 receptor blockade (parietal cell). *HCl,* hydrochloric acid.

steroidal anti-inflammatory agents) (Twedt and Wingfield, 1983). Anorexia, **hematemesis,** pain, and **melena** are common signs of gastric ulcers. Most cases of gastric ulceration involve increased gastric acid production and require treatment of the underlying cause as well as symptomatic therapy. Five classes of drugs are most commonly used to treat gastric ulcers: (1) H_2 receptor antagonists, (2) proton pump inhibitors, (3) antacids, (4) gastromucosal protectants, and (5) prostaglandin E-1 analogs.

H_2 Receptor Antagonists

One of the primary stimuli for secretion of hydrochloric acid by gastric **parietal cells** is activation of H_2 receptors by histamine. By blocking H_2 receptors, H_2 receptor antagonists reduce the release of hydrochloric acid, thus decreasing irritation of the eroded mucosa and promoting healing (Figure 8-7). H_2 blockers in current use include cimetidine and ranitidine.

Cimetidine

Cimetidine competitively inhibits histamine at H_2 receptors of gastric parietal cells, thereby reducing hydrochloric acid secretion by these cells.

Clinical Uses. Cimetidine is used for treatment or prevention of gastric, abomasal, or duodenal ulcers;

hypersecretory conditions of the stomach; esophagitis; gastric reflux; and experimentally as an immunomodulator.

Dosage Forms. Products approved for use in humans are also used in animals.

1. Cimetidine tablets (Tagamet), 100, 200, 300, 400, and 800 mg
2. Cimetidine oral solution (Tagamet), 60 mg/ml
3. Cimetidine HCl for injection (Tagamet)

Adverse Side Effects. These are rare in animals; however, cimetidine does inhibit microsomal enzymes in the liver and thus may alter the rate of metabolism of other drugs.

Ranitidine

Ranitidine is also an H_2 receptor antagonist that competitively inhibits histamine at parietal cell receptors and reduces hydrochloric acid secretion. Ranitidine has little effect on hepatic microenzymes and is unlikely to cause drug interactions. It is, however, more expensive than cimetidine at this time.

Clinical Uses. Clinical uses are identical to those of cimetidine.

Dosage Forms

1. Ranitidine HCl tablets (Zantac), 75, 150 and 300 mg
2. Ranitidine HCl oral syrup (Zantac), 15 mg/ml
3. Ranitidine injection (Zantac), 25 mg/ml

Adverse Side Effects. Adverse side effects are rare in animals.

Famotidine

Famotidine is an H_2 receptor that is more potent than ranitidine but less bioavailable. It is administered twice a day and may have fewer drug interactions than cimetidine or ranitidine.

Clinical Uses. The clinical uses are similar to cimetidine and ranitidine.

Dosage Forms

1. Famotidine film coated tablets (Pepcid or Pepcid AC), 10, 20, and 40 mg
2. Famotidine oral powder (Pepcid)
3. Famotidine injection (Pepcid IV)

Adverse Side Effects. Due to limited use, side effects have not been determined.

One other H_2 receptor antagonist called nizatidine (Axid) is available but has had limited use in veterinary medicine.

Proton Pump Inhibitors

Omeprazole and lansoprazole are benzimidazoles that act as proton pump inhibitors. These agents bind irreversibly at the secretory surface of the parietal cell to the enzyme Na-K ATPase. This enzyme is responsible for "pumping" hydrogen ions into the stomach against a concentration gradient. When bound in this way the enzyme is inactivated and the cell is unable to secrete acid until new enzyme is synthesized.

Clinical Uses. These agents are used to treat gastric or duodenal ulcers and esophagitis and may be useful in treating parietal hypersecretion associated with gastrinomas and mast cell tumors (Willard, 1998).

Dosage Forms

1. Omeprazole oral sustained release capsules (Prilosec), 10 and 20 mg
2. Omeprazole (Losec) (Canada)
3. Lansoprazole (Prevacid)

Adverse Side Effects. These are constipation, sedation, ileus, pancreatitis, and CNS effects.

Antacids

Antacids used in veterinary medicine are (relatively) non-absorbable salts of aluminium, calcium, or magnesium. Antacids are used to decrease the hydrochloric acid levels in the stomach as an aid in the treatment of gastric ulcers. In ruminants, antacids such as magnesium hydroxide are used to treat rumen acidosis (rumen overload syndrome) and are used as a laxative. Antacids may also be used in patients with renal failure to bind with (chelate) intestinal phosphorus and reduce hyperphosphatemia.

Clinical Uses. These include treatment of gastric ulcers, gastritis, esophagitis, and hyperphosphatemia in small animals. In ruminants, they are used to treat rumen overload.

Dosage Forms

1. Human label
   a. Aluminum/magnesium hydroxide (Maalox, Mylanta, WinGel)
   b. Aluminum carbonate (Basaljel)
   c. Aluminum hydroxide (Amphojel)
   d. Magnesium hydroxide (milk of magnesia)
2. Veterinary label: magnesium hydroxide (Magnalax, Rulax II)

Adverse Side Effects. Adverse side effects in monogastric animals include constipation (with aluminium- and calcium-containing products) and diarrhea (with magnesium-containing products).

Technician's Notes

1. Generally, do not give oral antacids within 1 to 2 hours of other oral medications because of their ability to decrease the absorption of drugs such as tetracycline, cimetidine, ranitidine, digoxin, captopril, corticosteroids, and ketoconazole.
2. Magnesium-containing antacids are contraindicated in animals with renal disease.

Gastromucosal Protectants

Sucralfate is the only gastromucosal protectant in common use in veterinary medicine. This drug is a disaccharide that, when administered orally, forms a pastelike substance in the stomach that binds to the surface of gastric ulcers. This pastelike material forms a barrier over the ulcer to protect it from further damage and to allow healing to occur. Because sucralfate binds to ulcers better in an acidic environment, it should be administered before (30 minutes to 1 hour) H_2 receptor antagonists. It may also reduce the availability of some other drugs.

Clinical Uses. Sucralfate is used in the treatment of oral, esophageal, gastric, and duodenal ulcers.

Dosage Form

1. Sucralfate (Carafate), 1 g tablets

Adverse Side Effects. These are usually limited to constipation.

Prostaglandin E-1 Analogs

Misoprostol is a prostaglandin E-1 analog that directly inhibits the parietal cell from secreting hydrogen ions into the stomach. It also protects the gastric mucosa by increasing the production of mucus and bicarbonate.

Clinical Uses. Prostaglandin E-1 analogs are used primarily to prevent or treat gastric ulcers associated with the use of NSAIDs.

Dosage Form

1. Misoprostol oral tablets (Cytotec), 100 and 200 μg

Adverse Side Effects. Side effects include diarrhea, vomiting, flatulence, and abdominal pain.

DIARRHEA

Diarrhea is the passage of loose or liquid stools, often with increased frequency. Diarrhea can result from primary disease of the intestinal tract or may accompany non-GI disease. Explanation of the pathophysiology of diarrhea is beyond the scope of this text; however, categories of mechanisms described in veterinary references include hypersecretion, increased permeability, osmotic overload, and altered intestinal motility. Parasitism is a common cause of diarrhea in all domestic animal species and causes diarrhea due to a combination of the previously described mechanisms. Parasitism should always be ruled out when determining a diagnosis.

Increased secretion of fluid from the intestine may result from the action of bacterial endotoxins from microorganisms such as *Escherichia coli, Clostridium perfringens, Campylobacter jejuni,* and *Helicobacter.* Intestinal epithelium damaged by viruses or other organisms may lose fluid as a result of increased permeability. Osmotic overload may occur as a result of poorly digestible foods, maldigestion or malabsorption, or a rapid change in diet. Although diarrhea has often been associated with hypermotility of the GI tract, the current belief is that most patients with diarrhea actually have hypomotility.

Decreased segmental contractions (hypomotility) increase the lumen diameter and allow more rapid passage, resulting in diarrhea. Normal segmental constrictions narrow the diameter of the intestinal lumen and actually slow the passage of contents.

Diarrhea, if not controlled, can result in significant fluid and electrolyte (sodium, chloride, potassium, and bicarbonate) losses. Dehydration, acidosis, weakness, and anorexia may follow.

Acute diarrhea, like acute vomiting, in dogs and cats often responds to dietary management and conservative treatment. In cases that do not respond to conservative management, symptomatic and specific treatment are essential. A discussion of the medications used in the treatment of diarrhea follows.

 ANTIDIARRHEAL MEDICATIONS

Narcotic Analgesics

Narcotic analgesics (opiates) are effective agents in the control of diarrhea because of their ability to (1) increase segmental contractions, (2) decrease intestinal secretions, and (3) increase intestinal absorption. Many clinicians consider opiates to be the drugs of choice for the control of diarrhea in dogs. They are also used for the treatment of diarrhea in calves, but their use in cats and horses is controversial because of a tendency to cause CNS stimulation. Narcotic agents are sometimes prepared as combination products with other classes of antidiarrheals.

Clinical Uses. The opiates are used in GI therapy for the control of diarrhea.

Dosage Forms

1. Diphenoxylate (Lomotil). Diphenoxylate is a synthetic narcotic agent (class V) that is structurally similar to meperidine. Atropine sulfate is added to commercial preparations to discourage substance abuse.
2. Loperamide (Imodium). Loperamide is a synthetic narcotic that is available in a non-prescription preparation. Loperamide poorly penetrates the CNS in cats and is acceptable in this species (Willard, 1998).
3. Paregoric/kaolin/pectin (Parepectolin)
4. Opium/kaolin/pectin/anticholinergics (Donnagel)

Adverse Side Effects. Adverse side effects of all the opiates include constipation, ileus, sedation, and CNS excitement (cats, horses).

Anticholinergics/Antispasmodics

The anticholinergics and antispasmodics have been widely used in veterinary medicine for the treatment of diarrhea. Because hypomotility rather than hypermotility is now considered to be associated with most cases of diarrhea, anticholinergics and antispasmodics should be used with caution for the treatment of diarrhea. A few commercial antidiarrheal preparations contain an anticholinergic plus a CNS depressant.

Clinical Uses. Anticholinergics/antispasmodics are used for the treatment of diarrhea.

Dosage Forms

1. Aminopentamide (Centrine)
2. Methscopolamine (Pamine)
3. Hyoscyamine (Levsin)
4. Propantheline (Pro-Banthine)

5. Clidinium/chlordiazepoxide (Librax)
6. Hyoscyamine/phenobarbital (Donnatal)

Adverse Side Effects. Adverse side effects are addressed in the antiemetic section.

Protectants/Adsorbents

Products in this category may have protectant or **adsorbent** qualities in the GI tract. The coating action of these drugs protects inflamed mucosa from further irritation. Their adsorbent activity binds bacteria or their toxins to protect against the harmful effects of these organisms. Kaolin and pectin are two ingredients often used in protectant compounds. The ability of protectants to control diarrhea has been questioned by some clinicians.

Bismuth subsalicylate is a compound found in products such as Corrective Suspension and Pepto-Bismol. Bismuth subsalicylate is converted to bismuth carbonate and salicylate in the small intestine. The bismuth has a coating and antibacterial effect, and the salicylate (aspirin-like compound) has an anti-inflammatory effect and reduces secretion by inhibiting prostaglandins (Burrows, 1983).

Activated charcoal is an adsorbent that is used primarily to treat poisoning.

Clinical Uses. These agents are used to control diarrhea and act as an adsorbent.

Dosage Forms

1. Bismuth subsalicylate
   a. Corrective Mixture (veterinary approved)
   b. Pepto-Bismol (human label)
2. Kaolin/pectin
   a. Kaopectolin
   b. Kao-Forte
   c. K-Pek
3. Activated charcoal
   a. Toxiban Suspension and Granules
   b. SuperChar-Vet Powder and Liquid

Adverse Side Effects. Adverse side effects are rare and are usually limited to constipation.

Technician's Notes
1. Bismuth subsalicylate compounds should be used with caution in cats because of the conversion to aspirin.
2. Bismuth may appear opaque on radiographs.
3. Administration of bismuth subsalicylate can result in black stools that resemble melena.

LAXATIVES

Laxatives are substances that loosen the bowel contents and encourage their evacuation. Laxatives with a strong or harsh effect are called *cathartics,* or *purgatives.* Categories of laxatives include saline/hyperosmotic agents, bulk-producing agents, lubricants, surfactants/stool softeners, irritants, and miscellaneous agents.

Saline/Hyperosmotic Agents

Saline or hyperosmotic laxatives contain magnesium or phosphate anions that are very poorly absorbed from the GI tract. It is generally held that these anions hold water in the tract osmotically. The increased water in the GI tract then softens the stool and stimulates stretch receptors in the gut wall to enhance peristalsis.

Clinical Uses. These agents are used for the relief of constipation.

Dosage Forms. Dosage forms include suspensions, crystals, powders, and boluses.

1. Lactulose (Cephulac, Constulose or Enulose). Lactulose also reduces blood ammonia levels in certain hepatic diseases.
2. Magnesium hydroxide
   a. Milk of magnesia. A suspension for use in dogs and cats
   b. Carmilax-Powder and Bolets. For use in cattle (laxative/antacid)
   c. Magnalax Bolus and Powder. For cattle
   d. Poly Ox II Bolus. For cattle

3. Magnesium sulfate
   a. Epsom salts. Has been used in horses and birds
4. Sodium phosphate salts
   a. Fleet enema. For use in dogs and foals
   b. Gent-L-Tip Enema. Dog and foal use

Adverse Side Effects. These are rare but may include cramping or nausea. Overdose or overuse may result in hyperphosphatemia or hypocalcemia. Cats are especially susceptible to these electrolyte imbalances.

> **Technician's Notes**
> Phosphate enemas should not be used in cats because cats are especially sensitive to the electrolyte imbalances that may occur.

Bulk-Producing Agents

Bulk-producing agents are often indigestible plant material (cellulose or hemicellulose) that acts by absorbing water and swelling to increase the bulk of the intestinal contents, thereby stimulating peristalsis.

Clinical Uses. Bulk-producing agents are used for relief of constipation and for relief of certain types of impactions (sand primarily) in horses.

Dosage Forms. Dosage forms are primarily psyllium preparations. Psyllium is obtained from the ripe seed of species of *Plantago* (Plumb, 1999).

1. Metamucil
2. Equine Psyllium
3. Equi-Phar Sweet Psyllium
4. Equine Laxative
5. Bran. A bulk-producing agent often used in horses (bran mash)

Adverse Side Effects. Adverse side effects are rare.

Lubricants

Lubricants are typically oils or other hydrocarbon derivatives (petrolatum) that soften the fecal mass and make it easier to move through the GI tract.

Clinical Uses. These include treatment of constipation and fecal impaction.

Dosage Forms. Dosage forms are liquids (mineral oil) or a jellylike mass (petrolatum).

1. Mineral oil. Mineral oil is used in horses for the treatment of constipation, colic, and impactions. This substance is also used as a laxative in other species. Heavy mineral oil is preferred over light mineral oil.
2. Petrolatum. This is a jellylike mass that is insoluble in water and only slightly soluble in alcohol. Petrolatum is the principal ingredient in many of the oral laxatives for hairball treatment in cats.
   a. Laxatone
   b. Felaxin
   c. Kat-A-Lax

Adverse Side Effects. These are minimal when used appropriately.

> **Technician's Notes**
> When administering mineral oil orally to a patient, care should be taken to avoid aspiration. Mineral oil is very bland and may not readily stimulate a swallowing reflex.

Surfactants/Stool Softeners

Surfactants reduce surface tension and allow water to penetrate the GI contents and thus soften the stool. They may also increase intestinal secretions.

Clinical Uses. Clinical uses include the treatment of hard, dry feces in small animals, impactions in horses, and occasionally digestive upsets in cattle.

Dosage Forms. These products are available in liquid, syrup, capsule, tablet, and enema forms. Docusate sodium, also called dioctyl sodium sulfosuccinate, is the main ingredient.

1. Docusate Sodium (Colase)
2. Docusate Calcium (Surfak)
3. Disposject Enema

Adverse Side Effects. Adverse side effects are rare.

Technician's Notes

Docusate sodium given with mineral oil may result in some absorption of the mineral oil.

Irritants

Irritants act by irritating the gut wall, causing stimulation of GI smooth muscle and increased peristalsis. These drugs are seldom used in veterinary medicine. This category includes several agents that are sometimes used in the treatment of constipation in humans.

1. Bisacodyl (Dulcolax)
2. Castor oil
3. Emodin

GASTROINTESTINAL PROKINETICS/STIMULANTS

Prokinetic/stimulant drugs increase the motility of a part or parts of the gastrointestinal tract and by doing this enhance the transit of material through the tract. Several classes of drugs have the ability to enhance gastrointestinal motility, including the dopaminergic antagonists, the serotonergic drugs, the motilin-like drugs, the direct cholinergics, and the acetylcholinesterase inhibitors.

Dopaminergic Antagonists

The dopaminergic antagonists used as prokinetics in veterinary medicine include metoclopramide and domperidone (Hall and Washabau, 1997a). These agents stimulate motility of the gastroesophageal sphincter, stomach, and the small intestine. Domperidone has had limited use as a prokinetic in the United States.

Clinical Uses. Metoclopramide is used to treat gastroesophageal reflux and delayed gastric emptying, to stimulate the gastrointestinal tract in foals, and for gastrointestinal motility disorders in dogs and cats. Metoclopramide has been shown to increase the gastric emptying of liquids faster than solids. The use of metoclopramide as an antiemetic is discussed in a previous section.

Dosage Forms

1. Metoclopramide (Reglan) tablets, syrup, and injection
2. Domperidone (Motilium)

Adverse Side Effects. Side effects include behavioral changes in dogs, cats, and adult horses. Cats have shown frenzied behavior (Plumb, 1999), and adult horses have shown alternating periods of sedation and excitement.

Serotonergic Drugs

Cisapride is the serotonergic prokinetic used frequently in veterinary medicine. Cisapride stimulates motility of the proximal and distal gastrointestinal tract including the gastroesophageal sphincter, stomach, small intestine, and colon (Washabau and Hall, 1997). Cisapride is not effective as an antiemetic but may be better than metoclopramide in treating certain motility disorders and in promoting the gastric emptying of solid material.

Clinical Uses. Uses include the treatment of constipation (along with dietary and/or surgical considerations) in cats; gastroesophageal reflux; and gastrointestinal stasis in dogs, cats, and horses.

Dosage Form

1. Cisapride (Propulsid), 10 and 20 mg tablets or 1 mg/ml suspension

Adverse Side Effects. Side effects may include diarrhea and abdominal pain.

Motilin-Like Drugs

Erythromycin has been used by veterinarians to treat bacterial and mycoplasmal infections for many years. This drug has also been shown to stimulate gastrointestinal motility by mimicking the effect of the hormone **motilin** (Hall and Washabau, 1997b). Erythromycin stimulates motility in the esophageal sphincter, stomach, and small intestine at microbially ineffective doses.

Clinical Uses. Uses may include increasing the lower esophageal sphincter pressure, accelerating gastric emptying, or facilitating intestinal transit time.

Dosage Form

1. Erythromycin (Erythro)

Adverse Side Effects. Side effects can include anorexia, vomiting, diarrhea, and abdominal pain.

Direct Cholinergics

Clinical Uses. These include postoperative treatment of ileus or retention of flatus or feces and equine colic (without obstruction).

Dosage Forms

1. Veterinary approved: dexpanthenol (d-Panthenol Injectable, d-Panthenol Injection)
2. Human approved: dexpanthenol (Ilopan injection)

Adverse Side Effects. Adverse side effects are rare but can include cramping or diarrhea.

Technician's Notes

Dexpanthenol should not be used within 12 hours of the use of neostigmine, parasympathomimetic agents, or succinylcholine.

Acetylcholinesterase Inhibitors

These drugs increase the amount of acetylcholine available to bind smooth muscle receptors.

Clinical Uses. These agents are used to treat rumen atony, to increase gastric emptying (ranitidine), to stimulate peristalsis, to empty the bladder of large animals, and to aid in the diagnosis of myasthenia gravis (neostigmine) in dogs. They may also be used to treat curare overdose.

Dosage Forms

1. Neostigmine methylsulfate (Stiglyn injection)
2. Ranitidine (Zantac)

Adverse Side Effects. Adverse side effects are cholinergic and can include nausea, vomiting, diarrhea, drooling, sweating, lacrimation, bradycardia, and various others.

DIGESTIVE ENZYMES

Pancrelipase is a product containing pancreatic enzymes to aid in the digestion of fats, proteins, and carbohydrates. The powder containing the enzymes is mixed with the animal's food, which is allowed to stand for 15 to 20 minutes before feeding.

Clinical Uses. This product is used to treat pancreatic exocrine insufficiency.

Dosage Form

1. Pancrelipase (Viokase-V powder, Pancrezyme powder). Both are approved for use in dogs and cats.

Adverse Side Effects. Adverse side effects of high doses include cramping, nausea, or diarrhea.

Technician's Notes

1. Powder spilled on the skin should be washed off to prevent irritation.
2. Inhaled powder can cause nasal irritation or can precipitate an asthma attack.

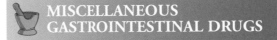

MISCELLANEOUS GASTROINTESTINAL DRUGS

The drugs discussed in this section include the antibiotics, the anti-inflammatory agents, and the antifoaming agents.

Antibiotics

Antibiotics are not routinely used in the treatment of GI tract disease in small animals because these agents may destroy the normal inhabitants of the GI tract and allow pathogenic bacteria (*Salmonella* species, *C. jejuni, C. perfringens, Helicobacter,* and others) to grow on the mucosal surface. Bloody diarrhea or signs of sepsis may indicate the need for aggressive antibiotic therapy with aminoglycosides and cephalosporins (Dimski, 1989). Other antibiotics that are sometimes used for treating bacterial overgrowth and other GI conditions are metronidazole, amoxicillin, and tylosin.

Metronidazole

Metronidazole is a synthetic antibacterial and antiprotozoal agent.

Clinical Uses

1. Treatment of giardiasis, trichomoniasis, balantidiasis, plasmacytic/lymphocytic enteritis, ulcerative colitis, hepatic encephalopathy, and anaerobic infections in dogs
2. Treatment of giardiasis and anaerobic infections in cats
3. Treatment of anaerobic infections in horses

Dosage Form

1. Metronidazole (Flagyl tablets, Flagyl IV powder for reconstitution, and Flagyl IV RTU injection)

Adverse Side Effects. These include anorexia, hepatotoxicity, neutropenia, vomiting, and diarrhea.

Technician's Notes

1. Metronidazole should not be given to debilitated, pregnant, or nursing animals.
2. Tylosin is a macrolide antibiotic that is sometimes used to treat chronic colitis in animals.

Anti-Inflammatory Agents

Anti-inflammatory agents are used in the treatment of idiopathic inflammatory bowel disease in animals. These diseases are characterized by increased numbers of lymphocytes, macrophages, plasma cells, or eosinophils in the intestinal wall. Treatment often involves the use of hypoallergenic diets and anti-inflammatory agents.

Dosage Forms. The anti-inflammatory agents used in the treatment of inflammatory bowel disease include prednisone, azathioprine, and sulfasalazine.

1. Prednisone. Many generic and trade name products are available.
2. Azathioprine (Imuran). A purine antagonist antimetabolite that may be used in the treatment of

inflammatory bowel diseases because of its immunosuppressive effects.
3. Sulfasalazine (Azulfidine). A drug that is converted by intestinal bacteria to a sulfa drug (sulfapyridine) and aspirin (salicylic acid). Aspirin is the active component that has an anti-inflammatory effect and is useful in many cases of colitis in dogs and cats. It should be used with care in cats because of their poor ability to metabolize aspirin.

Antifoaming Agents

Antifoaming agents are used to treat frothy bloat in ruminants. In this condition, gas bubbles form and become trapped in the rumen fluid as a result of the consumption of wheat pasture or legumes such as alfalfa or clover. The trapped bubbles cause a form of bloat that cannot be relieved by usual means.

The antifoaming agents act as surfactants (reduce surface tension) and cause the bubbles to break down so that the gas can be relieved by eructation or stomach tube. These products are given orally.

Clinical Uses. Antifoaming agents are used for the treatment of frothy bloat in ruminants.

Dosage Forms

1. Bloat Guard
2. Bloat Treatment
3. Bloat-Pac
4. Therabloat

Adverse Side Effects. These are rare if the products are given as directed.

ORAL PRODUCTS

An increased emphasis on dentistry in veterinary practice in recent years has fueled a demand for products that promote and maintain oral health. Many of these products help to remove food particles and plaque and assist in the maintenance of pleasant-smelling breath. Some are labeled as a **dentifrice,** and others may be applied as an oral rinse or with a toothbrush. They are prepared as solutions, gels, and premoistened gauze sponges. Various flavors are available, as well as products with fluoride. These products should not be considered a substitute for veterinary dental treatment.

Other oral products include grit-impregnated paste for polishing teeth and smoothing out rough surfaces left by scaling, as well as disclosing solution to assist in identifying plaque.

Dentifrice and Cleansing Products

1. C.E.T. Dentifrices. Contain various active ingredients, as well as mint, malt, and poultry flavors; should not be rinsed
2. Nolvadent oral cleansing solution. Chlorhexidine acetate is the active ingredient; also contains a peppermint flavor; may be used with a toothbrush or as a rinse
3. Oral Dent. Similar to Nolvadent but made by a different company
4. Oxydent. An effervescent dentifrice with various ingredients
5. VRx Oral Hygiene Pads
6. C.E.T. Oral Hygiene Spray
7. CHx Gel and Solution
8. PetDent
9. Maxi/Guard Oral Cleansing Gel
10. Fresh Mouth Oral Spray
11. C.E.T. Chews
12. Friskies Cheweez
13. C.E.T. Cat Toothbrush
14. Hills t/d Diet
15. Heinz Tarter Check
16. Friskies Dental Diet

Fluoride Products

1. SF04 Stannous Fluoride Gel
2. FluroFom
3. C.E.T. Oral Hygiene Spray with Fluoride

Perioceutic Agents

1. Heska Perioceutic. This agent is placed in the periodontal pocket after dental cleaning using a cannula. Upon contact with the aqueous environment

the product coagulates and releases doxycycline for several weeks.

Polishing Paste

1. C.E.T. Prophypaste

Disclosing Solution

1. Duo 128 Disclosing Solution

REFERENCES

Bill, R.: Drugs affecting the gastrointestinal system. In Bill, R. (ed.): Pharmacology for Veterinary Technicians. American Veterinary Publications, Goleta, CA, 1993.

Burrows, C.F.: The treatment of diarrhea. In Kirk, R.W. (ed.): Current Veterinary Therapy VII: Small Animal Practice. W.B. Saunders Company, Philadelphia, 1983.

Dimski, D.S.: How to choose the proper drug therapy for gastrointestinal disorders. In Dimski, D.S., Twedt, D.C., Tams, T.R., et al. (eds.): Managing Gastrointestinal Disorders. Veterinary Medicine Publishing Company, Lenexa, KS, 1989.

Ganong, W.: Regulation of gastrointestinal function. In Ganong, W. (ed.): Review of Medical Physiology. Appleton & Lange, Norwalk, CT, 1993.

Hall J.A., Washabau R.J.: Gastrointestinal Prokinetic Therapy: Dopaminergic Antagonist Drugs. Compend. Contin. Educ. Pract. Vet. 19(2):214-219, 1997a.

Hall J.A., Washabau, R.J.: Gastrointestinal Prokinetic Therapy: Motilin-Like Drugs. Compend. Contin. Educ. Pract. Vet. 19(3):281-286, 1997b.

Plumb, D.C.: Apomorphine. In Plumb, D.C. (ed.): Veterinary Drug Handbook. Iowa State University Press, Ames, 1999.

Twedt, D.C., Wingfield, W.E.: Diseases of the stomach. In Ettinger, S.J. (ed.): Textbook of Veterinary Internal Medicine, 2nd ed. W.B. Saunders Company, Philadelphia, 1983.

Upson, D.W.: Gastrointestinal system. In Upson, D.W. (ed.): Handbook of Clinical Veterinary Pharmacology, 3rd ed. Dan Upson Enterprises, Manhattan, KS, 1988.

Washabau R.J., Hall, J.A.: Gastrointestinal Prokinetic Therapy: Serotonergic Drugs. Compend. Contin. Educ. Pract. Vet. 19(4):473-478, 1997.

Willard, M.D.: Gastrointestinal Drugs. In Boothe, D.M. (ed.): The Veterinary Clinics of North America, Small Animal Practice. W.B. Saunders Company, Philadelphia, 1998.

■ Review Questions

1. List three general functions of the GI tract.

   _____

2. List three examples of monogastric animals.

   _____

3. What is the GI configuration of ruminant animals?

   _____

4. What is the difference between vomiting and regurgitation? _____

5. Ruminants are animals that use

   _____ to digest coarse plant material.

6. What are the three basic control mechanisms of the GI tract? _____

7. What is the significance of the presence of bacterial endotoxins in the GI tract?

   _____

8. The CRTZ stimulates vomiting when activated by

   _____

9. List two examples of centrally acting emetics and two examples of peripherally acting emetics.

   _____

10. Drugs that inhibit vomiting are called

    _____

11. H_2 receptor antagonists promote the healing of GI ulcers by _____

12. List two H_2 receptor antagonists.

    _____

13. What are the two types of intestinal motility patterns?

    _____

14. Acute vomiting and diarrhea in dogs and cats often respond to conservative management such as

    _____

15. List two species that do not vomit.

    _____

16. What is the mechanism of action of saline/hyperosmotic laxatives? _____

17. What is the active ingredient of Metamucil?

    _____

18. Direct cholinergic drugs stimulate the GI tract by what mechanism? _____

19. A synthetic antibiotic/anti-inflammatory agent used to treat giardiasis and anaerobic bacterial infections in animals is called _____

20. List four products used as dentifrice/oral cleansing agents. _____

Drugs Used in Hormonal, Endocrine, and Reproductive Disorders

LEARNING OBJECTIVES

After studying this chapter, you should be able to:

1. Discuss the control mechanisms (physiology) of the endocrine system
2. List the endocrine glands
3. List the reasons why hormones are clinically used
4. Describe the difference between an endogenous and an exogenous hormone
5. Describe the location and functions of the pituitary gland
6. Differentiate between a positive and a negative feedback control mechanism
7. Describe a neurohormonal reflex
8. Discuss the uses and classes of gonadotropins, gonadal hormones, progestins, and prostaglandins used in veterinary medicine
9. Describe the uses and classes of drugs that affect uterine contractility
10. Define pheromone and give an example
11. Describe the location, function, and hormonal products of the thyroid gland
12. Describe the hormonal treatment of hypothyroidism and hyperthyroidism
13. List the endogenous source of insulin and its metabolic effects
14. List the classes of insulin products and their general characteristics
15. Describe the method of action of the growth promoters
16. List the clinical uses for the anabolic steroids

157

KEY TERMS

Anabolism The constructive phase of metabolism in which body cells repair and replace tissue.

Analog A chemical compound having a structure similar to another but differing from it in some way.

Dystocia Difficult birth.

Endometrium The mucous membrane lining of the uterus.

Euthyroid A normal thyroid gland.

Feed efficiency The rate at which animals convert feed into tissue; expressed as the number of pounds or kilograms of feed needed to produce 1 pound or kilogram of animal.

Feedback The return of some of the output product of a process as input in a way that controls the process.

Gonadotropin Hormone that stimulates the ovaries or testes.

Hypophyseal portal system The portal system of the pituitary gland in which venules from the hypothalamus connect with capillaries of the anterior pituitary.

Involution A return of a reproductive organ to normal size after delivery.

Levo isomer A left-sided arrangement of a molecule that may exist in either a left- or right-sided configuration. Levo and dextro isomers have the same molecular formula.

Myofibril A muscle fibril composed of numerous myofilaments.

Nitrogen balance The condition of the body as it relates to protein intake and utilization. Positive nitrogen balance implies a net gain in body protein.

Primary hypothyroidism Hypothyroidism resulting from pathology in the thyroid itself.

Releasing factor (releasing hormone) A hormone produced by the hypothalamus and transported to the anterior pituitary to stimulate the release of trophic hormones.

Trophic hormone A hormone that results in production of a second hormone in a target gland.

INTRODUCTION

The traditional definition of the endocrine system states that it is composed of organs (glands) or groups of cells that secrete regulatory substances (hormones) directly into the bloodstream. This definition has now been extended to include regulatory substances that are distributed by diffusion across cell membranes.

The endocrine system and the nervous system constitute the two major control mechanisms of the body. These two control mechanisms are linked together through the complex integrating action of the hypothalamus (Figure 9-1). Coordination of these two systems allows an individual to adapt its reproductive and survival strategies to changes in the environment.

Endocrine glands include the pituitary, adrenals, thyroid, ovaries, testicles, pancreas, and kidneys. These glands produce hormones that are carried to target organs, where they influence the physiologic activity of these structures.

Hormones are generally administered to animals for one of two reasons: (1) to correct a deficiency of that hormone or (2) to obtain a desired effect (e.g., to postpone estrus). Hormones that are administered to an animal are called *exogenous* hormones, whereas those produced naturally in the body are *endogenous* hormones.

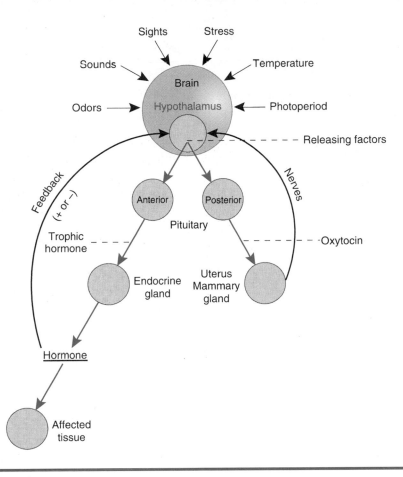

Figure 9-1

Hypothalamic integration of endocrine and nervous systems.

ANATOMY AND PHYSIOLOGY

PITUITARY GLAND

The pituitary gland has been called the master gland of the endocrine system because of the control it exerts over the regulation of this system. It is located at the base of the brain just ventral to the hypothalamus and is connected to the brain by a stalk. It is divided into two main lobes—an anterior lobe (adenohypophysis), which arises from the embryologic pharynx, and a posterior lobe (neurohypophysis), which arises from the brain (Figure 9-2).

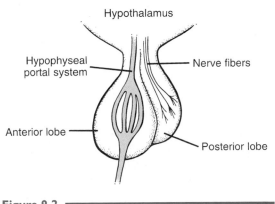

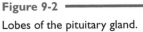

Figure 9-2

Lobes of the pituitary gland.

The hypothalamus exerts control over the anterior pituitary through the transport of **releasing hormones,** or **factors,** down the **hypophyseal portal system.** In the anterior pituitary, these releasing factors cause the secretion of **trophic hormones** into the circulation. The trophic hormones produced by the anterior pituitary include thyroid-stimulating hormone (TSH), adrenocorticotropic hormone (ACTH), luteinizing hormone (LH), follicle-stimulating hormone (FSH), prolactin (LTH), and growth hormone (GH, or somatotropin). These trophic hormones are sometimes called *indirect-acting hormones* because they cause their target organ to produce a second hormone, which in turn influences a second target organ or tissue (Table 9-1). For example, TSH stimulates the thyroid gland to produce triiodothyronine (T_3) and tetraiodothyronine (T_4), hormones that in turn influence the metabolic rate of all tissues in the body.

The two hormones of the posterior pituitary are vasopressin (antidiuretic hormone) and oxytocin. These hormones are produced in the hypothalamus and subsequently travel down nerve fibers to the posterior pituitary, where they are stored for release into the circulation. The hormones of the posterior pituitary are called *direct-acting hormones* because they produce the desired activity directly in the target organ (e.g., contraction of the uterus).

CONTROL OF THE ENDOCRINE SYSTEM

Feedback Mechanism

The nervous system is sensitive to levels of hormones through a mechanism called the **feedback** mechanism. By this mechanism, the plasma level of a particular hormone controls the activity of the gland that produces it. The type of feedback may be negative or positive (Figure 9-3).

With negative feedback, high plasma levels of a hormone are sensed by the hypothalamus, which then reduces the amount of the appropriate releasing factor (or hormone). A decreased amount of releasing factor reduces the amount of trophic hormone released from the pituitary, causing less activity in the organ that is producing the hormone in question. The overall effect is to lower the amount of the hormone in the plasma.

In the positive feedback scheme, low levels of a hormone are sensed by the hypothalamus, and release of the appropriate releasing factor increases. Increased amounts of the corresponding trophic hormone are

TABLE 9-1 Pituitary Hormones

Source and Name	Target and Actions
Anterior Lobe	
Thyroid-stimulating hormone (TSH)	Stimulates the thyroid to produce T_3/T_4
Follicle-stimulating hormone (FSH)	Stimulates ovarian follicle growth (female) and spermatogenesis (male)
Luteinizing hormone (LH)	Stimulates ovulation (female) and testosterone production (male)
Growth hormone (somatotropin)	Accelerates body growth and increases milk production
Adrenocorticotropic hormone (ACTH)	Stimulates production of corticosteroids by adrenal cortex
Posterior Lobe	
Oxytocin	Stimulates urine contraction and milk letdown
Vasopressin (antidiuretic hormone, ADH)	Stimulates water retention

then secreted, causing increased activity in the target organ and a corresponding rise in the plasma levels of the hormone.

Neurohormonal Reflex

The neurohormonal reflex applies to the release of oxytocin by the posterior pituitary. The first step in this reflex can be initiated by (1) stimulation of the udder by a nursing calf or by preparation of the udder for milking, (2) stimulation of the uterus and vagina in parturition, or (3) stimulation of the cerebral cortex by sensory stimuli associated with nursing or milking.

Control of the Reproductive System

The reproductive (estrus) cycle in animals has traditionally been divided into four stages called *proestrus,*

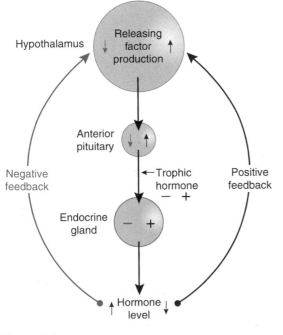

Figure 9-3

Feedback control mechanisms. Positive and negative feedback mechanisms control the amount of a particular hormone.

estrus, diestrus, and *anestrus.* The cycle may also be divided into a follicular phase and a luteal phase. In the follicular phase, the cycle is under the influence of estrogen produced by a developing follicle, and in the luteal phase it is under the influence of progesterone made by the corpus luteum.

Control of the reproductive system is coordinated in the hypothalamus, where gonadotropin-releasing hormone (GnRH) is produced in response to various stimuli (Figure 9-4). These stimuli can include the day-night length (photoperiod), pheromones, and positive and negative internal feedback mechanisms. GnRH causes the release of FSH and LH from the anterior pituitary.

FSH causes the growth and maturation of a follicle, which begins to produce increasing amounts of estrogen as it matures. Estrogen causes the changes that occur in proestrus and estrus and include the behavioral characteristics associated with estrus (e.g., standing to be mounted). The follicle also produces inhibin, which, along with estrogen, serves as negative feedback to the hypothalamus to inhibit the release of GnRH.

LH release causes ovulation of the mature follicle and the formation of a corpus luteum in its place. This event signals the beginning of diestrus and the beginning of the luteal phase of the cycle. The corpus luteum produces progesterone, which prepares the uterus for pregnancy and, once pregnancy occurs, maintains a uterine environment conducive to normal progression of pregnancy. Progesterone levels in the blood serve as negative feedback to prevent the release of GnRH and the development of new follicles during pregnancy.

When the gestation period nears its end, the fetus begins to produce increasing amounts of ACTH. ACTH causes increased amounts of cortisol to be produced by the adrenal glands. The increased cortisol levels result in increased production of estrogen and prostaglandin by the uterus. These two substances sensitize the uterus to the contraction-producing effects of oxytocin and allow parturition to begin. Prostaglandin also causes breakdown (lysis) of the corpus luteum at the end of pregnancy and at the end of diestrus if pregnancy does not occur.

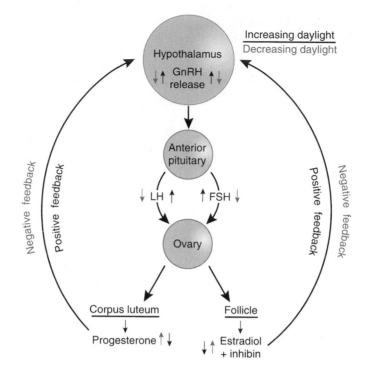

Figure 9-4

Control of the reproductive system is primarily through feedback mechanisms and the photoperiod. *GnRH,* gonadotropin releasing hormone; *LH,* luteinizing hormone; *FSH,* follicle-stimulating hormone.

HORMONAL DRUGS ASSOCIATED WITH REPRODUCTION

GONADOTROPINS AND GONADAL HORMONES

Products in this category are used in veterinary medicine for various reasons. Some of these include synchronization of estrus, suppression of estrus, induction of estrus, treatment of cystic ovaries, and termination of pregnancy.

Gonadotropins

Gonadotropins are drugs that act like GnRH, LH, or FSH. Gonadotropins cause the release of LH and FSH or cause activity like that of LH or FSH. LH may be prepared from the pituitary glands of slaughtered animals or obtained from the urine of pregnant women in the form of human chorionic gonadotropin (hCG). FSH may be obtained from pituitary glands (FSH-P) and from the serum of pregnant mares (PMS) between the 40th and 140th day of pregnancy. GnRH is prepared synthetically.

FSH that is released endogenously by the anterior pituitary causes growth and maturation of the ovarian follicle in females and spermatogenesis in males. LH, also released by the anterior pituitary, causes ovulation in females and production of testosterone in males.

Gonadorelin

Gonadorelin (GnRH) is produced endogenously by the hypothalamus. Gonadorelin causes the release of FSH and LH by the anterior pituitary.

Clinical Uses. Gonadorelin is used to treat cystic (follicular) ovaries in dairy cattle. It has also been used in cats and horses (with limited success) to induce estrus.

Dosage Forms

1. Cystorelin. Gonadorelin for injection
2. Factrel. Gonadorelin for injection
3. Fertagyl. Gonadorelin for injection

Adverse Side Effects. These are minimal with use of this product.

Chorionic Gonadotropin

Chorionic gonadotropin (hCG) is a hormone secreted by the uterus and obtained from the urine of pregnant women. It mimics the effect of LH, although it has limited FSH activity. In males, it stimulates the production of male hormone by the testicles and may facilitate descent of the testicles.

Clinical Uses. Chorionic gonadotropin is used to treat cystic ovaries (nymphomania) in dairy cattle. In males, it has been used to treat cryptorchidism and infertility caused by low testosterone levels.

Dosage Forms

1. Follutein. hCG injection
2. P.G. 600. Combination of hCG and PMS. Contains both LH and FSH activity
3. Chorulon. hCG injection
4. Chorionic gonadotropin injection (generic)
5. APL

Adverse Side Effects. These are limited but may include hypersensitivity reactions and abortions in mares if given before the 35th day of pregnancy.

Follicle-Stimulating Hormone–Pituitary

FSH–P is obtained from the pituitary glands of slaughtered animals. FSH causes growth and maturation of the ovarian follicle.

Clinical Uses. FSH–P is used in veterinary medicine to induce superovulation and for out-of-season breeding.

Dosage Form

1. FSH–P

Adverse Side Effects. These include endometrial hyperplasia, superovulation, and follicular cysts.

Estrogens

Estrogens are a group of hormones synthesized by the ovaries and to a lesser extent by the testicles, adrenal cortex, and placenta. The estrogens are classified as sex steroids and are synthesized from a cholesterol precursor. Estrogens are necessary for normal growth and development of the female gonads. They cause secondary female characteristics and are responsible for female sex drive. These hormones inhibit ovulation, increase uterine tone, and cause proliferation of the **endometrium.**

Clinical Uses. In cattle, estrogens are used to treat persistent corpus luteum, to expel purulent material from the uterus, to expel retained placentas and mummified fetuses, and to promote weight gain. In dogs, estrogens are used to induce abortion and to control urinary incontinence. In horses, they may be used for induction of estrus in the non-breeding season.

Dosage Forms

1. Estradiol cypionate (ECP) injection
2. Estradiol cypionate (generic)
3. Diethylstilbestrol (DES) tablets
4. Implants to promote weight gain (discussed in a following section)

Adverse Side Effects. These include severe anemia, prolonged estrus, genital irritation, and follicular cysts.

Technician's Notes

1. Estrogens should not be given during pregnancy.
2. Estrogen administration can cause severe anemia.
3. Synthetic DES has been banned from use in food-producing animals because of its possible link with cervical cancer in women.

Androgens

Androgens are male sex hormones produced in the testicles, ovaries, and the adrenal cortex. Like the other gonadal hormones, they have a steroidal parent molecule. These hormones are necessary for growth and development of the male sex organs. They cause secondary male sex characteristics and produce male libido. The androgens promote tissue **anabolism,** weight gain, and red blood cell formation.

Testosterone Cypionate, Testosterone Enanthate, and Testosterone Propionate

These injectable testosterone products are available under a human label.

Clinical Uses. These androgens are used to treat urinary incontinence in male dogs and to increase libido and fertility in domestic animals (with generally poor results).

Dosage Forms

1. Danocrine (Danazol-derivative of ethinyl testosterone) (human label)
2. Testosterone cypionate injection (generic)
3. Testosterone enanthate (generic)
4. Testosterone propionate (generic)
5. Depo-Testosterone

Adverse Side Effects. These are uncommon when used as directed.

> **Technician's Notes**
> Testosterone products are now C-III controlled substances.

Mibolerone

Mibolerone is an androgen used for prevention of estrus in dogs. Mibolerone blocks the release of LH by the pituitary and prevents complete development of the follicle. Ovulation does not occur.

Clinical Uses. This product is used for prevention of estrus in adult female dogs and for treatment of pseudocyesis.

Dosage Forms

1. Cheque Drops. Oral liquid preparation
2. Implants to promote weight gain (discussed later)

Adverse Side Effects. Adverse side effects reported in the insert include premature epiphyseal clo-

sure and vaginitis in immature females. In mature females, vulvovaginitis, clitoral hypertrophy, riding behavior, increased body odor, and various other side effects have been reported. It is further reported that the side effects usually resolve with discontinuation of therapy.

> **Technician's Notes**
> Mibolerone should not be used in cats because of a very low margin of safety in this species.

Progestins

Progestins are a group of compounds that are similar in effect to progesterone. Endogenous progestins are produced by the corpus luteum. They cause increased secretions by the endometrium, decreased motility in the uterus, and increased secretory development in the mammary glands. They also inhibit the release of gonadotropins by the pituitary to produce an inactive ovary. In some situations, they can cause elevated blood glucose levels (antiinsulin effect) or serious suppression of the adrenal glands. These hormones are used clinically to suppress estrus and to treat false pregnancy, behavioral disorders, and progestin-responsive dermatitis. The root *gest* often allows name recognition of the progestins.

Megestrol Acetate

Megestrol acetate is a synthetic progestin labeled for use in dogs. It is used, however, in cats for some behavioral and dermatologic conditions.

Clinical Uses. Megestrol acetate is labeled for use in dogs to control estrus, treat false pregnancy, prevent vaginal hyperplasia, treat severe galactorrhea, and control unacceptable male behavior. Megestrol acetate has been used in cats for various dermatologic and behavioral problems as well as for suppression of estrus.

Dosage Forms

1. Ovaban. Megestrol acetate tablets in bottles or foil strips
2. Megace. Oral tablet preparation of megestrol acetate approved for use in humans

Adverse Side Effects. These can include hyperglycemia, adrenal suppression, endometrial hyperplasia, and increased appetite.

> **Technician's Notes**
>
> Clients should be made aware of the potential dangers associated with the use of this drug and should be asked to report any changes in their pet's health status after initiation of therapy.

Medroxyprogesterone Acetate

Medroxyprogesterone acetate (MPA) is a human label progestin that has been used to treat certain behavioral and dermatologic problems and to suppress estrus in dogs and cats.

Clinical Uses. MPA is used for (1) treatment of behavioral problems such as aggression, roaming, spraying, or mounting in males and (2) for treatment of certain dermatologic conditions.

Dosage Forms

1. Depo-Provera. MPA for injection (human label)
2. Provera tablets (human label)
3. Cycrin tablets (human label)

Adverse Side Effects. These are potentially numerous and include pyometra, personality changes, depression, lethargy, mammary changes, and increased appetite.

> **Technician's Notes**
>
> Progestins should be administered with strict adherence to accepted protocol to minimize side effects such as pyometra.

Altrenogest

Altrenogest is an oral progestin labeled for use in horses. This drug is used to suppress estrus in mares (mares stop cycling within 3 days of treatment and begin cycling again 4 to 5 days after treatment is stopped) and to manage other reproductive conditions that are listed later.

Clinical Uses

1. To suppress estrus for synchronization
2. To suppress estrus for long periods
3. To maintain pregnancy in mares with low levels of progesterone

Dosage Form

1. Regu-Mate. Altrenogest in oil oral solution

Adverse Side Effects. These have been reported as minimal when used correctly.

> **Technician's Notes**
>
> Altrenogest can be absorbed through the skin and should be used with great caution by pregnant women or anyone with vascular disorders. Read the label carefully before using.

Norgestomet

Norgestomet is a synthetic progestin that is used in combination with an estrogen (estradiol valerate) for synchronization of estrus in beef cows and nonlactating dairy cows. A treatment consists of one implant and an injection at the time of implantation.

Clinical Uses. Norgestomet is used for synchronization of estrus in cattle.

Dosage Form

1. Syncro-Mate-B

Adverse Side Effects. Adverse side effects are not reported in the insert.

Melengestrol Acetate

Melengestrol acetate is a progestin used in implants that promote weight gain (discussed in a separate section).

PROSTAGLANDINS

Prostaglandins are a group of naturally occurring long-chain fatty acids that mediate various physiologic events in the body. The primary use of prostaglandins in veterinary medicine is for regulation of activity in and treatment of conditions of the female reproductive tract. Of the six classes (A, B, C, D, E, and F), only prostaglandin F_{2alpha} has significant clinical application in the reproductive system.

Prostaglandin F_{2alpha} causes lysis of the corpus luteum, contraction of uterine muscle, and relaxation of the cervix. Lysis of the corpus luteum results in a decline in plasma levels of progesterone and, through the negative feedback mechanism, initiation of a new estrus cycle. Contraction of uterine muscle can facilitate evacuation of uterine contents (pus or a mummified fetus) or produce an abortion.

Bronchoconstriction, increased blood pressure, and smooth muscle contraction have been reported in other species, including humans. For these reasons, pregnant women and asthmatic individuals should handle prostaglandin products with extreme caution, because exposure (through injection or skin contact) can cause abortion or an asthma attack.

Name recognition of the prostaglandins is made easier by looking for *prost* in the drug name.

Dinoprost Tromethamine

Dinoprost tromethamine is a salt of the naturally occurring prostaglandin F_{2alpha} and is labeled for use in cattle, horses, and swine. It also has accepted clinical use in dogs, cats, sheep, and goats. It is effective only in animals with a corpus luteum.

Clinical Uses. Labeled clinical uses are as follows:

1. For estrus synchronization, treatment of silent estrus, and pyometra in cattle
2. For abortion of feedlot and other non-lactating cattle
3. For induction of parturition in swine
4. For controlling the timing of estrus in cycling mares and in anestrous mares that have a corpus luteum
5. For treatment of pyometra and endometrial hyperplasia and as an abortion-producing agent in dogs and cats
6. In sheep and goats: basically the same uses as for cattle

Dosage Form

1. Lutalyse. Dinoprost tromethamine for injection

Adverse Side Effects. These can include sweating (horses), abdominal pain (horses, dogs, cats, and swine),

urination/defecation (dogs, cats, and swine), dyspnea and panting (dogs and cats), tachycardia (dogs), and increased vocalization (cats and swine). Most of the side effects are self-limiting and disappear within a short time.

Technician's Notes

1. Lutalyse should be handled with extreme care by pregnant women, asthmatic persons, and people with bronchial disease.
2. Skin accidentally exposed should be washed off immediately.

Fenprostalene

Fenprostalene is a synthetic **analog** of prostaglandin F_{2alpha}. Fenprostalene produces effects similar to those of dinoprost and the other class F prostaglandins. It is labeled for synchronization of estrus and as an agent to induce abortion (150 days or fewer of gestation) in cattle.

Clinical Uses. Fenprostalene is used for induction of abortion in feedlot heifers and for synchronization of estrus in beef and non-lactating dairy cows. It should be administered subcutaneously.

Dosage Form

1. Bovilene. Fenprostalene for injection

Adverse Side Effects. These can include infections at the injection site and abortion (when not an indication for use).

Technician's Notes

1. Do not administer by intramuscular injection.
2. Skin exposure should be washed off immediately.
3. Pregnant women, asthmatics, or people with bronchial disease should handle this product with great caution.

Fluprostenol

Fluprostenol is a synthetic analog of prostaglandin F_{2alpha} for use in mares.

Clinical Uses

1. Estrus synchronization in cycling mares
2. To establish estrus cycles in anestrus mares
3. To induce parturition in mares
4. To treat lactational anestrus
5. For facilitation of postpartum (after foal-heat) breeding

Dosage Form

1. Equimate. Fluprostenol for injection

Adverse Side Effects. These can include sweating, increased respiration, abdominal discomfort, and defecation.

> **Technician's Notes**
> See the sections on dinoprost and fenprostalene.

Cloprostenol Sodium

Cloprostenol sodium is an analog of prostaglandin F_{2alpha} for use in cattle. This product is chemically very similar to dinoprost and fenprostalene and is labeled for uses (for cattle) that are very similar to those of dinoprost and fenprostalene. The same precautions should be taken when using this drug as with the other prostaglandins.

Clinical Uses. This drug is used for treatment of luteal cysts and mummified fetuses, termination of pregnancy, and estrus synchronization.

Dosage Form

1. Estrumate. Cloprostenol for injection

Adverse Side Effects. At high doses, adverse side effects may include uneasiness, frothing at the mouth, and milk letdown.

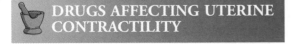

DRUGS AFFECTING UTERINE CONTRACTILITY

Several drugs have the ability to increase the contractility of uterine muscle. Some are used during pregnancy to cause abortion, and others are used at term to induce parturition, to aid in delivery of the fetus or the placenta, and to cause **involution** of the uterus after delivery. Great care should be taken to ensure that the cervix is dilated before administering these drugs.

One of these drugs, oxytocin, also causes contraction of the myoepithelial cells in the mammary glands to facilitate milk letdown.

Oxytocin

Oxytocin is a polypeptide made in the hypothalamus and stored in the posterior pituitary for release in response to appropriate stimuli from the reproductive tract or mammary glands. This hormone causes stronger uterine contractions by increasing the contractility of uterine **myofibrils.** The uterus must be primed for a period by progesterone and estrogen before oxytocin is effective in stimulating the uterus.

Oxytocin is used clinically to cause more forceful uterine contractions as an aid in delivery of a fetus. It is also used to assist delivery of the placenta, to cause uterine involution, and to reduce bleeding of the uterus after delivery. It should be used only when the cervix is sufficiently dilated and when it can be determined that the fetus can be delivered through the pelvic canal normally.

This hormone is responsible for milk letdown from the mammary glands through its stimulation of myoepithelial cells in the alveolar wall of the glands. It is released endogenously after stimulation of the udder or in response to environmental stimuli such as the sound of milking machines or other sights, sounds, or smells associated with nursing/milking.

Clinical Uses

1. To augment the force of uterine contractions during delivery
2. To aid in delivery of the placenta
3. To facilitate involution of the uterus (to reduce bleeding or to facilitate replacement of a prolapse)
4. To induce milk letdown
5. To assist in the treatment of agalactia in sows

Dosage Forms. Oxytocin injection is available in generic form from many sources.

Adverse Side Effects. These are minimal when used according to recommendations.

> **Technician's Notes**
> 1. Oxytocin should be used in **dystocia** only when the reproductive tract has been adequately examined. Inappropriate use can result in uterine torsion or rupture and can lead to death.
> 2. A single dose of oxytocin lasts approximately 15 minutes.

Ergot

Ergot is a fungus that grows on rye grass and possibly on some pasture grasses. It causes smooth muscle contraction and can cause intense vasoconstriction. If the vasoconstriction is severe enough, gangrene and sloughing may occur.

Ergonovine maleate has been used in veterinary medicine because it produces uterine contractions much like oxytocin. It results in very little vasoconstrictive action, however. This product is not commonly used.

Prostaglandins

Prostaglandins, as mentioned in a previous section, stimulate uterine smooth muscle and can be used to induce parturition or abortion.

Corticosteroids

Corticosteroids are a group of hormones produced by the adrenal cortex that are used primarily for their anti-inflammatory effect but can cause induction of parturition in the last trimester of pregnancy. This effect occurs because exogenous administration of the drug mimics the natural rise in the production of corticosteroids by the fetus as the time for delivery draws near. Induction of parturition or abortion is not a labeled use for the corticosteroids, but they have been applied clinically for this purpose.

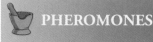

PHEROMONES

Pheromones are odors released by animals that influence the behavior of other animals of the same species. Although pheromones do not fit exactly into the endocrine category, they are considered in this section.

The first pheromone made commercially available was a boar odor aerosol called SOA (Sex Odor Aerosol). This product is a synthetic version of the natural pheromone that causes the typical boar odor and is used for heat detection in sows and gilts. Label instructions call for spraying the pheromone directly at the nostrils of the sow or gilt for 2 seconds. If the sow or gilt is in heat, she will demonstrate mating reflexes such as rigid posture, deviations of the tail, and erect ears.

Another pheromone that is commercially available is Feliway. Feliway is an analog of the feline facial pheromone. It is labeled for use in stopping or preventing urinary marking by the cat and to comfort the cat in an unknown or stressful environment. Cats deposit facial pheromones by rubbing an object with the side of the face. The manufacturer recommends spraying this product directly onto the places soiled by the cat and also on prominent objects that could be attractive to the cat. The product should be applied daily at a height of 8 inches from the floor until the cat is seen rubbing the area with its head. Feliway can also be used to familiarize cats with new environments, such as carriers and cages.

THYROID HORMONES

The thyroid gland is made up of two lobes (one on each side of the trachea) and is located near the thyroid cartilage of the larynx. Microscopically, the thyroid is composed of follicles that, on stimulation by TSH from the anterior pituitary, produce two metabolically active hormones. The thyroid synthesizes these hormones by first trapping iodide from the blood and then oxidizing the iodide to iodine. The iodine is then combined with the amino acid tyrosine to form (through several intermediary steps) T_3 and T_4. T_3 is considered to be the active form at the cellular level. Although both T_3 and T_4 are released from the thyroid gland, some of the T_4 is converted to T_3 after release. T_4, also called *thyroxine,* is found in higher levels than T_3 in **euthyroid** animals.

Thyroid hormones control many events in the body, including metabolic rate, growth and development, body temperature, heart rate, metabolism of nutrients, skin condition, resistance to infection, and others. Two abnormalities of thyroid function that are encountered in veterinary medicine are hypothyroidism and hyperthyroidism.

Hypothyroidism is noted most often in dogs and is characterized by lethargy, cold intolerance, dry haircoat, and bradycardia. Hyperthyroidism is encountered more often in older cats and is accompanied by weight loss, increased appetite, restlessness, hyperexcitability, and tachycardia. Diagnosis of thyroid conditions is made through the observation of clinical signs and by measuring serum levels of T_3 and T_4 before and after TSH administration.

Goiter is a condition caused by inadequate levels of iodide in the diet. Lack of iodide causes the thyroid to be unable to produce T_3 or T_4. The thyroid attempts to increase its output by enlarging, often to a size that can be palpated and visualized. Goiter is almost non-existent in animals receiving a commercial diet.

DRUGS USED TO TREAT HYPOTHYROIDISM

Treatment of hypothyroidism consists of supplementation of thyroid hormone on a daily basis. Clinical signs usually resolve within a short time of initiating treatment, but lifelong therapy is required.

Thyroid hormone can be extracted from collected thyroid glands or can be prepared synthetically. Purification of the animal source hormones is difficult and has led to the common use of the synthetic products. Synthetic thyroxine (T_4) is considered to be the compound of choice in the treatment of hypothyroidism. T_3 products are recommended only when a poor response to T_4 occurs.

Levothyroxine Sodium (T_4)

Levothyroxine is a synthetic **levo isomer** of T_4. It is the compound of choice in treating hypothyroidism in all species.

Clinical Uses. Levothyroxine is used for the treatment of hypothyroid conditions.

Dosage Forms

1. Soloxine. Levothyroxine tablets, approved for dogs
2. Thyro-Form. Levothyroxine chewable tablets, approved for dogs
3. Thyro-L. Levothyroxine powder, approved for horses
4. NUTRIVED T-4 Chewables. Levothyroxine chewable tablets, approved for dogs
5. Thyro-Tab. Levothyroxine tablets for dogs
6. Thyrosyn Tablets. Levothyroxine tablets for dogs
7. Thyrozine Tablets. Levothyroxine tablets for dogs
8. Synthroid. Levothyroxine tablets approved for humans

Adverse Side Effects. These are rare when used according to recommendations.

Liothyronine Sodium

Liothyronine sodium (T_3) is a synthetic salt of endogenous T_3. T_3 is not the compound of choice when treating hypothyroidism. It may be useful, however, in cases that do not respond well to T_4.

Clinical Uses. T_3 is used for treatment of hypothyroidism in cases that respond poorly to T_4.

Dosage Form

1. Cytobin Tablets. Liothyronine sodium tablets, approved for dogs

Adverse Side Effects. These are probably minimal with careful use.

Thyroid-Stimulating Hormone

Thyrotropin is a purified form of TSH obtained form the anterior pituitary of cattle. It is used as an aid in the diagnosis of hypothyroidism.

Clinical Uses. In veterinary medicine, thyrotropin is used for diagnosis of **primary hypothyroidism** in the TSH stimulation test.

Dosage Forms

1. Dermathycin. TSH approved for use in dogs
2. Thyotropar. TSH approved for use in humans

Adverse Side Effects. Allergic reactions may occur in animals sensitive to bovine protein.

DRUGS USED TO TREAT HYPERTHYROIDISM

Treatment of hyperthyroidism is directed at lowering blood levels of T_3 and T_4. This can be accomplished by destruction or removal of the overproducing thyroid or by blocking production of the hormones. The thyroid can be removed surgically or destroyed with radioactive iodine. Drug therapy to block hormone production can be effective but is continuous and not curative.

The two antithyroid drugs used most often are methimazole and carbimazole. These compounds are used for long-term therapy and for presurgical preparation of patients. Hyperthyroid cats are often high surgical risks, primarily because of tachycardia and other potential cardiac abnormalities.

Methimazole

Methimazole is a compound that interferes with incorporation of iodine into the precursor molecules of T_3 and T_4. It does not alter thyroid hormones already released into the bloodstream.

Clinical Uses. Methimazole is used for the treatment of feline hyperthyroidism.

Dosage Form

1. Tapazole. Methimazole tablets (human approved)

Adverse Side Effects. These include anorexia, vomiting, and skin eruptions.

Propylthiouracil

Propylthiouracil has been used as an antithyroid drug but is considered dangerous to use in cats because of potential hematologic complications.

Radioactive Iodine

Radioactive iodine (I-131) may be given intravenously to destroy overproductive thyroid tissue. I-131 is concentrated by the thyroid, where it remains and destroys thyroid tissue. This method has appeal because it is performed only once and is not especially stressful to patients; however, it must be done at facilities that can handle radioactive materials.

Propranolol

Propranolol (Inderal) may be used preoperatively to treat the tachycardia associated with hyperthyroidism in cats.

AGENTS FOR THE TREATMENT OF DIABETES MELLITUS

Insulin

The pancreas produces two principal hormones, insulin and glucagon, in special cells of the islets of Langerhans. Insulin is made by beta cells, and glucagon is produced by alpha cells. Insulin causes a decrease in blood glucose levels, and glucagon promotes an increase. Only insulin is used clinically.

Insulin facilitates cellular uptake of glucose and its storage in the form of glycogen and fat. It inhibits the breakdown of fat, protein, and glycogen into forms that may be used as energy sources. Further, it promotes synthesis of protein, fatty acids, and glycogen. In the absence of insulin, the body cannot use glucose and must break down its own fat and protein to use for energy.

Diabetes mellitus is a complex disease that results from inability of the beta cells of the pancreas to produce enough insulin or from altered insulin action in cells. Diabetes mellitus that results from inadequate secretion of insulin is called *type I,* or *insulin-dependent diabetes mellitus.* This is the most common type of diabetes mellitus in dogs and cats. Diabetes mellitus that results from resistance of tissues to the action of insulin is called *type II,* or *non–insulin-dependent diabetes mellitus (NIDDM).* NIDDM is rare in dogs but is occasionally encountered in cats.

Both forms of diabetes mellitus eventually cause polydipsia, polyuria, polyphagia, and weight loss. Untreated diabetes mellitus proceeds to the condition called *diabetic ketoacidosis,* in which body fat is metabolized as a substitute energy source. Metabolism of body fat results in accumulation of byproducts of this process called *ketone bodies,* which promote a metabolic acidosis that can lead to death.

Because blood glucose levels can be increased by corticosteroids, epinephrine, and progesterone, these drugs should be given with caution to diabetic animals. Sudden changes in diet and exercise level should also be avoided because they can alter blood glucose levels and cause an imbalance in the ratio of insulin to glucose.

Insulin is not effective when given orally because the digestive tract breaks down the protein molecule before it can be absorbed. Insulin is usually administered by subcutaneous injection; however, some forms may be given intravenously or intramuscularly.

Sources of insulin have traditionally included beef or pork pancreas and preparations comprised of a purified (pure beef source or pure pork source) form or a combination beef/pork form. The beef/pork form is best suited to treat diabetes mellitus in dogs and cats. Pork insulin is very close in structure to dog and human insulins, whereas beef insulin is very similar to cat insulin.

All human insulin products are now prepared through recombinant DNA or synthetic processes. Beef source insulin products have been discontinued by insulin manufacturers; this situation could cause difficulty in treating diabetes in small-animal patients in the future since the human DNA insulins do not work as well in animals. Technicians should always consult current information when dealing with diabetic patients because the availability of insulin products is subject to change.

Insulin concentration is measured in units of insulin per milliliter. It is available in concentrations of 40 (U-40), 100 (U-100), and 500 (U-500) U/ml. All products for human use are U-100 concentrations.

A U-40 concentration makes administering the small amounts of insulin needed for cats and small dogs much easier. When insulin is drawn into the syringes, each mark on the syringe barrel denotes 1 U of insulin. Drawing up 5 U on a scale of 40, for example, is easier than drawing up 5 U on a scale of 100. Small-volume U-100 syringes are available, however, to facilitate administration of small doses of U-100 insulin.

U-40 syringes must be used with U-40 insulin, and U-100 syringes must be used with U-100 insulin. Table 9-2 lists insulin syringes that are available.

Insulin Classifications

Insulin is usually classified according to its duration of action as short acting, intermediate acting, or long acting. Short-acting insulins include regular crystalline and Semilente. NPH and Lente are intermediate-acting insulins. PZI and Ultralente are long-acting products. Two different forms are sometimes combined in the same preparation.

The onset of effect and route of administration are other important characteristics of insulin preparations to be considered (Table 9-3). For an in-depth discussion of insulin forms and characteristics, consult *Canine and Feline Endocrinology and Reproduction* (Feldman and Nelson, 1987).

REGULAR CRYSTALLINE INSULIN/SEMILENTE
Regular insulin is a fast-acting insulin that is made from zinc insulin crystals and is a clear solution that may be administered intravenously, intramuscularly, or subcutaneously. It is used mainly to treat diabetic ketoacidosis until blood glucose levels are reduced and the animal is metabolically stable. At that time, the animal is usually switched to a longer-acting form.

Semilente insulin is similar in effect to regular insulin but is prepared by a different process.

Clinical Uses. Semilente is primarily used for the treatment of diabetic ketoacidosis.

TABLE 9-2   Insulin Syringes

Name and Manufacturer	Insulin	Needle Gauge	Needle Size	Packaging
1-ml Syringes				
B-D Microfine IV	U-100	28	½ inch	100 (10 packs of 10)
B-D Microfine	U-100	27	⅝ inch	100 (10 packs of 10)
B-D Microfine IV	U-40	28	½ inch	100 (10 packs of 10)
Can-Am E-Z Ject	U-100	27	½ inch	100 (individually wrapped)
Can-Am E-Z Ject	U-100	28	½ inch	100 (individually wrapped)
Monoject Ultra Comfort 28	U-100	28	½ inch	100 or 30 (individually wrapped)
Pharma-Plast	U-100	28	½ inch	100 (10 packs of 10)
Terumo	U-100	29	½ inch	100 (individually wrapped)
Terumo	U-100	27	½ inch	100 (individually wrapped)
¼-ml Syringes				
Terumo	U-100	29	½ inch	100 (individually wrapped)
½-ml Syringes				
B-D Microfine IV	U-100	28	½ inch	100 (10 packs of 10)
Can-Am E-Z Ject	U-50	28	½ inch	100 (individually wrapped)
Monoject Ultra Comfort 28	U-100	28	½ inch	100 or 30 (individually wrapped)
Pharma-Plast	U-100	28	½ inch	100 (10 packs of 10)
Terumo	U-100	29	½ inch	100 (individually wrapped)
Terumo	U-100	27	½ inch	100 (individually wrapped)
³⁄₁₀-ml Syringes				
B-D Microfine IV	U-100	28	½ inch	100 (10 packs of 10)

From Peterson, M.E.: Insulin and insulin syringes. In Kirk, R.W., Bonagura, J.D. (eds.): Current Veterinary Therapy XI: Small Animal Practice. W.B. Saunders Company, Philadelphia, 1992, p. 358.

TABLE 9-3   Properties of Beef/Pork Insulin Preparations Used in Dogs and Cats*

Type of Insulin	Route of Administration	Duration of Effect (Hours) Dog	Cat
Regular crystalline,	IV	1–4	1–4
Semilente	IM	3–8	3–8
	SC	4–10	4–10
NPH (isophane)	SC	6–24	4–12
PZI	SC	6–28	6–24
Lente†	SC	8–24	6–18
Ultralente‡	SC	8–28	8–24

From Birchard, S.J., Sherding, R.G.: Saunders Manual of Small Animal Practice. W.B. Saunders Company, Philadelphia, 1994, p. 254.
*Purified pork and recombinant human insulins appear to be more potent, act faster, and have a shorter duration of effect than beef/pork insulins. Major manufacturers of insulin include Eli Lilly Co., E.R. Squibb and Sons, and Novo Nordisk.
†Initial insulin of choice for diabetic dogs.
‡Initial insulin of choice for diabetic cats.

Dosage Forms. Many products approved for humans are available. The following is a partial listing:

1. Regular Iletin I (pork/beef source) (discontinued)
2. Regular Iletin II (purified pork)
3. Purified Pork R (purified pork) (see Table 9-4 for an inclusive list)
4. Humilin R
5. Novolin R

Adverse Side Effects. These are usually related to overdose and may include weakness, ataxia, shaking, and seizures.

Technician's Notes

1. Although not required by label in the newer products, refrigeration probably enhances storage life. Do not freeze.
2. Do not use regular insulin preparations if discolorations or precipitates are present.
3. Clients should be given thorough written instructions on the use of insulin products and the signs/treatment of overdose.

NPH (Isophane) Insulin/Lente

NPH insulin is a cloudy suspension of zinc insulin crystals and protamine zinc. It is longer acting than regular insulin and takes effect faster than PZI insulin. It is a commonly used insulin for the control of uncomplicated diabetes in dogs and cats.

Lente insulin is similar in activity to NPH insulin but is made without the use of protamine.

Clinical Uses. NPH insulin is used for treatment of uncomplicated diabetes mellitus.

Dosage Forms. A partial listing follows:

1. NPH Iletin I (beef/pork source) (discontinued)
2. NPH Insulin (discontinued)
3. Lente Iletin II (purified pork) (see Table 9-4)
4. NPH Iletin II (pork)
5. Lente Purified Pork
6. Humilin N
7. Novolin N

Adverse Side Effects. These are similar to those of regular insulin.

Technician's Notes

1. Resuspension by gently rolling the bottle is required before withdrawing the product from the bottle.
2. Store like regular insulin. Do not freeze.
3. NPH insulin is usually administered once a day.

Protamine Zinc Insulin (PZI)/Ultralente

PZI insulin is a cloudy suspension of a protamine-insulin-zinc precipitate that has poor solubility and is poorly absorbed from tissue. Because of this relative insolubility, this preparation is slowly absorbed from the injection site and therefore maintains a long-lasting blood level. The human label product was removed from the market in 1991 by the manufacturer because of a declining market in human medicine. Since PZI insulin is unavailable, some veterinarians are substituting ultralente unit for unit while others are reducing the ultralente by 25% (Plumb, 1999).

Ultralente insulin is similar in effect and duration to PZI insulin. Unlike PZI, ultralente does not contain protamine.

Clinical Uses. PZI is used for the treatment of uncomplicated diabetes mellitus.

Dosage Form

1. Ultralente (Humulin U)

Adverse Side Effects. These are similar to those of regular and NPH insulin.

Technician's Notes

1. PZI insulin is considered by some to be the insulin form of choice for use in cats.
2. Clients should be given thorough instructions on the use of insulin products and the signs/treatment of overdose.

TABLE 9-4   Insulins

Product	Manufacturer	Form	Strength
Rapid Acting (onset <15 minutes)			
Humalog	Lilly	Human	U-100
Humalog Cartridges	Lilly	Human	U-100
Short Acting (onset ½-2 hours)			
Humulin R (Regular)	Lilly	Human	U-100, U-500
Iletin I Regular DISCONTINUED/Supply Limited	Lilly	Beef/Pork	U-100
Iletin II Regular	Lilly	Pork	U-100
Humulin R Cartridges (1.5 ml)	Lilly	Human	U-100
Novolin R (Regular)	Novo Nordisk	Human	U-100
Novolin R PenFill (Regular)	Novo Nordisk	Human	U-100
Purified Pork R (Regular)	Novo Nordisk	Pork	U-100
Velosulin Human (Regular) (Buffered)	Novo Nordisk	Human	U-100
Novolin R (Regular) Prefilled	Novo Nordisk	Human	U-100
Intermediate Acting (onset 2-4 hours)			
Humulin L (Lente)	Lilly	Human	U-100
Humulin N (NPH)	Lilly	Human	U-100
Iletin Lente DISCONTINUED/Supply Limited	Lilly	Beef/Pork	U-100
Iletin I NPH DISCONTINUED/Supply Limited	Lilly	Beef/Pork	U-100
Iletin II Lente	Lilly	Pork	U-100
Iletin II NPH	Lilly	Pork	U-100
Humulin N Cartridges (1.5 ml)	Lilly	Human	U-100
Novolin L (Lente)	Novo Nordisk	Human	U-100
Novolin N (NPH)	Novo Nordisk	Human	U-100
Novolin N PenFill (NPH)	Novo Nordisk	Human	U-100
Novolin N Prefilled (NPH)	Novo Nordisk	Human	U-100
Purified Pork Lente	Novo Nordisk	Pork	U-100
Purified Pork N (NPH)	Novo Nordisk	Pork	U-100
Long Acting (onset 4-6 hours)			
Humulin U (Ultralente)	Lilly	Human	U-100
Mixtures			
Humulin 50/50 (50% NPH, 50% Regular)	Lilly	Human	U-100
Humulin 70/30 (70% NPH, 30% Regular)	Lilly	Human	U-100
Humulin 70/30 Cartridges (1.5 ml)	Lilly	Human	U-100
Novolin 70/30 (70% NPH, 30% Regular)	Novo Nordisk	Human	U-100
Novolin 70/30 PenFill (70% NPH, 30% Regular)	Novo Nordisk	Human	U-100
Novolin 70/30 Prefilled (70% NPH, 30% Regular)	Novo Nordisk	Human	U-100

From American Diabetes Association: 1999 Buyers Guide to Diabetes Products, Alexandria, VA, 1999.

Oral Hypoglycemic Agents

Oral hypoglycemic agents such as the sulfonyl-ureas are extensively used in human diabetic patients to control type II diabetes mellitus (NIDDM). They have little apparent effectiveness in diabetic dogs but may be useful in some cats with type II diabetes. Glipizide (Glucotrol) is the most commonly used drug in this category.

 HYPERGLYCEMIC AGENTS

As mentioned previously, several drugs such as corticosteroids, epinephrine, and progesterone can elevate blood glucose levels. The only product that is marketed for this purpose, however, is oral diazoxide (Proglycem and Eudemine). This drug is used to treat the low blood glucose levels associated with hypersecretion of insulin that occurs in tumors of the pancreas (insulinoma).

HORMONES THAT ACT AS GROWTH PROMOTERS

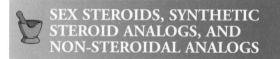 **SEX STEROIDS, SYNTHETIC STEROID ANALOGS, AND NON-STEROIDAL ANALOGS**

The factors that control growth, **feed efficiency,** and carcass composition in animals involve a complex interrelationship between genetic, metabolic, and hormonal mechanisms that are not always totally understood. It is possible, however, to increase growth (weight gain) in ruminants by administering sex steroid hormones (estrogen, testosterone, or progesterone), synthetic steroid hormone analogs (trenbolone), or certain non-steroidal hormone analogs (zeranol) that act like the first two substances.

The primary sex steroid used to promote weight gain is estrogen (estradiol). The mechanisms by which estradiol promotes weight gain include (1) increased water retention, (2) increased protein synthe-

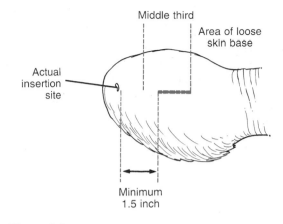

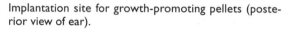

Figure 9-5

Implantation site for growth-promoting pellets (posterior view of ear).

sis, (3) increased fat deposition, and (4) possible increased release of growth hormone (bovine somatotropin).

Testosterone is used as an adjunct to estradiol in some growth promotion products because it is an anabolic agent in itself and because a second component in the compound slows down the release of the estradiol and prolongs its effective life span.

Progesterone is also added to growth promoters to slow the release of estradiol. It apparently has little anabolic effect of its own.

Trenbolone is a synthetic anabolic agent that improves feed efficiency and promotes weight gain in steers. It is used as the sole agent in some growth-promoting preparations.

Zeranol is an analog of a naturally occurring plant estrogen that increases feed efficiency, protein synthesis, and growth rate.

All of the growth-promoting products for use in cattle and sheep are prepared as compressed pellets that are implanted in the subcutaneous tissue of the dorsal, middle third of the ear (Figure 9-5). These pellets are designed to be used with corresponding needle devices and should be implanted with close adherence to product instructions (failure to do so is a violation of federal law in some cases).

The growth promotion products are considered here as a group, and minimal information is provided about each product.

Clinical Uses. These drugs are used to promote feed efficiency and weight gain in calves, steers, heifers, or sheep (depending on the product).

Dosage Forms

1. Synovex C. Estradiol/progesterone implant for use in calves older than 45 days
2. Synovex H. Estradiol/testosterone implant for use in heifers
3. Synovex S. Estradiol/testosterone implant for use in steers
4. Compudose. Estradiol implant for use in steers
5. Implus-H. Estradiol/testosterone implant for use in heifers
6. Implus-S. Estradiol/progesterone for use in steers
7. CALF-oid Implant. Progesterone/estradiol implant for calves older than 45 days
8. Finaplix-H. Trenbolone implant for use in feedlot heifers
9. Finaplix-S. Trenbolone implant for steers
10. Revalor-S. Trenbolone and estradiol implant for use in feedlot steers
11. Ralgro beef cattle implant. Zeranol implant for use in growing cattle, feedlot heifers, feedlot steers, suckling and weaned calves
12. Ralgro feedlot lamb implant. Zeranol implant for feedlot lambs

Adverse Side Effects. These may include mounting, elevated tailheads, rectal prolapse, and udder development.

Technician's Notes

1. Most growth-promoting implants should not be given to animals intended for breeding purposes or to dairy cattle.
2. Product insert instructions should be read and followed carefully with these products.

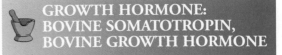

GROWTH HORMONE: BOVINE SOMATOTROPIN, BOVINE GROWTH HORMONE

Growth hormone, also called *somatotropin,* is a hormone produced by the anterior pituitary; its function before the onset of puberty is to stimulate growth. It is released throughout life to promote anabolic activity (e.g., increase protein synthesis). It has been shown to increase growth rate and feed efficiency in farm animals. Many of the growth-promoting agents listed in the previous section may work by stimulating the release of somatotropin. Somatotropin is a potent stimulator of milk production as well. Claims of a 20% boost in milk production of dairy cows after administration of somatotropin have been made.

The Food and Drug Administration (FDA) approved a recombinant (genetically engineered) bovine somatotropin (BST) for commercial production in 1993. This product, Posilac, is manufactured by the Monsanto company. Its market availability has sparked intense debate between certain groups. Some dairy producers have opposed its use because of their fear that increased production would drive milk prices down and reduce their overall income. Other groups have resisted the use of BST because of their concerns about residues of the hormone in milk products, even though the FDA has stated that milk from cows receiving BST is completely safe. Time and the workings of the marketplace should resolve the debates.

ANABOLIC STEROIDS

Anabolic steroids are steroids that cause a tissue-building (anabolic) effect. Testosterone is a naturally occurring anabolic steroid that produces masculinization in addition to the anabolic effects. Synthetic anabolic steroids are designed to prevent most of the masculinizing effects.

Anabolic steroid administration causes positive **nitrogen balance** and reverses processes that break down tissue. An increase in appetite, weight gain, improved overall condition, and recovery are promoted. These products are labeled for clinical use in dogs, cats, and horses for anorexia, weight loss, and debilitation. In working animals, they may be used in cases of overwork or overtraining. Anabolic steroids also promote red blood cell formation and are used to treat some forms of anemia. The product insert states that "anabolic therapy is intended primarily as an adjunct to other specific and supportive therapy, including nutritional therapy."

Because of the potential for abuse by bodybuilders and other athletes, the FDA has now classified anabolic steroids as controlled substances.

Stanozolol

Stanozolol is an anabolic steroid found to have an unusual pattern of biologic activity in that its anabolic effect far outweighs its weak androgenic influence.

Clinical Uses. Stanozolol is used for treatment of anorexia, debilitation, weight loss, overwork, and anemia.

Dosage Forms

1. Winstrol-V. Stanozolol sterile suspension for injection in dogs, cats, and horses
2. Winstrol-V. Stanozolol tablets for use in dogs and cats

Adverse Side Effects. These may include mild androgenic effects after prolonged use or overdose.

Technician's Notes

1. Winstrol-V should not be used in pregnant dogs or mares or in stallions.
2. Winstrol-V should not be given to horses intended for food.
3. All stanozolol products are now C-IV controlled substances.

Boldenone Undecylenate

Boldenone undecylenate is a steroid ester that possesses marked anabolic activity and a minimal amount of androgenic activity. It is labeled for use in horses.

Clinical Uses. Boldenone undecylenate acts as an aid in the treatment of debilitated horses.

Dosage Form

1. Equipoise. Boldenone injection for horses

Adverse Side Effects. These include androgenic effects such as overaggressiveness.

Technician's Notes

1. Boldenone should not be used in horses intended for food.
2. Boldenone should not be used in stallions or pregnant mares.

Nandrolone Decanoate

Nandrolone decanoate is an injectable anabolic steroid sold under the human label Deca-Durabolin. It has activity similar to the other anabolic agents.

REFERENCES

Feldman, E.C., Nelson, R.C.: Diabetes mellitus. In Feldman, E.C., Nelson, R.C. (eds.): Canine and Feline Endocrinology and Reproduction. W.B. Saunders Company, Philadelphia, 1987.
Plumb, D.C.: Insulin. In Veterinary Drug Handbook. Iowa State University Press, Ames, 1999.

■ Review Questions

1. Describe the relationship between hormonal releasing factors, trophic hormones, and the hormones produced by specific tissues or glands. _____

2. List the major endocrine glands. _____

3. What are the reasons for using hormonal therapy in veterinary medicine? _____

4. Endogenous hormones are those produced _____ , whereas exogenous hormones come from _____ sources.

5. Where is the pituitary gland located, and what are its functions? _____

6. Describe the difference between a negative and a positive feedback control mechanism in the endocrine system. _____

7. The release of oxytocin by the posterior pituitary is controlled through the _____ mechanism.

8. GnRH is classified as a/an _____.

9. Hormonal products with **gest** in their name are classified as _____.

10. List three potential uses of the prostaglandins in veterinary medicine. _____

11. Human skin contact or injection with prostaglandins can be a serious health risk to _____ women and _____.

12. Before oxytocin can exert its effects on the uterus, the uterus must first be primed by _____.

13. What precautions should be taken before oxytocin is administered? _____

14. What are the two active hormones produced by the thyroid gland? _____

15. List two drugs used in the treatment of hypothyroidism. _____

16. List the three major classes of insulin. _____

17. Which form of insulin is used in the treatment of diabetic ketoacidosis? _____

18. Which form(s) of insulin must be resuspended before administration? _____

19. What are some signs of insulin overdose? _____

20. Growth promoters generally should not be used in animals intended for _____.

21. Why are anabolic steroids classified as controlled substances? _____

Drugs Used in Ophthalmic and Otic Disorders

LEARNING OBJECTIVES

After studying this chapter, you should be able to:

1. Understand the clinical indications for the common ophthalmic and otic agents
2. Identify the different classes of ophthalmic and otic agents
3. Identify the possible adverse reactions and contraindications of many commonly used agents

KEY TERMS

Closed-angle glaucoma A type of primary glaucoma of the eye characterized by a shallow anterior chamber and a narrow angle that compromises filtration due to the iris's blocking the angle and causing an increase in intraocular pressure.
Conjunctivitis Inflammation of the conjunctiva.
Cycloplegia Paralysis of the ciliary muscle.
Glaucoma A group of eye diseases characterized by increased intraocular pressure that results in damage to the retina and the optic nerve.

Keratitis Inflammation of the cornea.
Miosis Contraction of the pupil.
Mydriasis Dilation of the pupil.
Open-angle glaucoma A type of primary glaucoma of the eye in which the angle of the anterior chamber remains open but filtration of the aqueous humor is gradually reduced, causing an increase in intraocular pressure.
Uvea The vascular layer of the eye, composed of the iris, ciliary body, and choroid.
Uveitis Inflammation of the uvea.

OPHTHALMIC AGENTS

Topical administration of eye drops or ointment is the most common method of treating disorders of the eye. Products used for this purpose are usually available as solutions or ointments. Drug penetration is one factor that veterinarians must consider when choosing a topical ophthalmic agent. Topical agents are more readily absorbed into the anterior chamber than the posterior chamber. For this reason, these agents have limited use in posterior eye disorders, and systemic agents are more effective. Lipid-soluble agents readily penetrate the corneal epithelium and endothelium layers. Water-soluble agents readily penetrate the corneal stroma layer (Figure 10-1). Therefore, drugs with both lipid-soluble and water-soluble characteristics achieve maximum corneal penetration (Gelatt, 1981). Most topical ophthalmic medications require several applications per day because the eye continuously secretes tears that wash away the medication. Ointments tend to necessitate less frequent applications than do drops, but they blur an animal's vision for a short period after application. When educating clients about topically treating the eyes, it is important to point out these factors. When clients understand why something needs to be done, they are usually more willing to make the extra effort to ensure that it is done properly.

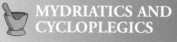

MYDRIATICS AND CYCLOPLEGICS

Mydriatic agents are used to dilate the pupils (Figure 10-2). This action facilitates examination of the posterior segment and the fundus of the eye. Cycloplegic agents paralyze the accommodative muscle of the ciliary body. In some cases, this action can minimize pain associated with ciliary spasms. These agents are often used before and after ophthalmic surgery.

Phenylephrine Hydrochloride

Phenylephrine hydrochloride is used to produce **mydriasis** but does not produce **cycloplegia**.

Clinical Uses. Phenylephrine HCl is used in the evaluation of uveitis, glaucoma, or scleritis. It may also be used before conjunctival surgery to reduce hemorrhage or used in combination with atropine before cataract or intraocular surgery. It can be used to determine the presence of Horner's syndrome.

Dosage Form
1. Mydfrin (human label)

Adverse Side Effects. These include local discomfort after application. Chronic use may lead to inflammation.

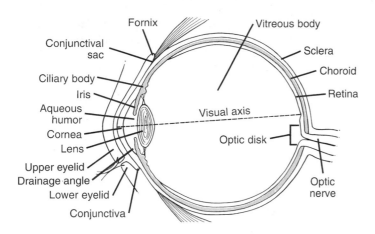

Figure 10-1

Internal structures of the eyeball.

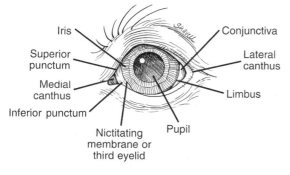

Figure 10-2

External structures of the eye.

Technician's Notes

Phenylephrine HCl is also used in cough preparations but at a higher concentration.

Atropine Sulfate

Atropine sulfate is one of the ophthalmic agents most commonly used to produce mydriasis and cycloplegia.

Clinical Uses. Atropine sulfate is used for refraction or for the treatment of acute inflammatory conditions of the anterior uveal tract.

Dosage Form

1. Atrophate

Adverse Side Effects. These include salivation. Atropine is contraindicated in **glaucoma** and keratoconjunctivitis sicca (KCS, or dry eyes).

Homatropine Hydrobromide

Homatropine hydrobromide produces mydriasis and cycloplegia but is less potent than atropine.

Clinical Uses. Homatropine hydrobromide is used for refraction and the treatment of **uveitis**.

Dosage Forms

1. Homatrocel Ophthalmic (human label)
2. Isopto Homatropine (human label)

Adverse Side Effects. These are the same as for atropine.

Cyclopentolate Hydrochloride

Cyclopentolate hydrochloride produces mydriasis and cycloplegia.

Clinical Uses. Cyclopentolate hydrochloride is used for refraction.

Dosage Form

1. Cyclogyl (human label)

Adverse Side Effects. These are the same as for atropine.

Tropicamide

Tropicamide is a rapid-acting mydriatic but has less cycloplegic effect than the previously mentioned drugs.

Clinical Uses. Tropicamide is used for ocular fundus examination.

Dosage Form

1. Mydriacyl (human label)

Adverse Side Effects. These include local discomfort after application and salivation. Contraindications are the same as for atropine.

Epinephrine

Epinephrine is administered topically and is available as epinephrine and dipivalyl epinephrine. Dipivalyl epinephrine more readily penetrates the corneal barrier and is converted to epinephrine in the cornea.

Clinical Uses. Epinephrine is used to reduce intraocular pressure, produce mydriasis, or aid in the diagnosis of Horner's syndrome.

Dosage Form

1. Epifrin (human label)

Adverse Side Effects. These include local irritation. Epinephrine is contraindicated in **closed-angle glaucoma.**

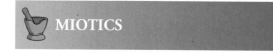

MIOTICS

Miotic agents produce pupillary constriction. These drugs are commonly used in the treatment of chronic **open-angle glaucoma,** acute and chronic closed-angle glaucoma, and some cases of secondary glaucoma. Miotics reduce intraocular pressure by increasing the outflow of aqueous humor.

Pilocarpine

Pilocarpine is a cholinergic drug that is commonly used to treat chronic open-angle glaucoma.

Clinical Uses. These include stimulation of tear production in some cases of keratoconjunctivitis sicca.

Dosage Form

1. Piloptic

Adverse Side Effects. These include local irritation and discomfort. Repeated use may cause vomiting, diarrhea, and salivation.

Carbachol

Carbachol is a cholinergic drug, and it is used less commonly than pilocarpine.

Clinical Uses. Carbachol is used to treat glaucoma.

Dosage Form

1. Carbacel (human label)

Adverse Side Effects. These are uncommon.

Echothiophate Iodide

Echothiophate iodide is an organophosphate that also produces **miosis** when applied topically to the eyes. This solution has a longer duration of action than pilocarpine.

Clinical Uses. These include the treatment of open-angle glaucoma.

Dosage Forms

1. Echodids (human label)
2. Phospholine Iodide (human label)

Adverse Side Effects. Systemic organophosphate toxicity is possible in smaller patients.

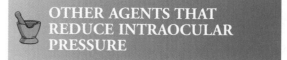

OTHER AGENTS THAT REDUCE INTRAOCULAR PRESSURE

Carbonic Anhydrase Inhibitors

Carbonic anhydrase inhibitors reduce intraocular pressure by reducing the production of aqueous humor. These products, like those previously mentioned, are used to control glaucoma, but some are administered orally and intravenously rather than topically.

Dosage Forms

1. Dichlorphenamide (Daranide—human label)
2. Acetazolamide (Diamox—human label)
3. Methazolamide (Neptazane—human label)
4. Dorzolamide (Trusopt—human label)

Adverse Side Effects. These include vomiting, diarrhea, panting, and weakness.

Timolol Maleate

Timolol maleate is an ophthalmic beta blocker with action that results in decreased production of aqueous humor.

Clinical Uses. Timolol maleate is used in the contralateral eye of a dog with primary glaucoma to prevent the development of bilateral disease. It does reduce intraocular pressure some but is not as effective in the treatment of glaucoma.

Dosage Form

1. Timoptic (human label)

Adverse Side Effects. Adverse side effects are uncommon. See the Technician's Notes below.

> **Technician's Notes**
> Timolol may be contraindicated in some patients with cardiovascular disease or bronchoconstrictive disease.

Mannitol

Mannitol is an osmotic diuretic that is administered intravenously to reduce intraocular pressure in emergency situations.

Dosage Form

1. Mannitol injection

Adverse Side Effects. These include fluid and electrolyte imbalance, nausea, vomiting, pulmonary edema, congestive heart failure, and tachycardia.

Glycerol

Glycerol (glycerin) is an osmotic diuretic that is administered orally to reduce intraocular pressure in emergency situations.

Dosage Form

1. Osmoglyn (human label)

Adverse Side Effects. Vomiting may occur after administration.

> **Technician's Notes**
> Glycerol acts more slowly than mannitol.

TOPICAL ANESTHETICS

Topical anesthetics anesthetize the corneal surface and are commonly used to allow removal of a foreign body or sutures, to allow the use of instruments to measure intraocular pressure, or to aid in the application of a hydrophilic contact lens.

Proparacaine Hydrochloride

Proparacaine hydrochloride is a commonly used topical anesthetic. Anesthesia lasts 5 to 10 minutes.

Dosage Form

1. Ophthaine

Adverse Side Effects. These are very uncommon.

> **Technician's Notes**
> Unopened bottles may be stored at room temperature, but opened bottles should be refrigerated. Any discolored solutions should be discarded.

Tetracaine and Tetracaine Hydrochloride

Tetracaine and tetracaine hydrochloride are also used for anesthetizing the cornea.

Dosage Forms

1. Pontocaine (human label)
2. Pontocaine hydrochloride (human label)

Adverse Side Effects. These include irritation that usually resolves within a short period after administration.

> **Technician's Notes**
> Unlike proparacaine, tetracaine inhibits the growth of microorganisms, and cultures should be obtained before its administration.

OPHTHALMIC STAINS

Ophthalmic stains are used as diagnostic aids for detecting disease in both the anterior and posterior segments and in the nasolacrimal system.

Fluorescein strips are the most commonly used dye for the detection of corneal epithelial defects. The strip is placed in the lower conjunctival sac until adequate moistening occurs, allowing the stain to cover the eye. A drop of sterile saline may be used if tear production is insufficient to moisten the strip. Excess dye is rinsed from the eye with sterile eye wash. Fluorescein stain is a water-soluble agent. The outer (epithelial) layer of the cornea is a fat-soluble layer, and the stroma, just beneath the epithelium, is a water-soluble layer. If the epithelium is intact, the stain does not adhere because of the difference in solubilities. If the epithelium is eroded as in the case of a corneal ulcer, the stain gains access to the water-soluble stroma where it adheres and remains after the eye is rinsed. Appearance of fluorescein stain at the nostril opening indicates functional patency of the nasolacrimal drainage system.

> **Technician's Notes**
> Fluorescein stains the hair if allowed to drain on the face. By using gauze or a paper towel to absorb the dye during rinsing, staining is minimal.

COLLAGEN SHIELDS

Collagen shields are biodegradable contact lens–shaped films made from porcine or bovine collagen. They dissolve in 12 to 72 hours because of the naturally occurring enzymes found in tears.

Clinical Uses. A collagen shield may be used in the treatment of superficial corneal ulcers.

Dosage Form

1. Vet-Shield 72

> **Technician's Notes**
> A topical ophthalmic anesthetic should be used before placing the shield onto the eye. It may be necessary to sedate the animal with a short-acting general anesthetic.

TOPICAL OPHTHALMIC ANTI-INFECTIVES

Antiviral Agents

Antiviral agents may be used to treat viral infections of the eye, such as herpes simplex **keratitis** (e.g., feline ocular herpes).

Dosage Forms

1. Idoxuridine (Stoxil—human label)
2. Trifluridine (Viroptic ophthalmic solution—human label)
3. Vidarabine (Vir-A Ophthalmic—human label)

ANTIFUNGAL AGENTS

Antifungal agents are used to treat ophthalmic fungal infections such as mycotic keratitis, mycotic endophthalmitis, and blepharodermatomycosis. Mycotic keratitis occurs most commonly in horses.

Dosage Forms

1. Natamycin (Natacyn—human label)
2. Miconazole injection (Monistat–IV—human label)

Technician's Notes
Miconazole injection is applied topically to the cornea in the treatment of mycotic keratitis (Plumb, 1999).

ANTIBACTERIAL AGENTS

Antibacterial agents are used to treat superficial ocular infections resulting from bacterial organisms. These drugs are often used in combination with each other to provide broad-spectrum activity.

1. **Bacitracin** is used topically to treat superficial ocular infections resulting from primarily gram-positive bacteria and is often combined with other antibacterial agents such as neomycin and polymyxin B.
2. **Chloramphenicol** is available for topical ophthalmic administration and provides broad-spectrum activity. This agent is antagonistic with aminoglycosides.
3. **Gentamicin** is used topically to treat **conjunctivitis** caused by susceptible bacterial agents.
4. **Polymyxin B sulfate** is effective against gram-negative organisms and may be combined with other antibacterial agents to provide broad-spectrum activity.
5. **Oxytetracycline** is used to treat superficial ocular infections and provides broad-spectrum activity. It may be used in combination with other agents such as polymyxin B.
6. **Neomycin** provides broad-spectrum activity and is often used in combination with other topical ophthalmic antibacterials.
7. **Fluroquinolone** ophthalmic antibiotics are used to treat established gram-negative corneal infections. Ciprofloxacin, Norfloxacin, and ofloxacin are available as human products. They are not recommended for prophylactic use before or after surgery (Plumb, 1999).

Technician's Notes
Chloramphenicol must not be used in animals raised for food production.

TOPICAL OPHTHALMIC ANTI-INFLAMMATORY AGENTS

Non-Steroidal Agents

Non-steroidal anti-inflammatory agents are used in the treatment of uveitis. They are commonly used for postsurgical inflammation after cataract surgery.

Dosage Forms

1. Flurbiprofen sodium (Ocufen—human label)
2. Ketorolac tromethamine (Acular—human label)
3. Diclofenac sodium (Voltaren—human label)

Adverse Side Effects. These are uncommon, but flurbiprofen can cause immunosuppression.

Topical Corticosteroid Agents

Corticosteroid agents are used to treat inflammatory conditions of the cornea, iris, conjunctiva, sclera, and anterior uvea. Topical corticosteroids have poor penetration into the eyelid and the posterior segment of the eye (Plumb, 1999). They may be combined with antibacterial agents to manage ocular infections. Some common corticosteroid agents for ophthalmic use include prednisolone, hydrocortisone, dexamethasone, betamethasone, and flumethasone.

Dosage Forms

1. Prednisolone acetate drops—human label
2. Prednisolone sodium phosphate drops—human label
3. Gentocin durafilm solution
4. Anaprime ophthalmic solution
5. Neo-Predef

Adverse Side Effects. Topical corticosteroids can cause problems similar to systemic corticosteroids.

These include delayed healing, steroid dependency, and corneal complication such as ulcerative keratitis.

> **Technician's Notes**
>
> Ophthalmic products containing corticosteroids are contraindicated in the treatment of deep corneal ulcers, fungal infections, and viral infections.

AGENTS FOR THE TREATMENT OF KERATOCONJUNCTIVITIS SICCA

Keratoconjunctivitis sicca (KCS) is a common ocular disorder in dogs. With this disorder there is reduced secretion of the lacrimal glands resulting in corneal dryness. If left untreated, corneal ulceration and eventual perforation may occur (Tizard, 1992).

Cyclosporine

Cyclosporine is used for the management of KCS and chronic superficial keratitis (CSK, or German shepherd pannus). It stimulates increased tear production although its mechanism of action is not fully understood.

Dosage Form

1. Optimmune Ophthalmic Ointment

Adverse Side Effects. Adverse side effects are uncommon.

> **Technician's Notes**
>
> It may take several days to a few weeks before the effects of cyclosporine therapy are evident.

Artificial Tear Products and Ocular Lubricants

Before the availability of cyclosporine, artificial tears were used in the treatment of KCS and CSK. These products serve as lubricants for dry eyes and are commonly used in conjunction with cyclosporine therapy. Ocular lubricants are petroleum-based products used to lubricate and protect the eyes. They are commonly used during anesthetic procedures in which the eyes may remain open and may become dry.

Dosage Forms

1. Bion Tears (human label)
2. Liquifilm Tears (human label)
3. Lacri-Lube S.O.P. (human label)

Adverse Side Effects. These are uncommon.

OTIC DRUGS

INTRODUCTION

"My dog is shaking his head" is a common complaint that is heard all too often, unfortunately. Many breeds of dogs such as the spaniels, Chinese sharpei, and poodles have predisposing factors that make them likely candidates for chronic ear problems. Ear problems commonly treated topically range from parasitic infection caused by *Otodectes cyanotis* to chronic otitis externa. Systemic medications may be necessary in some cases of infection or inflammation. Topical preparations for the ears are often combinations of different types of drugs such as an antibacterial, antifungal, antipruritic and anti-inflammatory (e.g., Panalog ointment). Other preparations include cleansers, drying agents, and parasiticides. These preparations are often indicated for other uses such as superficial skin infections. When educating clients about cleaning the ears and using otic medications, show them how to properly clean the vertical canal of the ear at home. Assure them that because of the anatomy of the ear, they cannot easily reach the eardrum, and emphasize that preventive ear care is much easier in dogs predisposed to such problems than having to treat infections continually (Figure 10-3).

TOPICAL OTIC ANTI-INFECTIVE AGENTS

Many topical otic preparations with antibacterial or antifungal properties are available. These preparations often contain anti-inflammatory agents to reduce inflammation and decrease pruritus. Before using these medications, it is often necessary to clip the hair on the inside of the pinna and any hair that may block the external canal. Cleansers are often used before medicating to remove wax and debris from the external canal so that the medicine can work effectively. After the ear is cleaned, it should be dried before treatment.

Gentamicin Sulfate

Gentamicin sulfate is an antibacterial agent found in otic preparations. It is commonly combined with a corticosteroid such as betamethasone valerate. Some products also have antifungal properties because of the addition of clotrimazole.

Clinical Uses. These include the treatment of acute and chronic otitis in dogs, and in cats it may be used to treat superficial infected lesions caused by bacteria susceptible to gentamicin.

Dosage Forms
1. GentaVed Otic Solution
2. Gentocin Otic Solution
3. Otomax
4. Tri-Otic

Adverse Side Effects. These include possible ototoxicity because gentamicin is an aminoglycoside.

Technician's Notes

1. Patients should be carefully monitored for signs of ototoxicity. Products that lower the pH, producing an acidic environment in the ear, reduce the efficacy of gentamicin.
2. Do not use these products with other agents that may cause ototoxicity.
3. Do not use in the presence of a ruptured eardrum.

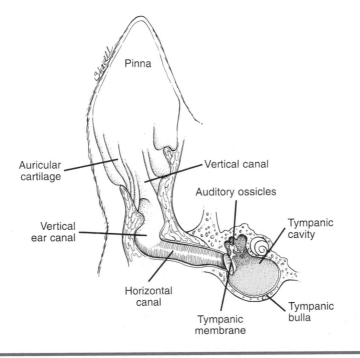

Figure 10-3

Structures of the ear.

Chloramphenicol

Chloramphenicol is an antibacterial agent often combined with a corticosteroid such as prednisolone. Products may also contain an anesthetic (tetracaine) and squalane (cerumene). Squalane enhances the product by speeding up percutaneous penetration of the active ingredients.

Clinical Uses. These include treatment for acute otitis externa and pyodermas in dogs and cats.

Dosage Forms

1. Liquichlor
2. Chlora-Otic

Technician's Notes

Products containing chloramphenicol cannot be used in animals raised for food production.

Neomycin Sulfate

Neomycin sulfate is an antibacterial agent often combined with drugs such as corticosteroids, antifungals, and/or anesthetics.

Clinical Uses. Clinical uses of this antibacterial, antifungal/antiparasitic, and anti-inflammatory combination include the treatment of otitis externa and certain bacterial, fungal, and inflammatory skin disorders.

Dosage Forms

1. Tresaderm
2. Tritop
3. Panalog

Adverse Side Effects. These include sensitivity resulting from the neomycin. If such signs (e.g., erythema) develop after treatment, the medication should be discontinued. Ototoxicity is also a potential side effect.

Technician's Notes

1. Do not use in the presence of a ruptured eardrum membrane.
2. Observe the patient for signs of ototoxicity.

ANTIPARASITICS

Ear mites are the most common parasite affecting the ears of dogs, cats, and rabbits. These mites are macroscopic, white, and freely motile. They are highly contagious, and often the entire pet household requires treatment. Because of the life cycle of the ear mite, treatment should continue for at least 3 weeks. The spinose ear tick *(Otobius megnini)* affects the external ear canal of cattle and horses and occasionally dogs and cats. The immature ticks pack the ear canal and cause discomfort. The ticks should be removed, and periodically treating the animal with an insecticide such as a flea and tick spray prevents reinfection. Cattle and horses can be treated with topical sprays such as Catron IV. This product should not be used in lactating dairy animals or on household pets.

Pyrethrins

Some products containing pyrethrins are indicated for the treatment of ticks and mites in the ears of dogs and cats.

Dosage Forms

1. Cerumite
2. Aurimite
3. Mita-Clear

Rotenone

Rotenone is an effective agent for the treatment of ear mites in dogs, cats, and rabbits.

Dosage Forms

1. Ear miticide
2. Mitaplex-R

Ivermectin

Ivermectin has been indicated as an effective treatment for ear mites in dogs and cats. This is an extralabel use of the bovine injectable product Ivomec. The dose is most often given by subcutaneous injection.

DRYING AGENTS

Drying agents are used to reduce moisture in the ears. Excess moisture provides a warm, moist environment that is ideal for the growth of certain bacterial and yeast agents that can cause infection or inflammation. These preparations may also contain an antimicrobial or a corticosteroid. Tannic acid, salicylic acid, acetic acid, and boric acid are commonly used in drying solutions.

Dosage Forms

1. Dermal Dry
2. Ace-Otic Cleanser
3. Clear$_x$ Ear Drying Solution

Technician's Notes

1. It is recommended that the ears be cleaned before applying a drying agent or other medication.
2. Some ear cleansing products also contain drying agents.

CLEANING AGENTS

Ear cleansers are used to clean the ears and provide odor control. In the presence of otitis externa, they help to remove necrotic tissue, debris, and wax. Many breeds, as mentioned before, are predisposed to ear problems, and routine cleaning can often reduce or prevent these problems. These cleansers may also contain an antimicrobial agent, anesthetic, or drying agent. Many cleansers contain an agent such as squalane (cerumene) that helps to break up and soften wax and debris and facilitate cleaning. If wax and debris are impacted in the horizontal canal, it may be necessary to flush the ear canal to remove the wax and debris before starting routine cleaning. The ear is usually too painful for this type of cleaning to be done on an unanesthetized patient. A common solution for flushing the ear canal is a mixture of warm water and chlorhexidine surgical scrub diluted 1:100. Flushing may be accomplished using a bulb syringe, a soft rubber feeding tube, or a regular-tip syringe. It is very important to use gentle pressure when flushing the ear canal to reduce the possibility of damaging the eardrum. Thorough drying of the canal after flushing provides better visualization of the eardrum.

Dosage Forms

1. Epi-Otic ear cleanser
2. Fresh-Ear
3. Oti-Clens

REFERENCES

Gelatt, K. N.: Textbook of Veterinary Ophthalmology. Lea & Febiger, Philadelphia, 1981.

Plumb, Donald C.: Veterinary Drug Handbook, 3rd ed. Iowa State University Press, Ames, 1999.

Tizard, I.: Veterinary Immunology: An Introduction, 4th ed. W.B. Saunders Company, Philadelphia, 1992.

■ Review Questions

1. What factors affect absorption of topical ophthalmic agents? _____

2. Why must most ophthalmic medications be applied several times a day? _____

3. Describe the difference between mydriatics, miotics, and cycloplegics. _____

4. What contraindication is common with the mydriatics/cycloplegics? _____

5. When might corticosteroids be contraindicated for use in treating ophthalmic conditions? _____

6. What preparation may be needed before applying medication to the ear? _____

7. What are some contraindications and side effects of aminoglycosides used in otic preparations? _____

8. How long should the treatment for ear mites last and why? _____

9. When might an otic drying solution be indicated? _____

10. What is a common solution for flushing the ear canal to remove impacted wax and debris? _____

Chapter 11

Drugs Used in Skin Disorders

LEARNING OBJECTIVES

After studying this chapter, you should be able to:

1. Develop a basic understanding of the anatomy and physiology of the skin
2. Be knowledgeable about the common ingredients of topical antiseborrheics
3. Understand the use of topical antipruritics
4. Understand the use of fatty acid supplements
5. Understand the use of astringents
6. Understand the use of skin antiseptics
7. Develop a basic understanding of wound healing
8. Understand the use of topical wound dressings
9. Understand the use of irritants

KEY TERMS

Angiogenesis The development of blood vessels.

Astringent An agent that causes contraction after application to tissue.

Callus Hypertrophy of the horny layer of the epidermis in a localized area resulting from pressure or friction.

Collagen A fibrous substance found in skin, tendon, bone, cartilage, and all other connective tissues.

Comedo (pl. comedones) A plug of keratin and sebum within a hair follicle of the skin.

Dermatitis Inflammation of the skin.

Erythema Redness of the skin caused by congestion of the capillaries.

Exudation Leakage of fluid, cells, or cellular debris from blood vessels and their deposition in or on the tissue.

Granulation tissue New tissue formed in the healing of wounds of the soft tissue, consisting of connective tissue cells and ingrowing young vessels, ultimately forming a scar.

Keratolytic An agent that promotes loosening or separation of the horny layer of the epidermis.

Keratoplastic An agent that promotes normalization of the development of keratin.

Pruritus Itching.

Pyoderma Any skin disease characterized by the presence or formation of pus.

Seborrhea An increase in scaling of the skin; sebum production may or may not be increased.

Seborrhea dermatitis An inflammatory type of seborrhea characterized by scaling and greasiness.

Seborrhea oleosa Characterized by scaling and excess lipid production that forms brownish yellow clumps that adhere to the hair and skin.

Seborrhea sicca Characterized by dry skin and white to gray scales that do not adhere to the hair or skin.

INTRODUCTION

Dermatologic therapy can seem very confusing because of the great number of products available for treating skin disorders. This chapter focuses only on topical products for treating skin disorders. Previous chapters discuss various systemic and parasiticidal products and their uses. Topical skin products include shampoos, dips, soaks, lotions, creams, ointments, sprays, and powders. They may be used to treat a range of problems, from parasites to **pyoderma.** It is very useful for technicians to have an understanding of topical products and how they are commonly used. Many problems can affect the skin and haircoat, and many clients' complaints arise from such problems. Patients are often presented for skin disease when actually they have an underlying systemic illness. Veterinarians use various diagnostic procedures to deter-mine the cause of skin disease. Technicians can have a vital role by learning to obtain a complete history, knowing how to perform the diagnostic procedures used in a dermatologic workup, and providing client education. Client education is essential when treating skin disease. Clients must understand the purpose of medications and how they are properly used. Only then can clients be expected to conform to the necessary treatment protocol.

ANATOMY AND PHYSIOLOGY

The skin is composed of three layers (Figure 11-1). The epidermis is the outer layer, and it provides protection from injurious external agents. The dermis, or corium, lies beneath the epidermis and is made up of

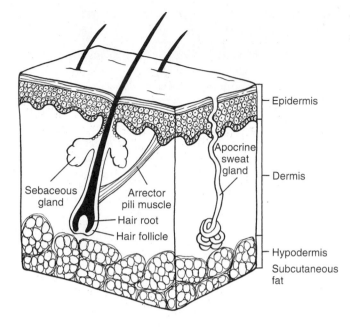

Figure 11-1

Schematic representation of the skin layers of normal canine skin.

connective tissue that contains blood vessels and nerves. Hair follicles, sebaceous glands, apocrine sweat glands, arrector pili muscles, and lymph glands are also located within this layer. The hypodermis consists of fat cells interwoven with connective tissue. The skin has several functions, including protection, temperature regulation, storage, immunoregulation, sensory perception, secretion, and vitamin D production. How well the skin is able to perform its functions is determined not only by its external health but also by the health of the body's internal systems.

 TOPICAL ANTISEBORRHEICS

Keratolytics and **keratoplastics** are known as *antiseborrheic drugs*. These drugs are most often found in medicated shampoos and are available in combinations. Table 11-1 compares products and their uses.

Sulfur

Sulfur is commonly found in shampoos and is also available in ointments. It is nonirritating, nonstain-ing, and safe for cats. Primarily it is keratolytic and keratoplastic. It is also antipruritic, antibacterial, antifungal, and antiparasitic. It is a mild follicular flusher but is not degreasing.

Clinical Uses. Sulfur is used to treat **seborrhea sicca.**

Dosage Forms

1. SebaLyt Shampoo
2. NuSal-T Shampoo
3. Sebolux Shampoo
4. Allerseb-T Shampoo

Adverse Side Effects. These include local irritation resulting from excessive and prolonged treatment. Sulfur is not recommended for routine bathing.

Technician's Notes

1. Products that contain sulfur are not recommended for routine bathing.
2. Manufacturers of most products recommend allowing the shampoo to remain on the coat for 3 to 5 minutes before rinsing.

TABLE 11-1 Common Skin Disorders with Suggested Treatments and Various Products Available

Disease	Sulfur	Salicylic Acid	Coal Tar	Benzoyl Peroxide	Chlor-hexidine	Hydro-cortisone	Therapeutic Products
Seborrhea sicca	✓	✓					SebaLyt Shampoo Sebolux Shampoo Allerseb-T Shampoo
Seborrhea oleosa	✓	✓	✓	✓			LyTar Shampoo Pyoben Shampoo Sulf/OxyDex Shampoo
Hot spots				✓	✓	✓	ChlorHex Shampoo Pyoben Gel Gentocin Topical Spray
Skinfold dermatitis				✓			OxyDex Gel Pyoben Gel
Deep pyoderma				✓			Pyoben Shampoo Sulf/OxyDex Shampoo Systemic antibiotics
Superficial pustular dermatitis				✓			Pyoben Shampoo OxyDex Shampoo Sulf/OxyDex Shampoo
Superficial folliculitis				✓	✓		ChlorHex Shampoo Pyoben Shampoo Sulf/OxyDex Shampoo
Atopy/allergic contact dermatitis	✓	✓	✓			✓	Micro Pearls Advantage Seba-Moist Moisturizing Shampoo DermaCool-HC Spray
Schnauzer comedo syndrome				✓			Micro Pearls Advantage Benzoyl Plus Shampoo OxyDex Shampoo

Salicylic Acid

Salicylic acid is a common ingredient also found in many antiseborrheic products. It is non-irritating, non-staining, and safe for cats. It is primarily keratoplastic, but it also has keratolytic, antipruritic, and antibacterial properties.

Clinical Uses. These include its combination with sulfur to treat seborrhea sicca. It may also be used to treat hyperkeratotic skin disorders such as **calluses,** thickened foot pads, and planum nasale. It is also an ingredient in many otic preparations.

Dosage Forms

1. SebaLyt Shampoo
2. Micro Pearls Advantage Seba-Moist Shampoo
3. KeraSolv Gel

Adverse Side Effects. Adverse side effects are uncommon.

Technician's Notes

Products containing salicylic acid as an active ingredient are not recommended for routine bathing.

Coal Tar

Coal tar is potentially irritating and may stain some light-colored haircoats. It is primarily keratolytic and keratoplastic and is mildly degreasing. The refining process used to produce coal tar solutions helps to decrease the staining effect, strong odor, and potential carcinogenic effect.

Clinical Uses. Coal tar is used to treat seborrhea sicca.

Dosage Forms

1. LyTar Shampoo
2. LyTar Therapeutic Spray
3. Mycodex Tar and Sulfur Shampoo

Adverse Side Effects. These include toxicity in cats.

Technician's Notes

1. Products containing coal tar should not be used on cats.
2. Manufacturers of most products recommend allowing the shampoo to remain on the haircoat for 3 to 5 minutes before rinsing.

Benzoyl Peroxide

Benzoyl peroxide is primarily keratolytic, antipruritic, follicular flushing, and degreasing. It is also antibacterial.

Clinical Uses. Benzoyl peroxide is used to treat **seborrhea oleosa,** hot spots, skinfold **dermatitis,** deep pyoderma, superficial pustular dermatitis, superficial folliculitis, schnauzer **comedo** syndrome, tail gland hyperplasia, and stud tail.

Dosage Forms

1. OxyDex Gel and Shampoo
2. Micro Pearls Benzoyl Plus Shampoo
3. Pyoben Gel and Shampoo
4. Sulf/OxyDex Shampoo

Adverse Side Effects. These include hypersensitivity in some humans.

Technician's Notes

1. Manufacturers of most products recommend allowing the shampoo to remain on the haircoat for 5 to 10 minutes before rinsing.
2. Benzoyl peroxide is safe for cats.
3. Benzoyl peroxide may bleach colored fabrics.

Selenium Sulfide

Selenium sulfide is primarily keratolytic, keratoplastic, and degreasing. It is also antifungal.

Clinical Uses. Selenium sulfide is used to treat dry eczema and **seborrhea.**

Dosage Forms

1. Seleen Plus Medicated Shampoo
2. Selsun Blue (human label) Shampoo
3. Selsun (human label) Shampoo

Adverse Side Effects. These include possible rash or irritation after use.

Technician's Notes

1. Selenium sulfide can be irritating and may stain.
2. Do not use selenium sulfide on cats.
3. Manufacturers of most products recommend allowing the shampoo to remain on the haircoat for 5 to 15 minutes before rinsing.
4. Human label products tend to be less irritating and tend to stain less.

TOPICAL MEDICATIONS MIXED WITH WATER

These products may be used in baths or applied with compresses. They possess a range of uses in veterinary medicines.

Aluminum Acetate

Aluminum acetate (Burow's solution [USP]) is drying, **astringent,** and mildly antiseptic.

Clinical Uses. Aluminum acetate is used in cool water soaks to prevent **exudation** resulting from inflammation and to relieve itching.

Dosage Forms

1. Domeboro powder
2. Domeboro tablets

Adverse Side Effects. Adverse side effects are uncommon.

Technician's Notes

One pack of powder or one tablet is mixed with ½ to 1 L of water.

Magnesium Sulfate

Magnesium sulfate is mixed with water to produce a mildly hypertonic solution for wet dressings.

Clinical Uses. Wet dressings that contain magnesium sulfate are used to dehydrate or "draw" water from tissues.

Dosage Form

1. Epsom salt

Adverse Side Effects. Adverse side effects are uncommon.

Technician's Notes

To produce a 1:65 solution, mix 1 tbsp of magnesium sulfate with 1 L of water.

Bath Oils

Bath oils may be used to manage seborrhea sicca by normalizing keratinization. These may be applied as sprays or diluted and used as a bath rinse. They contain ingredients such as sodium lactate, lanolin, and mineral oil.

Clinical Uses. Bath oils are used in the treatment of dry skin and haircoat.

Dosage Forms

1. HyLyt efa Bath Oil/Coat Conditioner
2. Alpha Keri Therapeutic Bath Oil (human label)
3. Humilac

Adverse Side Effects. Adverse side effects are uncommon.

Technician's Notes
1. Excessive use makes the haircoat greasy and causes it to collect dirt.
2. Humilac is an oil-free humectant and does not cause the haircoat to become greasy.

TOPICAL ANTIPRURITICS

Non-Steroidal Antipruritics

Topical antipruritics provide only temporary relief of itching. They are often used in conjunction with systemic or topical corticosteroids or systemic antihistamines. Colloidal oatmeal provides a soothing effect and may be beneficial for a few hours to days. Pramoxine HCl is also used topically as a palliative treatment for itching. These products provide safe and often effective alternatives to corticosteroids.

Clinical Uses. Topical antipruritics are used to provide relief of itching discomfort.

Dosage Forms
1. Epi-Soothe Shampoo
2. Epi-Soothe Bath Treatment
3. Relief Shampoo
4. Relief Spray
5. Relief Lotion

Adverse Side Effects. Adverse side effects are uncommon.

Topical Corticosteroids

Topical corticosteroids provide relief from itching, burning, and inflammation. They are often combined with other ingredients such as antimicrobial agents and astringents. Hydrocortisone, triamcinolone, fluocinolone, and betamethasone are corticosteroids commonly used in topical preparations. These steroids differ in their potency and duration of action.

Clinical Uses. They are used in the treatment of inflammation and pruritus associated with conditions such as moist dermatosis (hot spots) and allergic dermatitis.

Dosage Forms
1. Gentocin Topical Spray
2. DermaCool-HC
3. Vetalog Cream

Adverse Side Effects. Adverse side effects are uncommon.

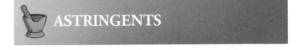
ASTRINGENTS

Astringents have very little penetration and act to precipitate proteins. They may be used alone or combined with other ingredients. Tannic acid, iodine, alcohol, and phenol are common astringents used in veterinary medicine.

Clinical Uses. These include the treatment of moist dermatitis in dogs and cats and weeping skin wounds in large animals. They also are used to toughen the foot pads of dogs.

Dosage Forms
1. Tanisol
2. Tanni-Gel
3. Stanisol

Adverse Side Effects. Astringents may cause irritation.

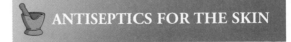
ANTISEPTICS FOR THE SKIN

Antiseptics inhibit the growth of bacteria and are found in many dermatologic preparations. They are used in the cleansing and treatment of wounds and may be found in products such as surgical scrubs and shampoos.

Alcohols

Alcohols are bactericidal, astringent, cooling, and rubefacient.

Dosage Forms

1. 70% ethyl alcohol
2. 70% to 90% isopropyl alcohol

Adverse Side Effects. Alcohols may cause irritation of denuded skin surfaces.

Propylene Glycol

Propylene glycol is antibacterial and antifungal. Concentrations greater than 50% are keratolytic. Propylene glycol is primarily used as a solvent and a vehicle for other drugs.

Dosage Forms

1. Propylene glycol
2. Topical preparations

Adverse Side Effects. **Erythema** can result when using propylene glycol concentrations greater than 50%.

Chlorhexidine

Chlorhexidine is bactericidal, fungicidal, and effective against many viruses. It is nonirritating, is not affected by organic debris, and is safe for cats. Concentrations of 0.5% to 2% may be found in forms such as shampoos, ointments, surgical scrub, and solution.

Dosage Forms

1. ChlorhexiDerm Maximum Shampoo
2. Nolvasan Antiseptic Ointment
3. Chlor-Scrub 40

Adverse Side Effects. Adverse side effects are uncommon.

Acetic Acid

Acetic acid may be found in many otic preparations. It is effective against superficial *Pseudomonas* spp. infections of the skin and ears.

Dosage Forms

1. Fresh-Ear
2. Clear$_x$ Ear Cleansing Solution and Drying Solution

Adverse Side Effects. Adverse side effects are uncommon.

Iodine

Iodine is bactericidal, fungicidal, virucidal, and sporicidal. It may be found in shampoos, surgical scrubs, surgical preparations, ointments, and sprays.

Dosage Forms

1. Iodine Tincture
2. Lugol's Solution
3. Betadine
4. Xenodine Spray

Adverse Side Effects. Iodine can be irritating and sensitizing, especially in cats. Most products stain.

Technician's Notes
1. Providone-iodine is non-staining.
2. Xenodine is not as irritating as other iodines.

Benzalkonium Chloride

Benzalkonium chloride is antifungal and antibacterial but is not effective against *Pseudomonas* spp. Soap or other anionic compounds inactivate it.

Dosage Forms

1. Topical wound spray
2. Myosan Cream
3. Dermacide

Adverse Side Effects. Toxicity can occur in cats.

Technician's Notes

This product is not approved for use in food-producing animals or animals intended for food.

WOUND HEALING

Normal wound healing can be divided into four stages. In stage I, inflammation begins and hemorrhage is limited by vessel contraction and constriction. Serum leakage into the wound deposits fibrinogen and other clotting elements. Later, this serum provides enzymes, proteins, antibodies, and complement. Stage II begins as neutrophils and monocytes migrate to the wound. Neutrophils phagocytize bacteria and then die and lyse. Monocytes become macrophages and phagocytize necrotic debris. During stage III, fibroblasts produce **collagen** and other connective tissue proteins. Capillaries infiltrate the wound to provide blood supply and oxygen. This process forms **granulation tissue.** Epithelial cells proliferate beneath the scab, and the wound begins to contract. Stage IV is a period of remodeling. During this time, the wound consolidates and strengthens. Many factors contribute to proper wound healing. For a patient, these factors include age, nutritional status, rest, environment, and general health. For a wound, these factors include size, location, environment, infection, inflammation, and contamination (Muller, et. al., 1989). A veterinarian must consider all factors when determining how to treat a wound and how well it will heal.

TOPICAL WOUND DRESSINGS

The treatment of wounds may include systemic therapy, bandages, topical medications, or a combination of these treatments. Topical dressing are commonly used in the treatment of wounds. These wound dressings are available as ointments, solutions, gels, creams, lotions, sprays, powders, and dressing sheets. The type of dressing used and the length of therapy is dependent on the previously mentioned factors that affect wound healing. For example, a de-gloving injury will take weeks to months for complete healing to occur, whereas a small laceration will heal in a few days.

Healing Stimulators

Some dressings will stimulate the activities of wound healing. These products may be used on simple wounds or are most helpful during the later stages of the healing of large wounds when there is less exudate produced. Some products may be used alone or in combination with other products. Depending on the wound, a bandage may be applied. Advances in products that stimulate healing include the addition of products containing acemannan or bovine collagen. Acemannan promotes fibroblast proliferation, collagen deposition, **angiogenesis,** and epithelialization. Products containing bovine collagen also promote fibroblast proliferation and collagen deposition (Swaim and Gillette, 1998).

Dosage Forms

1. Scarlet Oil
2. Zinc oxide
3. Carravet Wound Dressing
4. BioDres
5. Collamend

Adverse Side Effects. Adverse side effects are uncommon.

Technician's Notes

1. It is very important to follow manufacturer recommendations regarding application frequency.
2. Keep bandages dry and clean.
3. Some products may not be suitable for deep or puncture wounds.

Wound Cleansers

Wound cleansers are used to irrigate wounds to remove necrotic tissue, debris, and bacteria. Some products also act as healing stimulants. These products may be used in the initial cleansing of a wound before applying a wound dressing. More extensive wounds will require cleansing at every treatment because of the large amounts of exudate that may be produced during the early stages of healing. It is important that necrotic tissue and purulent debris be removed during the cleansing. Some products are applied directly to the wound after cleansing and the removal of necrotic tissue. A nonadherent bandage is then applied, and the product absorbs exudate and stimulates the healing process.

Dosage Forms

1. Oti-Clens
2. C-Stat
3. Intracell
4. Dakin's solution—a 0.5% solution of sodium hypochlorite (bleach)
5. Granulex-V

Adverse Side Effects. These are uncommon, but some products may cause temporary stinging after application.

Technician's Notes

1. These products should not be used on fresh arterial clots.
2. Keep bandages dry and clean.
3. Some products may not be suitable for deep or puncture wounds.

Protectants

Protectants provide a protective environment to assist healing of non-infected wounds. Some products protect the skin from irritation caused by urine, feces, and tape. They act as a barrier that prevents irritation and allows healing of previously irritated intact skin.

Dosage Forms

1. Dermal Wound Gel
2. Thuja-Zinc Oxide Ointment
3. Nexaband
4. No Sting Barrier Film

Technician's Notes

1. These products should be applied to clean, dry skin.
2. These products are not suitable for deep or puncture wounds.
3. Products containing zinc oxide may cause zinc toxicity if ingested.

OTHER DRUGS USED IN DERMATOLOGIC THERAPY

Systemic Corticosteroids

It is often necessary to use systemic corticosteroids in the treatment of some dermatosis and dermatitis. These drugs affect immunologic and inflammatory activity. Systemic steroids are available for oral and parenteral administration. The effect of systemic steroids may last from a few hours up to several weeks depending on the type of steroid used. Chapter 9 provides an in-depth discussion of systemic corticosteroids and their effects on the body.

Clinical Uses. In the treatment of dermatologic conditions, systemic corticosteroids are indicated for allergic reactions (e.g., flea bite hypersensitivity, atopy); moist dermatosis (hot spot); **seborrheic dermatitis;** and acral lick dermatitis.

Dosage Forms

1. Dexamethasone injection
2. Depo-Medrol injection
3. Predisone generic tablets
4. Medrol tablets

Adverse Side Effects. Adverse side effects are numerous. Many occur with misuse and long-term use. Side effects most commonly seen with doses used in the treatment of skin inflammation and **pruritus** include polyuria, polydipsia, and polyphagia, which may result in weight gain.

> **Technician's Notes**
> The technician should alert clients to the side effects seen with systemic corticosteroids. Polyuria and polydipsia may be problematic for some household pets.

Topical Antibacterial Agents

Topical antibacterial agents are used in the treatment and prevention of superficial bacterial infections of wounds. These products may also contain corticosteroids and antifungal agents. They may require frequent application (i.e., two to three times daily) and can be used under bandages.

Dosage Forms

1. Bactoderm
2. Nitrofurazone dressing
3. Forte-Topical
4. Prodine solution

> **Technician's Notes**
> To achieve good contact with the skin surface, clipping the hair before application is often necessary.

Topical Antifungal Agents

Topical antifungal agents are used in the treatment of superficial fungal infections. They are effective in the treatment of ringworm and for thrush in horses or ponies. They are often found in combination with antibacterial agents and corticosteroids. They may necessitate frequent application (i.e., two to three times daily) and can be used under bandages. Local treatment of fungal infections is not always effective, and the use of systemic antifungal agents may be necessary.

Dosage Forms

1. Conofite
2. Kopertox
3. Panalog
4. Iodine Shampoo

> **Technician's Notes**
> 1. To achieve good contact with the skin surface, clipping the hair before application is often necessary.
> 2. Kopertox and products containing iodine will stain clothes and light-colored hair.

Fatty Acid Supplements

Fatty acids consist of long chains of carbon atoms with a methyl group ($-CH3$) at one end. Polyunsaturated fatty acids have varying numbers of double bonds connecting the carbon atoms. Formulas used to identify fatty acids give the number of carbon atoms, followed by the number of double bonds, and last the distance of the first double bond from the methyl group. The formula for arachidonic acid is (20:4N-6); the formula indicates that this fatty acid has 20 carbon atoms and four double bonds and that the first double bond is six carbon atoms from the methyl group.

Fatty acids that have the first double bond six carbons atoms away from the methyl group are called *omega-6 (N-6) fatty acids,* and those that have the first double bond three carbons atoms away are called the *omega-3, (N-3) fatty acids.* (Scott, Miller, and Griffin, 1995). Linoleic acid (18:2N-6) and linolenic acid (18:3N-3) cannot be synthesized by the dog and must be supplied in the diet. For this reason linoleic and linolenic acids are called *essential fatty acids.* Arachidonic is also an essential fatty acid in the cat.

Fatty acids are responsible for the shine of the haircoat and the smooth texture of the skin. It has also been well-documented that fatty supplementation can play an important role in managing the itching dog or cat. The exact mechanism by which the fatty acids help to control itching is not known, but it has been proposed that the fatty acids may tie up cyclooxygenase and/or phospholipase (see Chapter 14) and therefore inhibit prostaglandin formation in the skin. A synergistic effect may be achieved by combining fatty acid therapy with the administration of antihistamines or glucocorticosteroids.

Fatty acid supplements are usually derived from fish oil and vegetable oil and may be combined with antioxidant vitamins such as A and E.

Clinical Uses. Fatty acid supplements are used to control itching (pruritis) associated with certain dermatologic conditions of dogs and cats. They may also be used to improve the luster of the skin.

Dosage Forms

1. Dermcaps
2. Dermcaps ES
3. Dermcaps ES liquid
4. EFA-Caps

Adverse Side Effects. Side effects may include vomiting, diarrhea, or increased bleeding times.

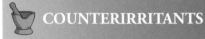 **COUNTERIRRITANTS**

Counterirritants are substances that are applied to the skin of horses to produce local irritation and inflammation. These compounds are sometimes used to treat chronic inflammatory conditions of bone, joints, ligaments, tendons, or other tissue below the surface. The rationale for their use is that creating an acute inflammatory condition increases blood supply to the inflamed area as well as adjacent tissue. This increased blood supply brings with it more oxygen, white blood cells, antibodies, complement, and other factors to promote healing. The proper use of counterirritants is complicated because underuse may have little effect and overuse may cause severe tissue damage. The beneficial effects of counterirritant use is controversial, and many clinicians claim that the period of enforced rest (1 to 3 months) for treated animals is actually responsible for the healing effect.

When counterirritants are applied to the skin, three stages of irritation result, depending on the agent applied, the quantity applied, or the way in which it is applied. The three stages are listed in the following:

1. Rubefaction
2. Vesication
3. Blistering

Rubefaction (reddening) indicates mild irritation accompanied by an increase in blood congestion in the skin. Liniments and "braces" are alcohol-based products that produce a rubefacient effect when massaged into the skin. Liniments and braces usually have alcohol as the primary ingredient and may include camphor, turpentine, oil of wintergreen, thymol, menthol, or ammonia. The major benefits of these products may be a result of the massage used in their application rather than the medicinal effect. A *tightener* is a rubefacient compound similar to a liniment or a brace that is applied under a cotton leg wrap in an effort to reduce edema around tendons or joints. A *sweat* usually contains alcohol and glycerin and is applied under a moisture-proof bandage to reduce edema.

Clinical Uses. Counterirritants are used for reducing "filling" (edema) around joints or tendons and the associated soreness.

Dosage Forms

1. White Liniment
2. Isopropyl alcohol
3. Lin-O-Gel
4. Shin-O-Gel
5. Tuttle Elixir
6. Absorbine Veterinary Liniment
7. Equ-Lin
8. BIGEOIL
9. SU-PER Sweat
10. Antiphlogistine Poultice
11. SU-PER Poultice

Adverse Side Effects. Tissue irritation may be caused by counterirritants.

Vesication is the second stage of counterirritation, and it is achieved by applying irritating substances under a bandage. Severe irritation accompanied by capillary damage results in vesication or blister formation. Mercuric oxide and cantharide ointments are commonly used as blisters. Because the application of vesicants is a painful process that can lead to self-mutilation, they should be applied only under the supervision of a veterinarian.

Clinical Uses. Vesication is used in the treatment of chronic inflammatory musculoskeletal conditions in horses.

Dosage Forms

1. Mercuric oxide
2. Cantharide

Adverse Side Effects. These may include severe tissue damage, worsening of the original condition, and self-mutilation.

> **Technician's Notes**
>
> Petroleum jelly should not be applied around the site where a vesicant is applied to prevent damage to adjacent tissue.

 CAUSTICS

Caustics are substances that destroy tissue at the application site. They are used to destroy excessive granulation tissue (proud flesh), superficial tumors (warts), or horn buds. They should be applied by knowledgeable persons because they can cause damage to adjacent tissue.

Clinical Uses. Caustics are used for the control of proud flesh, the removal of warts, and the removal of horn buds in calves.

Dosage Forms

1. Copper sulfate
2. Silver nitrate
3. Proudsoff
4. Wartsoff
5. Caustic Powder
6. Acidified Copper Sulfate
7. Caustic Dressing Powder
8. Equi-Phar Proud Blue Liquid
9. Dehorning Paste

Adverse Side Effects. These may include damage to adjacent tissue, especially the eye when used on the horn buds.

REFERENCES

Muller, G.H., Kirk, R.W., Scott, D.W.: Small Animal Dermatology, 4th ed. W.B. Saunders Company, Philadelphia, 1989.

Scott, D.W., Miller, W.H., Griffin, C.E.: Dermatologic therapy. In Small Animal Dermatology, 5th ed. W.B. Saunders Co., Philadelphia, 1995.

Swaim, S.F., R.L. Gillette: An Update on Wound Medications and Dressings. Compend. Cont. Educ. Prac. Vet. 20(10):1133-1145, 1998.

■ Review Questions

1. Discuss the functions of the skin layers.
   _____

2. Describe the action of antiseborrheics.
   _____

3. How do bath oils contribute to the management of seborrhea sicca? _____

4. Why are topical antipruritic products beneficial in relieving itching? _____

5. How are astringents used in treating skin disorders?
   _____

6. List common antiseptics used on the skin.
   _____

7. Discuss the stages of wound healing.
   _____

8. Discuss the contributing factors that determine proper wound healing. _____

9. How are topical corticosteroids used in treating skin disorders? _____

10. When are wound protectants contraindicated?
    _____

11. Describe the stages of irritation that occur after the application of counterirritants.
    _____

12. Describe the uses of counterirritants and caustics.
    _____

Anti-Infective Drugs

LEARNING OBJECTIVES

After studying this chapter, you should be able to:

1. Identify the classes of the anti-infective drugs
2. Understand the adverse side effects of the anti-infective drugs
3. Understand the clinical uses of the anti-infective drugs
4. Be familiar with the antiviral drugs
5. Be familiar with the disinfectants and antiseptics and their uses

KEY TERMS

Antibacterial An agent that inhibits bacterial growth, impedes replication of bacteria, or kills bacteria.

Antibiotic An agent produced by a microorganism or semi-synthetically that has the ability to inhibit the growth of or kill microorganisms.

Antimicrobial An agent that kills microorganisms or suppresses their multiplication or growth.

Bacteria Single-celled microorganisms that usually have a rigid cell wall and a round, rodlike, or spiral shape.

Bactericidal An agent with the capability to kill bacteria.

Bacteriostatic An agent that inhibits the growth or reproduction of bacteria.

Beta-lactamase Enzymes that reduce the effectiveness of certain antibiotics; beta-lactamase I is penicillinase; beta-lactamase II is cephalosporinase.

Dermatophytosis A fungal skin infection.

Detergent An agent that cleanses.

Disinfect To make free of pathogens or make them inactive.

Fungicidal An agent that kills fungi.

Fungistatic An agent that inhibits the growth of fungi.

In vitro Within an artificial environment.

In vivo Within the living body.

Iodophor An iodine compound with a longer activity period resulting from the combination of iodine and a carrier molecule that releases iodine over a period of time.

Microorganism An organism that is microscopic (e.g., bacterium, protozoan, *Rickettsia*, virus, and fungus).

Sporicidal An agent capable of killing spores.

INTRODUCTION

Hundreds of **antimicrobial** drugs have been developed since the early 1900s. These drugs have saved many lives, both human and animal. Antimicrobials vary in their degree of effectiveness against different **microorganisms.** A drug's spectrum of activity is the range of bacteria affected by its action. Once a drug's spectrum is determined, it may be classified as active against gram-positive, gram-negative, or acid-fast bacilli. These classifications are determined by laboratory testing. The Gram stain is the most common laboratory method for distinguishing the different types of **bacteria** (Figure 12-1). The Gram stain uses dyes to stain the organisms. If the cell wall is stained by the Gram stain, the organism is considered to be gram-positive and appears dark blue to purple; if no reaction occurs, the organism is gram-negative and appears pink to red.

Some bacteria (e.g., mycobacteria) cannot be identified with a Gram stain. These may be stained with carbolfuchsin and then decolorized with ethyl alcohol and hydrochloric acid, and if they retain stain, they are classified as acid-fast bacilli. Other bacteria may require identification by special techniques, such as dark-field examination or Gimenez stain. Giemsa's stain and Wright's stain may be used to identify parasites and intracellular microorganisms. These laboratory tests are important for determining bacteria's staining properties. Bacteria with similar staining properties tend to be susceptible to the same antimicrobial therapy. Another classification for bacteria is determined by an organism's ability to survive with or without oxygen. Aerobes are bacteria that must have oxygen to live and multiply. Some bacteria are able to live and multiply without available oxygen. These organisms are anaerobes, and they can be very difficult to eradicate.

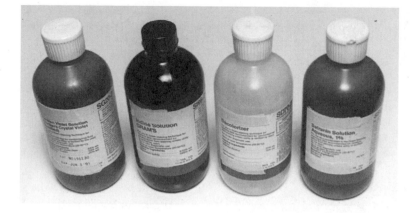

Figure 12-1

The Gram stain is a common laboratory test for distinguishing different types of bacteria. This procedure is as follows: (1) After preparing the slide and heat fixing, flood smear with crystal violet solution and let stand 1 minute. (2) Rinse gently with tap water. (3) Flood smear with Gram's iodine and let stand 1 minute. (4) Rinse gently with tap water and flood with Gram's decolorizer for 5 to 10 seconds. (5) Wash gently with tap water. (6) Flood smear with safranin counterstain for 30 to 60 seconds. (7) Wash gently with tap water, blot dry, and examine under oil immersion (100). The staining solutions are shown above in the order in which they are used.

MECHANISM OF ACTION

A drug's mechanism of action is determined by the drug's ability to be **bactericidal** or **bacteriostatic** for certain organisms. This action is sometimes altered by the formation of mutant strains of bacteria that have higher resistance to some antimicrobials. When a resistant strain has developed, determining a successful antimicrobial therapy can be difficult. To help prevent mutant strains of bacteria from forming, it is important not to use antimicrobial drugs indiscriminately, and when an antimicrobial drug has been prescribed, it should be given at a high enough dose and for an appropriate duration to lessen the occurrence of mutant strain formation. An antimicrobial drug occasionally is used in conjunction with another antimicrobial drug to treat an infection caused by two or more different types of organisms. When using antimicrobial drugs together, it is important that the chosen drugs work together and that they are not antagonists to each other. After a laboratory determines the type of organism causing an infection, a sensitivity test is often performed. Several tests are available to determine the susceptibility of an organism to a specific antimicrobial drug. The agar diffusion test is most commonly used in small laboratories (Figure 12-2). This test involves placing disks impregnated with different antimicrobial drugs onto agar plates containing the infective organism. After a specified time, the plate is observed for zones of inhibition. These zones show which antimicrobial agents are most effective **in vitro.** The broth dilution susceptibility test is used in larger laboratories (Figure 12-3). An organism is inoculated into a series of tubes or wells in a microculture plate. These tubes or wells contain different concentrations of antimicrobials. The lowest concentration that macroscopically inhibits growth of an organism is the minimal inhibitory concentration (MIC). The MIC represents the degree of susceptibility of the organism to a specific concentration of a particular antimicrobial drug. The antimicrobials that are effective in vitro may not always be the best choice to use **in vivo.** A clinician chooses which agent to use by considering the diagnosis and knowing each agent's pharmacodynamics and pharmacokinetics. This information allows a clinician to choose the most efficient and efficacious drug to treat the specific condition.

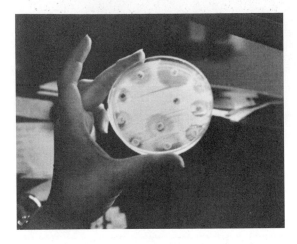

Figure 12-2

The agar diffusion test measures the in vitro susceptibility of a microorganism to specific antibiotics. Note the zones of inhibition surrounding the antibiotic disks.

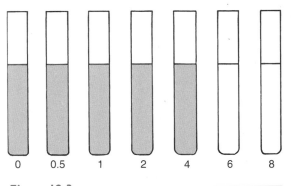

Figure 12-3

The broth dilution susceptibility test. Note that the organism grew in broth containing 0, 0.5, 1, 2, and 4 mg/ml of antibiotic. The organism was inhibited in the tube containing 6 mg/ml. The minimal inhibitory concentration is 6 mg/ml.

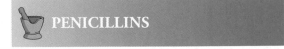
PENICILLINS

Although penicillin was developed during the 1940s, it still remains a very important and useful antimicrobial drug despite the introduction of many other an-timicrobials. Today researchers have developed natural and semi-synthetic compounds that display varied antimicrobial spectrums (Table 12–1).

PHARMACOKINETICS

Most absorption of penicillins given orally takes place in the stomach and upper small intestine. Most injectable penicillins are rapidly absorbed at the injection sites. Once absorbed, penicillins are rapidly distributed through most tissues. Some penicillins are metabolized by the liver, but the kidneys are the primary organs for excretion of penicillins. Penicillins are excreted through the milk in small amounts; therefore, withdrawal times for dairy animals must be adhered to.

PHARMACODYNAMICS

Research has shown that penicillins bind reversibly with enzymes, called *penicillin-binding proteins (PBPs),* outside the bacterial cytoplasmic membrane. These enzymes are involved in cell-wall synthesis and cell division, and when this binding occurs it increases the internal osmotic pressure and ruptures the cell. Some bacteria produce **beta-lactamase** (penicillinase), which increases the bacteria's resistance by converting penicillin to inactive penicillic acid. Some penicillins are more resistant to beta-lactamase hydrolysis and are referred to as *beta-lactamase–resistant* or *penicillinase-resistant penicillins.* Penicillins are usually very effective against gram-positive bacteria, but gram-negative bacteria have an outer membrane around the cell wall that limits the PBPs' permeability. Some penicillins that have been developed have an increased ability to penetrate this outer membrane and have more activity against the gram-negative bacteria.

Clinical Uses. Penicillins are used to treat bacterial infections resulting from penicillin-susceptible microorganisms.

Dosage Forms

1. Polyflex injection
2. Penicillin G procaine injection
3. Ambi-Pen injection
4. Amoxi-Tabs (dogs and cats)

TABLE 12-1 Penicillin Preparations, Indications, and Antagonistic Drugs

Drug	Indications	Antagonist	Comments
Narrow-Spectrum Penicillins			
Penicillin G sodium	Infections caused by penicillin-sensitive organisms. Bacterial pneumonia, upper respiratory tract infections, equine strangles, blackleg, infected wounds, urinary tract infections (at high doses)	Tetracyclines, chloramphenicol, and paromomycin	May add to sodium load.
Penicillin G potassium	Same as for penicillin G sodium	Same as for penicillin G sodium	May produce hyperkalemia (IV). Delayed absorption in horse (IM). Unreliable absorption.
Penicillin G procaine	Same as for penicillin G sodium	Same as for penicillin G sodium	Never give IV. Contraindicated in some exotics and horses that race. Preslaughter withdrawal and milk withholding periods.
Penicillin G benzathine	Same as for penicillin G sodium	Same as for penicillin G sodium	Never give IV. Preslaughter withdrawal required, and may persist in dairy cattle milk for 2 weeks.
Narrow-Spectrum–Acid-Resistant Penicillins			
Penicillin V	Mild infections already controlled by parenteral therapy	Same as for penicillin G sodium	Should not be administered with food. Less active against gram-negative bacteria than penicillin G.
Beta-Lactamase–Resistant Penicillins			
Methicillin	Pyodermatitis, otitis externa, and other conditions caused by *Staphylococcus aureus*	Same as for penicillin G sodium	Not stable in solution. Many incompatibilities in vitro.
Cloxacillin	Same as for methicillin	Same as for penicillin G sodium	Frequently used in dry-cow intramammary preparations.

IV, Intravenous(ly); *IM,* intramuscular(ly); *GI,* gastrointestinal.
Courtesy Fort Dodge Laboratories, Fort Dodge, Iowa.

Continued

TABLE 12-1 Penicillin Preparations, Indications, and Antagonistic Drugs—cont'd

Drug	Indications	Antagonist	Comments
Beta-Lactamase–Resistant Penicillins—cont'd			
Dicloxacillin and floxacillin	Same as for methicillin	Same as for penicillin G sodium	Absorbed from GI tract better than cloxacillin.
Oxacillin	Same as for methicillin	Sulfonamides	Not absorbed as well as cloxacillin.
Broad-Spectrum Penicillins			
Ampicillin and hetacillin	Infection of organs and tissues caused by ampicillin-sensitive bacteria	Chloramphenicol, erythromycin, tetracyclines, cephaloridine	Incompatible with many drugs and solutions. Food impairs absorption. Milk withholding and preslaughter withdrawal times.
Amoxicillin	Same as for ampicillin	Same as for ampicillin	Absorbed from GI tract better than ampicillin.
Piperacillin	Same as for ampicillin	Aminoglycosides	
Carbenicillin sodium	Same as for ampicillin, but especially *Pseudomonas* infections	Same as for ampicillin	Freshly mixed solutions should be used.
Broad-Spectrum Penicillins			
Carbenicillin indanyl sodium	Same as for carbenicillin sodium	Same as for ampicillin	Absorbed rapidly from the GI tract.
Ticarcillin	Same as for carbenicillin sodium	Same as for ampicillin	Used as an intrauterine infusion in mares.
Potentiated Penicillins			
Amoxicillin-potassium clavulanate (4:1)	Wide range of infections when used in combination	Same as for ampicillin	Capsules/tablets that are not kept in air-tight containers lose activity. Do not give to patients allergic to penicillins or cephalosporins.
Inhibitor of Tubular Secretion of Penicillins			
Probenecid	Prolongs blood levels of penicillins that have very short plasma half-lives or that are extremely costly	Same as for ampicillin.	

Courtesy Fort Dodge Laboratories, Fort Dodge, Iowa.

Adverse Side Effects. These include possible sensitivity reactions (e.g., hives or respiratory distress) to penicillin or procaine. Epinephrine should be administered immediately if respiratory distress is severe.

> **Technician's Notes**
> 1. Penicillin should not be used in horses intended for food.
> 2. Carefully read labels concerning milk withholding times and treating animals to be slaughtered for food.
> 3. Penicillin G benzathine is long acting (48 hours) and is not approved for use in dairy animals.

 ## CEPHALOSPORINS

Cephalosporins are primarily used in small-animal medicine. A few are now available for use in large-animal medicine. This group of drugs is classified into generations according to the drug's spectrum of activity (Table 12-2).

PHARMACOKINETICS

Because of the lack of absorption into the gastrointestinal (GI) tract, most cephalosporins are administered parenterally. Once absorbed, cephalosporins are distributed to tissues and fluids, with the exception of the central nervous system (CNS). Some cephalosporins are absorbed into the cerebrospinal fluid, but this absorption is limited. Metabolism occurs in the liver, with elimination occurring in the kidneys by glomerular filtration and tubular secretion into the urine; therefore, doses must be modified for patients in renal failure. A few exceptions are excreted through the feces from the biliary system.

PHARMACODYNAMICS

Like penicillins, the cephalosporins interfere with cell-wall synthesis by binding to the bacterial enzymes (PBPs). A cephalosporin's spectrum of activity is determined by the drug's ability to penetrate the bacterial cell wall and bind with proteins in the cytoplasmic membrane. Once this penetration and binding occur, the cell wall has been damaged and the body is able to use its natural defense mechanisms to destroy the bacteria (Williams and Baer, 1990). Another similarity between cephalosporins and penicillins is the cephalosporins' susceptibility to beta-lactamases (cephalosporinases), which can be produced by certain bacteria. Some cephalosporins are more effective in treating infections caused by bacteria that produce beta-lactamase II. For example, third-generation cephalosporins are highly resistant to beta-lactamase II, but first-generation cephalosporins are fairly susceptible to beta-lactamase II.

Clinical Uses. Cephalosporins are used to treat cystitis; skin and soft tissue infections in dogs and cats; bovine mastitis; shipping fever; and other respiratory infections in cattle, horses, sheep, and swine. Ceftiofur sodium (Naxcel) is also approved for use in day-old chicks and day-old turkey poults for control of early mortality associated with *Escherichia coli* organisms.

Dosage Forms
1. Cefa-Drops
2. Cefa-Tabs
3. Cefa-Lak (mastitis therapy)
4. Naxcel powder for injection
5. Excenel injectable suspension

Adverse Side Effects. These are uncommon but include nausea, vomiting, diarrhea, and lethargy.

> **Technician's Notes**
> 1. Carefully read labels regarding milk withholding time after mastitis treatment and use in animals to be slaughtered.
> 2. Naxcel is approved for use in lactating dairy animals.

TETRACYCLINES

Tetracyclines are available for oral and parenteral administration. The most common tetracyclines used in

TABLE 12-2	Cephalosporin Preparations, Indications, and Antagonistic Drugs		
Drug	**Indications**	**Antagonist**	**Comments**
Cefadroxil	Infections caused by sensitive organisms in the respiratory tract, skin, urinary tract, soft tissue, bones, joints, etc.	All cephalosporins: gentamicin	Ingestion of food does not impair absorption.
Cephalexin	Urinary tract infections		Ingestion of food may delay absorption.
Cephalothin	Infections caused by sensitive organisms in the respiratory tract, skin, urinary tract, soft tissue, bones, joints, etc.		IM injection painful. Inactivated in liver.
Cefazolin	Same as for cephalothin		Highly protein bound. Very rarely nephrotoxic.
Cephapirin	Same as for cephalothin		Intramammary infusion for mastitis.
Cefamandole	Life-threatening gram-negative infections		Dose should be reduced in patients with renal failure.
Cefoxitin (a cephamycin)	Treatment of susceptible infections		Local reaction may occur at injection site.
Ceftiofur HCl	Treatment of respiratory disease in cattle and swine. Broad spectrum against gram-positive and gram-negative bacteria including beta-lactamase–producing strains		May be used in lactating dairy animals.
Ceftiofur sodium	Treatment of respiratory disease in cattle, sheep, horses, and swine; urinary tract infections in dogs; and for control of early mortality associated with *E. coli* organisms in day-old chicks and day-old turkey poults. Broad spectrum against gram-positive and gram-negative bacteria including beta-lactamase–producing strains		May be used in lactating dairy animals.

Courtesy Fort Dodge Laboratories, Fort Dodge, Iowa.

TABLE 12-3	Tetracycline Preparations, Indications, and Antagonistic Drugs		
Drug	**Indications**	**Antagonist**	**Comments**
Oxytetracycline	Infections of organs or tissues caused by tetracycline-sensitive strains. Anaplasmosis. Often ineffective for endocarditis, empyema, meningitis, septic arthritis, and osteomyelitis	Antacids, milk, diuretics, methoxyflurane, penicillins, ferrous sulfate	Long withdrawal times in cattle. Shock reaction may occur when given intravenously in horses. Diarrhea also common in horses.
Chlortetracycline	Same as for oxytetracycline	Antacids, milk, diuretics, methoxyflurane, penicillins	
Tetracycline	Same as for oxytetracycline	Same as for oxytetracycline	
Doxycycline, minocycline	Same as for oxytetracycline but much better tissue penetration. Doxycycline is especially useful for canine ehrlichiosis	Minocycline—same as for chlortetracycline. Doxycycline—same as for oxytetracycline as well as barbiturates, carbamazepine	These drugs are potent broad-spectrum tetracyclines.

Courtesy Fort Dodge Laboratories, Fort Dodge, Iowa.

clinical practice are tetracycline, oxytetracycline, doxycycline, and minocycline (Table 12-3).

PHARMACOKINETICS

Once administered, tetracyclines are quickly distributed throughout the tissues, and in some instances they penetrate into the CNS. Very little metabolism occurs with most tetracyclines, causing them to be eliminated in the active form. Elimination mostly occurs by glomerular filtration, but in some instances biliary excretion occurs.

PHARMACODYNAMICS

Tetracyclines work by inhibiting protein synthesis, thereby impeding bacterial cell division. They offer a broad spectrum of activity against gram-positive and gram-negative bacteria. They are bacteriostatic, although at high dose concentrations they may become bactericidal.

Clinical Uses. Tetracyclines are used to treat respiratory tract infections, bacterial enteritis, and urinary tract infections caused by tetracycline-susceptible microorganisms.

Dosage Forms

1. Panmycin Aquadrops
2. Tetracycline Soluble Powder-324
3. Aureomycin Tablets
4. Oxy-Tet 100 injectable

Adverse Side Effects. These include permanent staining of the teeth if received while in utero or as a juvenile, and the drug is deposited in growing bones, slowing their development.

Technician's Notes

1. Absorption of tetracyclines by the GI tract is dramatically decreased by the presence of food, milk products, and antacids.
2. Carefully read labels about use in animals to be slaughtered.
3. Not approved for use in lactating dairy animals or poultry that produce eggs for human consumption.

AMINOGLYCOSIDES

Aminoglycosides provide broad-spectrum activity, and those commonly used include amikacin, gentamicin, kanamycin, and neomycin. They are used for treatment of large, small, and exotic animals. When aminoglycosides are used in reptiles and birds, it is important that intravenous fluid therapy be administered along with the **antibiotic** therapy to reduce the nephrotoxic effects. Although aminoglycosides are effective against most gram-negative and many gram-positive bacteria, their use should be restricted to treating primarily gram-negative infections. Aminoglycosides have the potential to cause serious side effects such as nephrotoxicity, ototoxicity, and neuromuscular synaptic dysfunction (Table 12-4).

PHARMACOKINETICS

Because they are not readily absorbed through the GI tract, aminoglycosides are administered parenterally, except for neomycin, which is administered orally.

TABLE 12-4 Aminoglycoside Preparations, Indications, and Antagonistic Drugs

Drug	Indications	Antagonist	Comments
All aminogly-cosides	Infections caused by susceptible pathogens, pneumonias, urinary tract infections, endometritis, and septicemias that are resistant to other antibiotics	Dimenhydrinate and ethacrynic acid affect hearing loss; methoxyflurane Chloramphenicol	Monitor patient for hearing loss; do not administer with methoxyflurane.
Kanamycin, tobramycin, gentamicin, neomycin, streptomycin		Neuromuscular blocking agents	Administer calcium and anticholinergic agents as prescribed.
Gentamicin		Amphotericin B and cephalosporins produce nephrotoxicity	Monitor renal function test results frequently when combining these agents.
Neomycin		Digitalis glycosides, penicillin V	Dosages may need to be adjusted when combining these agents.
Gentamicin, tobramycin		Carbenicillin, ticarcillin, azlocillin, mezlocillin, piperacillin	Never mix these two types of antibiotics; if a patient is receiving combined therapy, administer the doses at least 1 hour apart.

Once administered, aminoglycosides are absorbed into the bloodstream and then distributed into extracellular fluid. After parenteral administration, aminoglycosides do not reach therapeutic levels in bile, cerebrospinal fluid, respiratory secretions, prostatic or ocular fluids, or fetal tissue (Beech et al., 1987). Elimination occurs by glomerular filtration into the urine. Because of their tendency to accumulate at high concentrations in the renal cortical tissue, adequate renal function is necessary for their use. Ettinger (1993) recommends monitoring nephrotoxicity by obtaining a pretreatment serum creatinine level and comparing that with samples taken during treatment. Any significant change in the serum cre-atinine level could indicate the need to terminate treatment. Another area of concentration is in the inner ear, in which concentration levels do not diminish until after treatment is concluded. The ototoxicity that occurs may be vestibular or auditory.

PHARMACODYNAMICS

Like tetracyclines, aminoglycosides work by inhibiting protein synthesis, thereby impeding bacterial cell division. As mentioned earlier, they have a broad spectrum but should be used only in specific cases of gram-negative infections. Streptococcal species of bacteria do not show much sensitivity to aminoglycosides (Ettinger, 1993). They are mostly ineffective against anaerobic bacteria.

Clinical Uses. Aminoglycosides are used to treat pneumonia, endometritis, urinary tract infections, bacterial enteritis, conjunctivitis, and skin and soft tissue infections caused by aminoglycoside-susceptible microorganisms.

Dosage Forms

1. Amfocol Tablets
2. Neo-128
3. Gentamicin Sulfate Injection
4. Gentocin Ophthalmic Solution
5. Amiglyde-V Injection

Adverse Side Effects. These include nephrotoxicity, ototoxicity, cardiotoxicity, and neuromuscular blockade.

Technician's Notes

1. Because aminoglycosides enhance the effects of neuromuscular blocking drugs, it is best to not use these drugs at the same time. Aminoglycoside blood levels can be determined before use of neuromuscular blocking drugs to prevent the development of muscular collapse.
2. Aminoglycosides are contraindicated in animals with renal insufficiency.
3. Aminoglycosides are not approved for use in food-producing animals.

FLUOROQUINOLONES

Fluoroquinolones are relatively new to veterinary medicine and have been approved for use in dogs, cats, turkeys, chickens, and cattle. Their use in horses continues to be controversial and is not approved (Plumb, 1999). The fluoroquinolones approved for use in veterinary medicine include enrofloxacin, difloxacin hydrochloride, orbifloxacin, sarafloxacin, and marbofloxacin. Fluoroquinolones have broad-spectrum activity against gram-positive and gram-negative bacteria.

PHARMACOKINETICS

Fluoroquinolones are available for oral and parenteral administration. After administration, they are readily absorbed into tissues and body fluids. Metabolism occurs in the liver, and elimination occurs by the kidneys into the urine or the bile into the intestines.

PHARMACODYNAMICS

The broad spectrum of activity offered by fluoroquinolones is bactericidal against many different pathogens. The effect of fluoroquinolones is achieved through inhibition or interference of the bacterial enzyme DNA-gyrase.

Clinical Uses. Clinical uses in dogs and cats include the treatment of bacterial skin and soft tissue infections, respiratory infections, and cystitis (dogs). Fluoroquinolones are used in cattle for the treatment of bovine respiratory disease, in chickens to control mortality associated with *E. coli,* and in turkeys to control mortality associated with *E. coli* and *Pasteurella multocida.*

Dosage Forms

1. Baytril Injectable and Tablets (dogs and cats)
2. Dicural Tablets (dogs)
3. Baytril 100 Injectable Solution (cattle)
4. Orbax Tablets (dogs and cats)
5. SaraFlox Injectable (turkeys and chickens)
6. Zeniquin (dogs)

Adverse Side Effects. Adverse side effects of fluoroquinolones include the formation of lesions in the joint articular cartilage during rapid growth phases of dogs. Fluoroquinolones have been associated with CNS stimulation and should be used with caution in animals with known or suspected CNS disorders.

Technician's Notes

1. The safety of fluoroquinolones in breeding or pregnant dogs and cats has not been determined.
2. Fluoroquinolones cannot be used in cattle intended for dairy production or in veal calves.
3. Fluoroquinolones cannot be used in laying hens that produce eggs for human consumption.
4. Carefully read labels regarding withdrawal periods for animals intended for slaughter.

OTHER ANTI-INFECTIVES

Chloramphenicol

Chloramphenicol is available in tablet, capsule, and ophthalmic formulations. It is a broad-spectrum antibiotic with action against gram-negative and gram-positive bacteria. It is readily absorbed into tissues and body fluids after administration. Chloramphenicol is metabolized by the liver and excreted through the kidneys into the urine.

Clinical Uses. Chloramphenicol is used to treat bacterial respiratory tract infections, urinary tract infections, enteritis, and bacterial conjunctivitis caused by chloramphenicol-susceptible organisms.

Dosage Forms

1. Chloramphenicol 1% Ophthalmic Ointment
2. Duricol Chloramphenicol Capsules

Adverse Side Effects. These include blood dyscrasias in cats after prolonged treatment.

Technician's Notes

1. Chloramphenicol is very stable and should not be used in food-producing animals because residual amounts of the drug can be left in meat, milk, or eggs.
2. Chloramphenicol is not recommended for dogs maintained for breeding purposes.
3. Chloramphenicol should not be administered simultaneously with penicillin, streptomycin, or cephalosporins.

Florfenicol

Florfenicol is available as an injectable solution. It has broad-spectrum activity against many gram-positive and gram-negative bacteria. It is primarily bacteriostatic and acts by inhibiting bacterial protein synthesis. Florfenicol is well-distributed in the body and can achieve therapeutic levels in the cerebrospinal fluid (Plumb, 1999).

Clinical Uses. Florfenicol is approved for the treatment of bovine respiratory disease associated with *Pasteurella haemolytica, P. multocida,* and *Haemophilus somnus.*

Dosage Form

1. Nuflor Injectable Solution

Adverse Side Effects. Adverse side effects include transient inappetence, decreased water consumption, or diarrhea.

Macrolides and Lincosamides

Macrolides and lincosamides are primarily effective against gram-positive organisms. The most common macrolides used in veterinary medicine are tilmicosin phosphate, erythromycin, and tylosin. The lincosamides include lincomycin, clindamycin, and pirlimycin. Clindamycin is also effective in treating anaerobic infections and is used to treat deep pyodermas, wounds, abscesses, and osteomyelitis.

Macrolides

Clinical Uses. Macrolides are used to treat upper respiratory tract infections, mastitis, metritis, and foot rot caused by microorganisms susceptible to macrolides.

Dosage Forms

1. Gallimycin-100 Injectable
2. Gallimycin-36
3. Tylan 200 Injection
4. Tylan Soluble
5. Micotil Injection

Adverse Side Effects. These include diarrhea, vomiting, and anorexia in small animals after oral administration of erythromycin and tylosin. Severe diarrhea may result after oral administration of erythromycin and tylosin in ruminants and horses. Intramuscular injection of erythromycin and tylosin is very painful. Adverse side effects are uncommon after subcutaneous injection of tilmicosin phosphate (Micotil) in cattle.

Lincosamides

Clinical Uses. Lincosamides are used to treat upper respiratory tract infections and skin infections in dogs, cats, and swine and mastitis in cattle. Lincomycin may also be found in combination with other agents for use in chickens. Clindamycin is approved for use in dogs and cats to treat deep pyoderma, wound infections, abscesses, dental infections, and osteomyelitis.

Dosage Forms

1. Antirobe Capsules
2. Antirobe Aquadrops
3. Lincocin Tablets
4. Lincocin Sterile Solution (swine)
5. Pirsue Aqueous Gel

Adverse Side Effects. These include occasional vomiting and diarrhea.

Vancomycin

Vancomycin is not commonly used in veterinary medicine. It is very effective against gram-positive pathogens, particularly coccus organisms. It is administered intravenously or orally. Oral administration (not absorbed) is only to control *Clostridium difficile*.

Clinical Uses. Vancomycin is used to treat resistant staphylococcal and streptococcal infections.

Dosage Forms
1. Vancocin Powder
2. Vancocin Injection

Adverse Side Effects. These include possible thrombophlebitis and febrile reactions (Beech et al., 1987). Ototoxicity, nephrotoxicity, and hypersensitivity are other possible side effects.

Spectinomycin

Spectinomycin is an aminocyclitol antibiotic that is primarily effective against gram-negative bacteria, some mycoplasma, and some gram-positive bacteria. Its action inhibits protein synthesis in susceptible bacteria. It is not generally effective against anaerobic bacteria.

Clinical Uses. These include for turkey poults and chicks control of airsacculitis and chronic respiratory disease caused by organisms sensitive to spectinomycin. In baby pigs, it is used to control and treat infectious diarrhea due to *Escherichia coli*. In cattle, it is indicated for the treatment of bovine respiratory disease associated with *Pasteurella haemolytica, Pasteurella multocida,* and *Haemophilus somnus.*

Dosage Forms
1. Spectam Injectable (turkey poults and chicks)
2. Spectam Scour-Halt (swine)
3. Adspec Sterile Solution (cattle)

Adverse Side Effects. These are uncommon. Mild swelling at the injection site may occur in cattle.

Technician's Notes
1. Do not use in female dairy cattle 20 months of age or older.
2. Do not use in veal calves.
3. Carefully read labels about use in animals for slaughter.
4. Approved only for use in swine younger than 4 weeks of age or weighing less than 15 pounds.

Polymyxin B and Bacitracin

Polymixin B and bacitracin are restricted to topical skin and ophthalmic applications. These drugs are of-ten combined with other drugs (e.g., neomycin) in topical skin and ophthalmic ointments.

Clinical Uses. These include treatment of superficial bacterial infections of the eye, conjunctiva, and skin.

Dosage Forms
1. Mycitracin Sterile Ointment
2. Forte Topical
3. Neobacimyx Ophthalmic Solution

Adverse Side Effects. Adverse side effects of polymyxin B include nephrotoxicity and neurotoxicity if administered parenterally (Beech et al., 1987). Bacitracin is limited to topical application because it causes nephrotoxicity.

Technician's Notes
Care should be taken to avoid contaminating the applicator tip.

Sulfonamides

Sulfonamides, or sulfa drugs, are **antibacterials** that offer a relatively broad spectrum of activity against gram-positive and gram-negative bacteria. The most common sulfonamides used in veterinary medicine are sulfadiazine, sulfisoxazole, and sulfadimethoxine. Trimethoprim, pyrimethamine, and ormetoprim are commonly combined with sulfonamides to enhance their therapeutic index.

Clinical Uses. Sulfonamides are used to treat acute urinary tract infections, respiratory tract infections, wound infections, coccidiosis, and foot rot.

Dosage Forms
1. Tribrissen 48% Injection
2. Primor Tablets
3. Albon Boluses
4. Albon Oral Suspension 5%
5. Sustain III Cattle Bolus

Adverse Side Effects. These include urticaria, hives, vomiting, diarrhea, anorexia, fever, and crystal formation within the kidneys, which can result in hematuria, proteinuria, and renal tubular damage.

Keratoconjunctivitis sicca has been reported in dogs. The use of these drugs has been limited in food-producing animals because of residues of the drug in meat, milk, and eggs.

Technician's Notes
Maintaining normal hydration can decrease the risk of crystal formation in the kidneys.

Nitrofurans

Nitrofurans are a group of antibacterials with broad-spectrum activity. The most common nitrofurans used in clinical practice are nitrofurazone, nitrofurantoin, and furazolidone.

Clinical Uses. These include treatment of superficial bacterial infections of wounds, necrotic enteritis in swine, coccidiosis in chickens, and bacterial enteritis in pigs less than 4 weeks old. Nitrofurazone may also be used to treat pink eye in cattle, sheep, and goats and eye and ear infections in dogs and cats.

Dosage Forms
1. NFZ Puffer
2. Nitrofurazone Soluble Dressing
3. Nitrofurazone 0.2% Solution

Adverse Side Effects. Adverse side effects are uncommon.

Technician's Notes
1. The use of nitrofurans has been prohibited in food-producing animals except for approved topical use.
2. Nitrofurans should not be used in veal calves.

ANTIFUNGAL DRUGS

Fungal infections, or mycoses, are classified into two types: topical (superficial), affecting the skin and mucous membranes, and systemic, affecting such areas as the blood, lungs, or CNS. The diagnosis of a topical fungal infection may be determined by direct microscopic examination for the presence of delicate hyphae in skin cells or the presence of spores on the surface of an infected hair. Dermatophyte test medium is available for topical fungal identification at in-hospital laboratories (Figure 12-4). Systemic mycosis is usually diagnosed in large laboratories by serologic testing. Fungal infections are treated by oral, topical, or parenteral administration of drugs that are suitable for these infections. The antifungal, or antimycotic, drugs are divided into four classes: (1) polyene, (2) imidazole, (3) antimetabolic, and (4) superficial agents.

Polyene Antifungal Agents
Amphotericin B
Amphotericin B is an antifungal drug that may be **fungistatic** or **fungicidal**.

Clinical Uses. These drugs are used to treat systemic mycotic infections in dogs and cats.

Dosage Form
1. Fungizone (human label)

Adverse Side Effects. Numerous toxicities such as anorexia, vomiting, seizures, anemia, and cardiac arrest have been reported with the use of amphotericin B. Nephrotoxicity also occurs in most patients that receive this drug (Beech et al., 1987.)

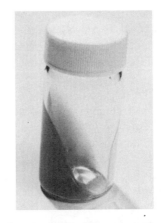

Figure 12-4

Dermatophyte test medium may be used to culture topical fungal infections. This medium contains a phenol red indicator that turns red as a dermatophyte grows and produces alkaline metabolic products.

Technician's Notes

1. Amphotericin B is administered intravenously by diluting in 5% dextrose.
2. Renal function should be monitored closely during treatment.

Nystatin

Nystatin may be fungistatic or fungicidal. It is often combined with other drugs such as neomycin, thiostrepton, and triamcinolone acetonide.

Clinical Uses. Nystatin is used to treat candidiasis infections of the skin, mucous membranes, and the intestinal tract in dogs and cats.

Dosage Forms

1. Animax Ointment
2. Dermalone Ointment
3. Panolog Cream

Adverse Side Effects. Adverse side effects are uncommon.

Imidazole Antifungal Agents

Ketoconazole and Miconazole

Ketoconazole and miconazole are two of the most commonly used drugs in this class. Ketoconazole is available in oral and topical preparations, and miconazole is available in parenteral and topical preparations.

Clinical Uses. These include the treatment of some systemic mycotic infections and some dermatophyoses and *Candida* infections in dogs and cats.

Dosage Forms

1. Nizoral Tablets (human label)—ketoconazole
2. Nizoral Cream (human label)—ketoconazole
3. Monistat (human label)—miconazole
4. Conofite Lotion or Spray—miconazole

Adverse Side Effects. Adverse side effects are not as severe as those of amphotericin B and are uncommon. Ketoconazole may produce hepatotoxicity. Miconazole may produce tachycardia, arrhythmias, fever, nausea, and thrombophlebitis after intravenous administration.

Technician's Notes

Ketoconazole may cause infertility in male dogs.

Itraconazole

Itraconazole is the most recent imidazole available for use in veterinary medicine.

Clinical Uses. Itraconazole is used to treat systemic mycotic infections in dogs and cats.

Dosage Form

1. Sporanox Capsules (human label)

Adverse Side Effects. These include anorexia associated with hepatotoxicity, ulcerative dermatitis resulting from vasculitis, and possible cardiotoxicity. Severe adverse reactions are uncommon.

Antimetabolic Antifungal Agents

Flucytosine

Flucytosine is a fungistatic oral antifungal agent. This drug may be used in combination with other antifungal agents for the treatment of some yeast infections.

Clinical Uses. Flucytosine is used to treat cryptococcal infections, but it inhibits the growth of other fungi as well.

Dosage Form

1. Ancobon (human label)

Adverse Side Effects. These include bone marrow depression, anemia, leukopenia, and thrombocytopenia. Severe reactions may occur in patients with renal insufficiency.

Superficial Antifungal Agents

Griseofulvin

Griseofulvin is primarily used in dogs, cats, and horses as an antifungal. It is administered orally in the form of a tablet or powder.

Clinical Uses. Griseofulvin is used to treat **dermatophytosis**.

Dosage Forms

1. Fulvicin-U/F Tablets
2. Fulvicin-U/F Powder

Adverse Side Effects. Adverse side effects are uncommon.

Technician's Notes

1. Griseofulvin should not be administered to pregnant or breeding animals.
2. Absorption of griseofulvin is enhanced by administering it with a fatty meal.

Other Antifungal Agents

Several agents that have other uses are also effective as topical antifungal drugs. A topical preparation is often used in conjunction with systemic antifungal drugs. Commonly used topical preparations include chlorhexidine, iodine, tolnaftate, benzoic acid, salicylic acid, and thiabendazole.

 ANTIVIRAL DRUGS

Antiviral drugs are used to treat viral infections. Their use in veterinary medicine is still limited, but research is increasing the use of these drugs for treatment of viral infections in animals. Since there are not any veterinary-approved antiviral agents, human-approved antiviral agents are used. Antivirals may be used for treating optic viral infections and non-neoplastic feline leukemia virus (FeLV)–associated disease. Antiviral drugs are available for topical and systematic use. Other antiviral drugs that also may be beneficial to veterinary medicine include amantadine, ganciclovir, idoxuridine, and azidothymidine.

Acyclovir

Clinical Uses. In veterinary medicine, acyclovir may be used in birds for the treatment of Pacheco's disease and in cats for confirmed feline herpes virus infection of the conjunctiva or cornea in which other treatments have failed (Plumb, 1999).

Dosage Forms

1. Zovirax tablets and capsules (human label)
2. Zovirax suspension (human label)
3. Zoviral injectable (human label)

Adverse Side Effects. Adverse side effects include leukopenia and anemias in treated cats. In birds, tissue necrosis can occur at the injection site if used parenterally for more than 72 hours (Oglesbee and Bishop, 1994).

Interferon Alfa-2A, Human Recombinant

Clinical Uses. In veterinary medicine interferon alfa-2A is administered orally to treat non-neoplastic FeLV disease in cats.

Dosage Form

1. Roferon-A

Adverse Side Effects. No adverse side effects have been noted (Plumb, 1999).

DISINFECTANTS/ANTISEPTICS

The use of disinfectants in a veterinary hospital ranges from table sprays to premise cleaners (Figure 12-5, p. 223). A disinfectant destroys disease-producing microorganisms or inactivates viruses. Its application is primarily for use on inanimate objects. Disinfection time is the time required for a particular agent to produce its maximum effect. This time varies with different agents but can be affected by a range of factors such as the type of material being disinfected, the amount of soil and microbial contamination, and the concentration of the disinfectant and its germicidal potency. Antiseptics are used on live tissue to destroy microorganisms. The terms *disinfectant* and *antiseptic* are commonly used inter-

TABLE 12-5 Disinfectant Preparations and Their Activity

Disinfectant Group	Proprietary Products	Recommen- dations	Bacteri- cidal	General Virucide	Fungicidal	Sporicidal at Room Temperature
Quaternary ammonium compounds	Q-Cide Roccal-D Plus D-128	Instruments, dairy equipment, rubber goods	M	M	M	N
Phenolics	Panteck Cleanser Lysol I.C. Disinfectant Spray Beaucoup	Laundry rinse, floors, walls, equipment	M	M	H	N
Halogens	*Chlorines:* Clorox Purex	Floors, spot disinfection	M	H	H	S
	Iodophors: Betadine Povidine Iosan	Presurgical skin preparation, thermometers, dairy operation	H	H	M	S
Glutaraldehyde	Cidex	Instruments	H	H	H	M
Chlorhexidine	Nolvasan Virosan	Instruments, surgical scrub, dairy operation	M	M	M	N
Alcohols	Isopropyl alcohol 70%	Instruments, thermometers, skin preparation	H	N	S	N

M, Moderate activity; *N,* no activity; *H,* high activity; *S,* slight activity.

changeably. Table 12-5 illustrates common products and their uses.

Alcohols

Alcohols, such as ethyl and isopropyl, work by protein coagulation and dissociation of membrane lipids. They are bactericidal, tuberculocidal, and active against some viruses, but they are not **sporicidal** or active against fungi. Alcohols do not penetrate organic material.

Clinical Uses. These include disinfection of ther-

mometers and instruments, for skin preparations, and for spot disinfections.

Adverse Side Effects. Alcohols can corrode metal and can be drying to skin.

Technician's Notes

1. Iodine (1% to 2%) can be added to alcohol for thermometer disinfection to increase its activity against spores and viruses.
2. Alcohols should not be applied to open wounds.

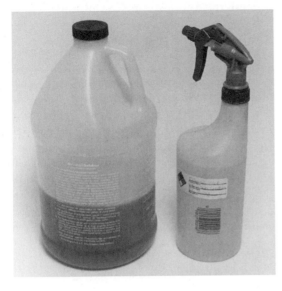

Figure 12-5

The concentrations of disinfectants vary from dilutions for disinfecting kennels, floors, and so forth to dilutions for use as table sprays.

Ethylene Oxide

Ethylene oxide works by substitution of the cell alkyl groups for labile hydrogen atoms. It sterilizes against bacteria, fungi, and viruses.

Clinical Uses. Ethylene oxide is used to sterilize inanimate objects such as blankets, pillows, mattresses, lensed instruments, rubber goods, thermolabile plastics, books, and papers.

Adverse Side Effects. Adverse side effects are uncommon.

> **Technician's Notes**
> Special equipment is required to use ethylene oxide as a sterilization gas.

Formaldehyde

The mode of action for formaldehyde is the same as for ethylene oxide. It is non-corrosive and is effective against bacteria, fungi, spores, and viruses.

Clinical Uses. Formaldehyde is used as a disinfecting gas or solution. The gas can be used to **disinfect** large areas such as a cabinet or incubator. The solution is appropriate for instrument disinfection. Delicate instruments may be vapor disinfected.

Adverse Side Effects. These include toxicity to skin and mucous membranes because of its strong odor.

> **Technician's Notes**
> 1. For adequate disinfection, formaldehyde requires long contact time.
> 2. Organic material inactivates its effectiveness.

Chlorines and Iodines

Chlorines and iodines are halogens that inactivate pathogens by oxidizing free sulfhydryl groups on bacterial enzymes. Chlorines are bactericidal, have high activity against viruses, and are fungicidal and tuberculocidal unless highly diluted. Iodines and **iodophors** are bactericidal, have high activity against viruses, are fungicidal and tuberculocidal, and are effective against bacterial spores.

Clinical Uses. Chlorines are recommended for floors, plumbing fixtures, spot disinfection, and fabrics not harmed by bleaching. Iodine tincture is used for skin preparations and thermometers (see the Alcohols section). Iodophors are used to disinfect thermometers, utensils, rubber goods, and dishes and for presurgical skin preparation.

Dosage Forms

1. Clorox bleach
2. Iodine tincture 7%
3. Betadine Surgical Scrub
4. Povidone Solution

Adverse Side Effects. The strong vapor of chlorines may irritate the eyes and mucous membranes. Skin irritation may result by failing to rinse a chlorine-disinfected surface. Chlorine bleaches colored fabrics and is corrosive to most metals (not to quality stainless steel). Tinctures of iodine contain alcohol and are drying to the skin. They stain and may corrode metal.

Iodophors may corrode metal; iodine solutions stain and may corrode metal, and high concentrations (3.5%) may irritate living tissue.

Technician's Notes

1. These compounds are inactivated by organic material.
2. Always check labels for dilution requirements.
3. Iodophors are less staining and irritating than other iodine compounds.

Phenolics: Saponated Cresol, Semi-Synthetic Phenols

The mode of action of phenolics is protein coagulation. They destroy selective permeability of cell membranes, and leakage of cell constituents results. They are effective against bacteria, fungi, and some viruses, but they are not sporicidal and are only weakly effective against non-enveloped viruses (e.g., parvovirus). Cresol must be used in soft water and is slow acting. Phenolics are not inactivated by organic matter, soap, or hard water (except cresol). They have high detergency and a residual effect if allowed to dry on surfaces.

Clinical Uses. These include use as a general disinfectant for laundry, floors, walls, and equipment.

Dosage Forms

1. Panteck Cleanser
2. Beaucoup
3. Lysol I.C. Disinfectant Spray

Adverse Side Effects. Adverse side effects are uncommon, but repeated and prolonged skin exposure may cause accumulation in tissues and eventual toxic effects such as neurotoxicity or teratogenic effects.

Technician's Notes

Some phenolics have objectionable odors.

Quaternary Ammonium Compounds: Cationic Detergents

Cationic **detergents** concentrate at the cell membrane and are thought to act by dissolving lipids in cell walls and membranes. They are more active against gram-positive than against gram-negative organisms. They are bacteriostatic at high dilutions, but spores, viruses, mycobacteria, and *Pseudomonas aeruginosa* are relatively resistant. Quaternary ammonium compounds are inactivated by organic debris, hard water, and anionic soaps and detergents.

Clinical Uses. These include cleaning instruments, utensils, inanimate objects, and rubber goods. They may be used for instrument soaks except for instruments with cemented lenses.

Dosage Forms

1. Roccal-D Plus
2. Q-Cide
3. D-128

Adverse Side Effects. Adverse side effects are uncommon.

Technician's Notes

Read labels carefully because some quaternary ammonium compounds do not effectively disinfect against some common viruses (e.g., parvovirus).

Biguanide Compounds

Chlorhexidine is the most common disinfectant in this group. In high dilutions, it is bactericidal, fungicidal, and active against enveloped viruses (e.g., feline infectious peritonitis virus and feline leukemia virus). Other viruses, spores, and mycobacteria are relatively resistant.

Clinical Uses. These include disinfecting surgical instruments, anesthetic equipment, and kennels. It is also available as a surgical scrub and teat dip.

Dosage Forms

1. Nolvasan Solution
2. Nolvasan Surgical Scrub
3. Virosan Solution

Adverse Side Effects. Adverse side effects are uncommon.

Other Disinfectants

Soaps. Soaps, or anionic detergents, have only slight bactericidal activity but are effective in the mechanical removal of organisms. They are not sporicidal or tuberculocidal and have limited virucidal activity. They often contain germicides such as triclosan to decrease the number of resident flora after washing. Their mode of action is the same as for cationic detergents.

Organic Mercury Compounds. These compounds, such as merbromin (Mercurochrome) and thimerosal (Merthiolate), may be used as antiseptics. These compounds have only slight bactericidal activity.

Alkalis. Alkalis such as lye and quicklime may be used for disinfecting stables and premises.

Hydrogen Peroxide. Hydrogen peroxide is an oxidizing agent available as a 3% aqueous solution that may be used for cleaning and disinfecting wounds and as a mouthwash for septic stomatitis.

Glutaraldehyde. Glutaraldehyde is a dialdehyde and is bactericidal, virucidal, fungicidal, and sporicidal. It is not inactivated by organic debris. Its uses include disinfecting surgical instruments, anesthetic equipment, floors, walls, and non-food contact surfaces.

REFERENCES

Beech, J., Bistner, S., Boothe, D.M., et al.: The Bristol Veterinary Handbook of Antimicrobial Therapy, 2nd ed. Veterinary Learning Systems Company, Trenton, NJ, 1987.

Ettinger, S.J.: Pocket Companion to Textbook of Veterinary Internal Medicine. W.B. Saunders Company, Philadelphia, 1993.

Oglesbee, B., Bishop, C.: Avian infectious diseases. In Birchard, S., Sherding, R (eds.): Saunders Manual of Small Animal Practice. W.B. Saunders Company, Philadelphia, 1994.

Plumb, D.C.: Veterinary Drug Handbook, 3rd ed. Iowa State University Press, Ames, 1999.

Williams, B.R., Baer, C.L.: Essentials of Clinical Pharmacology in Nursing. Springhouse Corporation, Springhouse, PA, 1990.

■ Review Questions

1. Name the most common classifications of bacteria.

   _____

2. What determines the susceptibility of an organism to an antibiotic on an agar diffusion test?

   _____

3. Define minimal inhibitory concentration.

   _____

4. Discuss the effect of beta-lactamase I on the effectiveness of penicillins. _____

5. What side effects are related to the use of tetracycline in pregnant animals? Juveniles?

   _____

6. Discuss the side effects of aminoglycosides.

   _____

7. How can the nephrotoxicity of aminoglycosides be monitored in a patient?

   _____

8. How is amphotericin administered for systemic mycosis?

   _____

9. What does *disinfection time* refer to?

   _____

10. What factors affect the disinfection time?

    _____

Antiparasitic Drugs

LEARNING OBJECTIVES

After studying this chapter, you should be able to:

1. Know the ingredients found in common anthelmintics and insecticides
2. Understand the delivery systems of insecticides
3. Educate clients about products covered in this chapter
4. Know the importance of reading and understanding product labels
5. Know the different classes of parasiticides and any contraindications for each particular class

INTRODUCTION

Veterinary technicians have an important role in the use of parasiticides. One of the most important aspects of this role is the responsibility for being familiar with products used in the hospital—how they are used and what to expect when using them. Clients rely on you to help them to choose which products will best suit their needs when trying to control **ectoparasites** such as ticks and fleas. They want to know how the dewormer is going to affect their new puppy, whether a product is safe to use in their pregnant queen, why their dog that only eats from the table continues to get tapeworms, and what those little yellow things are that are stuck on their horse's legs. After studying this chapter and taking a parasitology class, you will be able to help your clients answer these questions. Remember that data are continually changing, and it is important to keep up with these changes. Reading package inserts also helps you to understand how a particular drug works. Tables 13-1 to 13-5 will help you to identify products and their uses for various species.

ENDOPARASITES

Control of internal parasites is an important part of proper animal care. **Endoparasites** affect the well-being of all animals and can cause great economic loss in food animals. This section discusses some of the most common **anthelmintics** used in clinical practice today. Be aware that as a veterinary technician, you will probably come into contact with products not mentioned in this section. The charts in this section list various products, their proprietary names, and their effectiveness. Many veterinarians choose just a few products to meet their needs and to limit the amount of inventory used for anthelmintics. Some products are available under many different names. As you come into contact with these products during your work in a practice, you will become more familiar with the different brands available. The anthelmintics available today are more effective against parasites and less toxic to hosts (McCurnin, 1994). New product types have made administration easier for clients and veterinarians. Many products are available in several forms, such as powder mix for drinking water, liquid, paste, or tablets/capsules for oral administration. Some products are also available for parenteral administration.

 ANTINEMATODAL

Benzimidazoles

Dosage Forms. This class includes the following products:

1. Thiabendazole (Equizole, TBZ, Omnizole)
2. Oxibendazole (Anthelcide EQ)
3. Mebendazole (Telmin, Telmintic)
4. Febendazole (Panacur)
5. Cambendazole (Camvet)
6. Oxfendazole (Benzelmin, Synanthic)
7. Albendazole (Valbazen)

Clinical Uses. Benzimidazoles are used in the following species:

1. Horses. Effective against strongyli, pinworms, and ascarids.
2. Cattle. Ascarids, several species of strongyli and other stomach worms; albendazole is also effective against adult liver flukes and tapeworms; febendazole is also effective against lungworms.
3. Sheep and goats. Ascarids, several species of strongyli and other stomach worms; Panacur is also effective against lungworms.
4. Dogs. Hookworms, roundworms, whipworms; some are effective against *Taenia pisiformis* but not *Dipylidium caninum.*
5. Swine. *Strongyloides* and lungworms.
6. Many of the benzimidazoles are used as anthelmintics for exotics such as snakes and birds.

Adverse Side Effects. These are uncommon but include vomiting and diarrhea. Mebendazole has clinically produced hepatotoxicity in dogs.

Technician's Notes

1. Read labels carefully regarding use in lactating dairy animals and animals to be slaughtered.
2. None of these products are approved for use in cats.

Organophosphates

Dosage Forms. This class includes the following products:

1. Trichlorfon (Combot, Dyrex T.F., Equibot TC)
2. Coumaphos (Baymix, Dairy Dewormer BX Crumbles
3. Haloxon (Loxon)
4. Dichlorvos (Task, Atgard)

Clinical Uses. **Organophosphates** are used in the following species:

1. Horses. Effective against **bots,** roundworms, strongyli, and pinworms but less effective against *Strongyloides.*
2. Cattle, sheep, and goats. Strongyli.
3. Dogs and cats. Hookworms, roundworms, whipworms.
4. Swine. Ascarids, whipworms, nodule worms, strongyli.

Adverse Side Effects. Adverse side effects include those expected with any organophosphate poisoning: excessive salivation, vomiting, diarrhea, muscle tremors, and miosis.

Technician's Notes

1. It is very important that these anthelmintics not be administered concurrently or within a few days of the use of other cholinesterase inhibitors, other organophosphates, succinylcholine, or phenothiazine derivative agents.
2. Atropine and 2-PAM are antidotal.
3. Read labels carefully regarding use in lactating dairy animals and animals to be slaughtered.

TABLE 13-1 Parasiticides Used for Treatment and Control of Internal Parasites in Dogs and Cats

Drug (Trade Name)	Parasite		
	Toxocara-Toxascaris	Ancylostoma-Uncinaria	Strongyloides
Albendazole (Valbazen)	+	+	−
Amprolium (Corid)	−	−	−
Butamisole hydrochloride (Styquin)	−	+	−
Dichlorophene (many trade names)	−	−	−
Dichlorophene/toluene (many trade names)	+	+	−
Dichlorvos (many trade names)	+	+	−
Diethylcarbamazine (many trade names)	+	−	−
Epsiprantel (Cestex)	−	−	−
Febantel/praziquantel (Parasiticide-10)	+	+	−
Fenbendazole (Panacur)	+	+	−
Furazolidone (many trade names)	−	−	−
Ivermectin (Heartgard 30)	−	−	−
Ivermectin (Heartgard 30 Plus)	+	+	−
Ivermectin (Ivomec)	+	+	−
Mebendazole (Telmintic Powder)	+	+	−
Melarsomine dihydrochloride (Immiticide)	−	−	−
Metronidazole (Flagyl)	−	−	−
Milbemycin oxime (Interceptor)	+	+	−
N-Butyl chloride (many trade names)	+	+	−
Nitroscanate (Lopatol)	+	+	−
Oxibendazole/DEC (Filaribits Plus)	+	+	−
Piperazine salts (many trade names)	+	−	−
Praziquantel (Droncit)	−	−	−
Pyrantel pamoate (Nemex)	+	+	−
Praziquantel/pyrantel pamoate (Drontal)	+	+	−
Praziquantel/pyrantel pamoate/febantel (Drontal Plus)	+	+	−
Quinacrine hydrochloride (Atabrine)	−	−	−
Sulfadiazine/trimethoprim (many trade names)	−	−	−
Sulfadimethoxine (many trade names)	−	−	−
Thiabendazole (Mintezol)	−	−	+
Thiacetarsamide sodium (Caparsolate)	−	−	−
Tinidazole (available in England)	−	−	−

From McCurnin, D.M.: Clinical Textbook for Veterinary Technicians, 4th ed. W.B. Saunders Company, Philadelphia, 1998.
+, Indicated for use; −, not indicated for use.

| | | | Parasite | | | |
Trichuris	Dirofilaria Adults	Dirofilaria Microfilariae	Taenia	Dipylidium	Giardia	Coccidia
+	−	−	+	−	+	−
−	−	−	−	−	−	+
+	−	−	−	−	−	−
−	−	−	+	+	−	−
−	−	−	+	+	−	−
+	−	−	−	−	−	−
−	−	+	−	−	−	−
−	−	−	+	+	−	−
+	−	−	+	+	−	−
+	−	−	+	−	−	−
−	−	−	−	−	+	−
−	−	+	−	−	−	−
−	−	+	−	−	−	−
+	−	+	−	−	−	−
+	−	−	+	−	−	−
−	+	−	−	−	−	−
−	−	−	−	−	+	−
+	−	+	−	−	−	−
−	−	−	−	−	−	−
+	−	−	+	+	−	−
+	−	+	−	−	−	−
−	−	−	−	−	−	−
−	−	−	+	+	−	−
−	−	−	−	−	−	−
−	−	−	+	+	−	−
+	−	−	+	+	−	−
−	−	−	−	−	+	−
−	−	−	−	−	−	+
−	−	−	−	−	−	+
−	−	−	−	−	−	−
−	+	−	−	−	−	−
−	−	−	−	−	+	−

TABLE 13-2   Parasiticides Used for Treatment of Internal Parasites in Horses

Drug	Gaster-ophilus	Ascarids	Strongylus Vulgaris	Strongylus Edentatus	Small Strongyles	Pin-worms	Strongy-loides
Cambendazole (Camvet)	−	+	+	+	+	+	+
Dichlorvos (many trade names)	+	+	+	+	+	+	−
Fenbendazole (Panacur)	−	+	+	+	+	+	+
Ivermectin (Eqvalan)	+	+	+	+	+	+	+
Oxibendazole (Anthelcide EQ)	−	+	+	+	+	+	+
Oxifendazole (Benzelmin)	−	+	+	+	+	+	+
Phenothiazine (many trade names)	−	−	+	−	+	−	−
Piperazine salts (many trade names)	−	+	−	−	+	+	−
Pyrantel salts (many trade names)	−	+	+	+	+	−	−
Thiabendazole (many trade names)	−	−	+	+	+	+	+
Thiabendazole/ piperazine (Equizole A)	−	+	+	+	+	+	+
Thiabendazole/ trichlorfon (many trade names)	+	+	+	+	+	+	+
Trichlorfon (many trade names)	+	+	−	−	−	+	−
Trichlorfon/ phenothiazine/ piperazine (Dyrex)	+	+	+	−	+	+	−

From McCurnin, D.M.: Clinical Textbook for Veterinary Technicians, 4th ed. W.B. Saunders Company, Philadelphia, 1998.
+, Indicated for use; −, not indicated for use.

Tetrahydropyrimidines

Dosage Forms. This class includes the following products:

1. Pyrantel pamoate (Nemex, Strongid-T)
2. Pyrantel tartrate (Banminth 48)
3. Morantel tartrate (Nematel, Rumatel)

Clinical Uses. Tetrahydropyrimidines are used in the following species:

1. Horses. Ascarids, strongyli, pinworms.
2. Cattle, sheep, and goats. Strongyli.
3. Dogs and cats. Hookworms, roundworms.
4. Swine. Roundworms, strongyli.

Adverse Side Effects. These are uncommon but may include increased respiration, profuse sweating, or incoordination.

Imidazothiazoles

Dosage Forms. This class includes the following products:

1. Febantel (Rintal)
2. Levamisole (Tramisol, Levasole)

Clinical Uses. Imidazothiazoles are used in the following species:

1. Horses. Ascarids, strongyli.
2. Cattle, sheep, and goats. Strongyli, lungworms.
3. Dogs and cats. Febantel—hookworms, roundworms, whipworms; levamisole has been used in dogs as a microfilaricide.
4. Swine. Strongyli, *Strongyloides,* lungworms, nodule worms.
5. These products may also be used effectively in some exotic species.

Adverse Side Effects. These include transient foaming at the mouth.

Avermectins

Dosage Forms. This class includes the following products:

1. Ivermectin (Heartgard, Heartgard Plus, Heartgard for Cats, Eqvalan, Ivomec)
2. Moxidectin (ProHeart, Quest 2% Equine Oral Gel, Cydectin Pour-On)
3. Doramectin (Dectomax Injectable Solution, Dectomax Pour-On)

Clinical Uses

Ivermectin
1. Horses. Large and small strongles, pinworms, ascarids, hairworms, large-mouth stomach worms, neck threadworms, bots, lungworms, intestinal threadworms, and summer sores secondary to *Habronema* or *Draschia* spp.
2. Cattle. Gastrointestinal roundworms, lungworms, cattle grubs, sucking lice, and mites.
3. Swine. Gastrointestinal roundworms, lungworms, lice, and mage mites.
4. Dogs. Effective preventative for *Dirofilaria immitis;* Heartgard Plus contains pyrantel pamoate and is effective against hookworms and roundworms.
5. Cats. Effective preventative for *D. immitis* and for the removal of hookworms.
6. Birds and snakes. Effective against some endoparasites and ectoparasites.

Moxidectin
1. Horses. Large and small strongles, encysted cyathostomes, ascarids, pinworms, hairworms, large-mouth stomach worms, and bots.
2. Cattle. Gastrointestinal roundworms, lungworms, cattle grubs, mites, lice, and horn flies.
3. Dogs. Effective preventative for *D. immitis.*

Text continued on p. 238.

TABLE 13-3 Parasiticides Used for Treatment of Internal Parasites in Cattle, Sheep, and Goats

Drug	Hae-monchus	Oster-tagia	Tricho-strongylus	Cooperia	Nema-todirus	Strongly-loides
Albendazole (Valbazen)	+	+	+	+	+	−
Amprolium (Corid)	−	−	−	−	−	−
Chlorsulon (Curatrem)	−	−	−	−	−	−
Decoquinate (Deccox)	−	−	−	−	−	−
Doramectin (Dectomax)	+	+	+	+	+	−
Fenbendazole (many trade names)	+	+	+	+	+	+
Haloxon (Loxon)	+	+	+	+	−	−
Ivermectin (Ivomec)	+	+	+	+	+	+
Lasolacid (Bovatec)	−	−	−	−	−	−
Levamisole (many trade names)	+	+	+	+	+	+
Monensin (Rumensin)	−	−	−	−	−	−
Morantel tartrate (Rumatel)	+	+	+	+	+	+
Phenothiazine (many trade names)	+	+	+	−	−	−
Sulfonamides (many trade names)	−	−	−	−	−	−
Thiabendazole (many trade names)	+	+	+	+	+	+

From McCurnin, D.M.: Clinical Textbook for Veterinary Technicians, 4th ed. W.B. Saunders Company, Philadelphia, 1998.
+, Indicated for use; −, not indicated for use.

				Parasite			
Buno-stomum	Trichuris	Oesophago-stomum	Chabertia	Dictyo-caulus	Monezia	Fasciola	Coccidia
+	−	+	+	+	+	+	−
−	−	−	−	−	−	−	+
−	−	−	−	−	−	+	−
−	−	−	−	−	−	−	+
−	−	−	−	−	−	−	−
+	+	+	+	+	−	−	−
−	−	−	−	−	−	−	−
+	−	+	+	+	−	−	−
−	−	−	−	−	−	−	+
+	+	+	+	+	−	−	−
−	−	−	−	−	−	−	+
+	−	+	+	−	−	−	−
−	−	+	−	−	−	−	−
−	−	−	−	−	−	−	+
+	−	+	+	−	−	−	−

TABLE 13-4 Parasiticides Used for Treatment of Internal Parasites in Swine

Drug	Ascaris	Strongy-loides	Oesoph-agosto-mum	Trichuris	Hyo-stron-gylus	Meta-stron-gylus	Stepha-nurus	Coccidia
Dichlorvos (Atgard)	+	−	+	+	+	−	−	−
Fenbendazole (many trade names)	+	−	+	+	+	+	−	−
Hygromycin B (Hygromix)	+	−	+	+	−	−	−	−
Ivermectin (Ivomec)	+	+	+	−	+	+	+	−
Levamisole (many trade names)	+	+	+	−	+	+	+	−
Piperazine salts (many trade names)	+	−	−	−	−	−	−	−
Pyrantel tartrate (Banminth)	+	−	+	−	−	−	−	−
Sulfonamides (many trade names)	−	−	−	−	−	−	−	+
Thiabendazole (many trade names)	−	+	+	−	+	−	−	−

From McCurnin, D.M.: Clinical Textbook for Veterinary Technicians, 4th ed. W.B. Saunders Company, Philadelphia, 1998.
+, Indicated for use; −, not indicated for use.

TABLE 13-5 Drugs Used to Treat Internal Parasites in Reptiles

Drug	Parasite						
	Ecto-parasites	Nema-todes	Trema-todes	Cestodes	Crypto-sporidia	Coccidia	Amoebae and Tricho-monads
Metronidazole (Flagyl)	−	−	−	−	−	−	+
Humatin 400 (Paromomycin)	−	−	−	−	−	−	+
Praziquantel (Droncit)	−	−	+	+	−	−	−
Febantel plus Praziquantel (Vercom)	−	+	+	+	−	−	−
Dichlorvos (Task)	−	+	−	−	−	−	−
Levamisole (Tramisol, Ripercol)	−	+	−	−	−	−	−
Thiabendazole (Thibenzole)	−	+	−	−	−	−	−
Fenbendazole (Panacur)	−	+	−	−	−	−	−
Mebendazole (Telmin)	−	+	−	−	−	−	−
Ivermectin* (Ivomec)	+	+	−	−	−	−	−
Dithiazanine iodide (Dizan)	−	+	−	−	−	−	−
Vapona Strip	+	−	−	−	−	−	−
Sulfadiazine (many trade names)	−	−	−	−	−	+	−
Sulfamerazine (many trade names)	−	−	−	−	−	+	−
Sulfamethazine (many trade names)	−	−	−	−	−	+	−
Sulfadimethoxine (Albon)	−	−	−	−	−	+	−
Trimethoprim plus Sulfadiazine (Di-Trim, Tribrissen)	−	−	−	−	+	+	−

+Effective.
−Not effective.

*Do not use in chelonians. Contraindicated in animals that have been given diazepam or will receive diazepam within 10 days of administration of ivermectin.

Data from Frye, F.L.: Reptile Care, vol I. T.F.H. Publications, Neptune City, NJ, 1991.

Doramectin

1. Cattle. Gastrointestinal roundworms, lungworms, eyeworms, grubs, biting and sucking lice, horn flies, and mange mites.
2. Swine. Gastrointestinal roundworms, lungworms, kidney worms, sucking lice, and mange mites.

Adverse Side Effects. These are uncommon. Toxic signs include mydriasis, ataxia, tremors, and depression.

> **Technician's Notes**
> 1. Although not approved, Ivomec is sometimes used for the treatment of ear mites in cats and scabies in dogs.
> 2. Because of the small amount of medication in the heartworm preventatives, crumbling or breaking the tablets or chewables is not recommended.
> 3. Read labels carefully regarding use in lactating dairy animals and animals for slaughter. Moxidectin is approved for use in dairy cattle of all ages and stages of lactation, except for veal calves.

Other Agents

Piperazine (Pipa-tabs, Pip-pop 320)

1. Dogs and cats. Roundworms.
2. Used effectively in exotics such as birds and snakes.
3. Commonly combined in large-animal dewormers to broaden its spectrum and increase its efficacy.

Praziquantel/Pyrantel Pamoate/Febantel (Drontal Plus)

1. Dogs. Effective for the removal of tapeworms, hookworms, roundworms, and whipworms.

Adverse Side Effects. These are uncommon.

> **Technician's Notes**
> 1. Do not use in dogs weighing less than 2 pounds or puppies younger than 3 weeks old.
> 2. Do not use in pregnant animals.

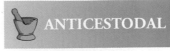
ANTICESTODAL

Drugs used for treating tapeworms have greatly improved over the years. These newer agents are more effective and do not require fasting before their administration.

Praziquantel (Droncit)

1. Dogs. *Taenia pisiformis, Dipylidium caninum, Echinococcus granulosus,* and *Echinococcus multilocularis.*
2. Cats. *D. caninum, T. taeniaeformis.*

Adverse Side Effects. These are uncommon but include vomiting, anorexia, diarrhea, and lethargy.

> **Technician's Notes**
> 1. No adverse reactions have been reported in pregnant or breeding animals.
> 2. Not for use in puppies younger than 4 weeks or kittens younger than 6 weeks old.

Epsiprantel (Cestex)

1. Dogs. *T. pisiformis* and *D. caninum.*
2. Cats. *T. taeniaeformis* and *D. caninum.*

Adverse Side Effects. These are uncommon.

> **Technician's Notes**
> 1. Safety in pregnant or breeding animals has not been established.
> 2. Not for use in puppies or kittens younger than 7 weeks old.

ANTITREMATODAL

Clorsulon (Curatrem)

1. Cattle. Liver flukes.
2. Effective against immature and adult flukes.

Adverse Side Effects. These are uncommon.

Albendazole (Valbazen)

1. Cattle. Liver flukes.
2. Effective against adult flukes and many intestinal worms.

Praziquantel (Droncit)

Praziquantel may be used for lung flukes in dogs and cats.

ANTIPROTOZOAL

Protozoa are single-celled organisms found at various body sites. Coccidia and *Giardia* are the most common protozoans associated with diarrhea in many species of animals. Both protozoans are most commonly transmitted via contaminated feed and/or water. Prevention of both diseases includes providing uncontaminated food and water and clean housing and avoiding overcrowding. A vaccine is also available for the prevention of giardiasis in dogs. *Babesia* is a hematozoan protozoa that is transmitted by ticks and also affects many species of animals. An injectable treatment for babesiosis is available for dogs.

Drugs for Treating Coccidia

1. Monensin (Coban 60). Turkeys and chickens
2. Amprolium (Corid). Calves
3. Clopidol (Coyden 25). Chickens
4. Maduramicin ammonium (Cygro Type A Medicated Article). Chickens
5. Decoquinate (Deccox). Cattle, calves, and goats
6. Narasin/nicarbazine (Maxiban 72). Chickens
7. Robenidine hydrochloride (Robenz Type A Medicated Article). Chickens
8. Sulfadimethoxine (Albon). Chickens, turkeys, dogs, and cats

Adverse Side Effects. These are uncommon.

Drugs for Treating *Giardia*

1. Metronidazole (Flagyl). Dogs and cats
2. Albendazole (Valbazen). Dogs and cats

Adverse Side Effects. These are uncommon, but vomiting and diarrhea may occur in some animals treated with metronidazole.

Drugs for Preventing *Giardia*

A vaccine for dogs is available as an aid in the prevention of *Giardia lamblia* infection and reduction in the duration of cyst shedding. The vaccine is administered subcutaneously with a booster given 2 to 4 weeks after the first vaccination. Annual revaccination is recommended.

Dosage Form
1. GiardiaVax

Adverse Side Effects. These are uncommon.

Drugs for Treating *Babesia*

Imidocarb dipropionate is available for the treatment of clinical signs of babesiosis and/or evidence of *Babesia* organisms in the blood. The product is indicated for use in dogs, and treatment consists of two injections given in a 2-week interval.

Dosage Form

1. Imizol

Adverse Side Effects. These may include injection pain and mild cholingeric signs such as salivation, nasal drip, or vomiting. Other less common side effects are panting, restlessness, diarrhea, and mild injection site inflammation.

Technician's Notes
1. Severe cholinergic signs may be reversed with atropine sulfate.

HEARTWORM DISEASE

Heartworm disease is commonly found throughout the United States. This disease primarily affects dogs and wild Canidae. *D. immitis* is the filarial **nematode** that causes heartworm disease. *Dipetalonema reconditum* is also a filarial nematode but does not require any therapeutic treatment because it is a harmless parasite. Prevention is the key word for controlling heartworm disease. Dogs not on an approved heartworm disease prevention program should be tested for the presence of adult heartworms before beginning preventative treatment. Clients should be educated about the importance of treating an existing infection if one exists, preventing infection or reinfection, and periodic testing that may be necessary. In the past several years, the number of cats diagnosed with heartworm disease has increased. The treatment and justification of prevention of heartworms in cats continues to be controversial (Smith,

1999). Products for the prevention of *D. immitis* infection in cats are available. There are not any adulticide products approved for use in cats.

ADULTICIDES

Melarsomine Dihydrochloride (Immiticide)

1. An arsenic compound administered by deep intramuscular injection in the third through fifth lumbar region.
2. Administration schedule is based on the classification of the severity of heartworm disease.
3. Melarsomine appears to be more efficacious than thiacetarsamide, less irritating to tissues, and does not cause hepatic necrosis (Plumb, 1999).

Adverse Side Effects. Some dogs experience reactions such as pain, swelling, and tenderness at the injection site. Firm nodules may form at the infection site. Coughing, gagging, depression, lethargy, anorexia, fever, lung congestion, and vomiting are also common reactions.

Technician's Notes
1. The manufacturer recommends using a 23-gauge 1-inch needle for dogs equal to or less than 22 pounds and a 22-gauge 1½-inch needle for dogs greater than 22 pounds.
2. The safety in breeding, lactating, or pregnant bitches has not been determined.
3. Melarsomine is contraindicated in dogs with very severe heartworm disease (Class 4, according to manufacturer disease classification).
4. Clients must be informed of the potential of morbidity and mortality associated with heartworm treatment.
5. Dogs should have exercise restricted after treatment.

MICROFILARICIDES

1. Given 6 weeks after administration of the adulticide.
2. Kill circulating **microfilaria.**
3. Although not approved as a microfilaricide, ivermectin and milbemycin oxime have been used.
4. Levamisole has also been used as a microfilaricide.

PREVENTATIVES

Ivermectin (Heartgard, Heartgard Plus, Heartgard for Cats)

1. Dogs. Monthly preventative; the Plus formula contains pyrantel pamoate and is effective against hookworms and roundworms.
2. Cats. Monthly preventative for *D. immitis* and for the removal of hookworms.
3. Eliminates the tissue stage of heartworm larvae.

Adverse Side Effects. These are uncommon. Toxic signs include mydriasis, depression, and ataxia.

> **Technician's Notes**
> 1. If replacing diethylcarbamazine citrate (DEC), the first dose should be given within a month after stopping DEC treatment.
> 2. This product is safe to use in pregnant and breeding animals.
> 3. Do not use in puppies or kittens younger than 6 weeks old.

Milbemycin Oxime (Interceptor, Sentinel)

1. Dogs. Monthly preventative; also controls hookworms, roundworms, and whipworms.
2. Eliminates the tissue stage of heartworm larvae.
3. Sentinel product contains lufenuron for flea control.

Adverse Side Effects. These are uncommon.

> **Technician's Notes**
> 1. If replacing DEC, the first dose should be given within 1 month after stopping DEC treatment.
> 2. This product is safe to use in pregnant and breeding animals.
> 3. Do not use in puppies younger than 4 weeks old.

Moxidectin (ProHeart)

1. Dogs. Monthly preventative for *D. immitis.*
2. Eliminates the tissue stage of heartworm larvae.

Adverse Side Effects. Adverse side effects may include lethargy, vomiting, ataxia, anorexia, diarrhea, nervousness, weakness, polydipsia, and itching.

> **Technician's Notes**
> 1. If replacing DEC, the first dose should be given within 1 month after stopping DEC treatment.
> 2. This product is safe to use in pregnant and breeding animals.
> 3. Do not use in puppies younger than 8 weeks old.

Selamectin (Revolution)

1. Dogs and cats. Monthly preventative.
2. Available as a solution for topical administration.
3. Indications include the prevention of heartworm disease caused by *Dirofilaria immitis*, prevention and control of flea infestations, treatment and control of earmite (*Otodectes cynotis*) infestation, treatment and control of sarcoptic (*Sarcoptes scabiei*) mange in dogs, and hookworm and roundworm treatment in cats.

Adverse Side Effects. These are uncommon but include transient, localized alopecia at the application site of some treated cats.

Technician's Notes

1. If replacing diethycarbamazine citrate (DEC), the first dose should be given within 1 month after stopping DEC treatment.
2. This product is safe to use in pregnant and breeding animals and in avermectin-sensitive collies.
3. Do not use in puppies or kittens younger than 6 weeks old.
4. This product should not be applied if the haircoat is wet. Bathing the animal 2 or more hours after treatment will not reduce the effectiveness.

Diethylcarbamazine Citrate (Carbam, Filaribits, Filaribits Plus)

1. Daily preventative; also controls roundworms.
2. Filaribits Plus also contains oxibendazole for the control of hookworms, whipworms, and roundworms.
3. Eliminates the tissue stage of heartworm larvae.

Adverse Side Effects. These include occasional vomiting. Filaribits Plus has been linked with hepatic dysfunction.

Technician's Notes

1. Administering with food or directly after a meal reduces the possibility of vomiting.
2. This product is safe to use in pregnant and breeding animals.
3. Missing just 2 to 3 days can affect the efficacy of this product.
4. Do not use in puppies younger than 8 weeks old.

ECTOPARASITES

Control of ectoparasites can be a troubling problem. Environmental factors such as housing (indoor or outdoor) and geographic location affect the incidence of many ectoparasites, such as fleas and ticks. When trying to control ectoparasites, the veterinary technician must be familiar with the products in order to educate clients about how to properly combat their problem. Not only do ectoparasites cause misery to their host, but many dermatologic problems arise from their infestation.

APPLICATION SYSTEMS

Prediluted Sprays

1. Consumers like the convenience of sprays.
2. Sprays are available for animal and environment use.
3. These formulations are for only the use specified on the label and should be used accordingly.
4. Sprays are available as water based or alcohol based.
   a. Water-based sprays do not penetrate oily coats or fabrics as well and do not dry as quickly as alcohol-based sprays.
   b. Alcohol-based sprays may be irritating and drying to the skin. They usually kill ectoparasites quickly.
5. Environmental sprays are usually residual. Most pet sprays require application daily or every 2 to 3 days for adequate parasite control.

Adverse Side Effects. These vary among products. Carefully read warning labels.

Technician's Notes

1. Spray the pet from head to tail, including the legs and abdomen. Avoid only the eyes, mouth, and nose. For best results, spray against the natural lay of the hair.
2. Educate clients about environment control as well as treating the pet.
3. Read labels before applying to young, sick, or pregnant animals. Some products are not safe for certain species (e.g., cats).

Emulsifiable Concentrates
Dips

1. Concentrates need to be diluted with water.
2. Dips are usually used after a shampoo.
3. Dips are generally considered residual.

Adverse Side Effects. These vary among products. Read labels carefully for animal and user safety and precautions.

Technician's Notes
1. Removing excess water or drying the coat before dipping is recommended to prevent further dilution of the product.
2. For best results, do not rinse after applying the dip.

Yard and Kennel Sprays

1. These are designed for environment use and should not be used on animals.
2. These products are residual.

Adverse Side Effects. These vary among products. Directions for application should be followed carefully for the safety of the user and animals.

Shampoos

1. These products may contain insecticides or medications or may be effective only for cleaning the coat.
2. Some shampoos are available as concentrates and require dilution before use.
3. Shampoos are not considered to be residual.
4. Rinse shampoos well; water hardness/softness affects how quickly some shampoos rinse away.

Adverse Side Effects. These vary among products. Shampoos containing carbamates or organophosphates should not be used with other products of the same origin.

Technician's Notes
1. Read labels carefully; shampoos may seem harmless, but they can be harmful if used improperly.
2. It is recommended that most shampoos be left on the haircoat for 5 to 10 minutes before rinsing.

Dusts

1. Popularity has decreased with the availability of effective sprays.
2. Dusts do not provide a quick kill.

Adverse Side Effects. These include irritation to mucous membranes and drying of the skin and haircoat.

Technician's Notes
Read labels carefully.

Foggers

1. Foggers work best in large, open rooms.
2. Remind clients that foggers do not go around corners, under couches, or into closets.
3. Combination use of foggers with a premises spray enhances results.
4. Read labels carefully.

Monthly Flea and Tick Products
Fipronil (Frontline Top Spot for Dogs, Frontline Top Spot for Cats)

1. Topical solution that provides flea and tick control; according to the manufacturer, the product collects in the oils of the skin and hair follicles.
2. Controls less severe flea infestations for up to 3 months.
3. Controls ticks for 1 month.
4. Kills newly emerged adult fleas and all stages of ticks.

Adverse Side Effects. Adverse side effects are uncommon.

Technician's Notes

1. Remains effective after bathing, water immersion, or exposure to sunlight.
2. Do not use on kittens younger than 12 weeks old or on puppies younger than 10 weeks old.
3. This product may be harmful to debilitated, aged, pregnant, or nursing animals.
4. Do not use more often than once every 30 days.
5. It is recommended that gloves be worn when applying the product.

Imidacloprid (Advantage)

1. Topical solution that provides flea control, and according to the manufacturer, is not absorbed into the bloodstream or other internal organs.
2. Controls less severe flea infestations for up to 4 weeks.
3. Kills newly emerged adult fleas.

Adverse Side Effects. Adverse side effects are uncommon.

Technician's Notes

1. Remains effective after bathing, water immersion, or exposure to sunlight.
2. Do not use on kittens younger than 8 weeks old or on puppies younger than 7 weeks old.
3. This product should not be used in pregnant animals.
4. May be used weekly for severe infestations.
5. It is not necessary to wear gloves when applying the product.

Lufenuron (Program Tablets, Program 6 Month Injectable for Cats, Program Suspension, Sentinel)

1. Monthly flea control administered orally; it is absorbed into fatty tissue and slowly released into the bloodstream.
2. Sentinel contains milbemycin for the prevention of heartworms and control of some intestinal parasites in dogs.
3. Controls fleas by preventing the development of flea eggs. Does not kill adult fleas.
4. Fleas must take a bloodmeal to ingest the product.

Adverse Side Effects. Adverse side effects are uncommon. Cats may develop a small lump at the injection site.

Technician's Notes

1. Do not use in puppies or kittens younger than 6 weeks old. Sentinel is approved for use in puppies 4 weeks old.
2. The oral products are considered to be safe for use in pregnant, breeding, or lactating animals.
3. The safety of the injectable product in reproducing animals has not been established.

Permethrin (Defend ExSpot Insecticide for Dogs)

1. Topical solution that provides flea and tick control, and according to the manufacturer, migration of the permethrin occurs on the skin surface.
2. Controls fleas, deer ticks, and brown dog ticks for up to 4 weeks.
3. Controls American dog ticks for 2 to 3 weeks.
4. Dogs should be tested for heartworm disease befor initial treatment with Sentinel.

Adverse Side Effects. Adverse side effects include skin sensitivity and lethargy.

Technician's Notes

1. Efficacy is reduced with bathing.
2. Do not use more often than once every 7 days.
3. Do not use on cats.

Selamectin (Revolution)

1. Topical solution applied monthly that provides prevention and control of flea infestations in dogs and cats.
2. Kills adult fleas and prevents flea eggs from hatching.
3. Also indicated for prevention of heartworm disease in dogs and cats, treatment and control of ear mite infestations in dogs and cats, and the treatment of hookworm and roundworm infections in cats.

Adverse Side Effects. These are uncommon but include transient, localized alopecia at the application site of some treated cats.

> **Technician's Notes**
> 1. This product is safe to use in pregnant and breeding animals and in avermectin-sensitive collies.
> 2. Do not use in puppies or kittens younger than 6 weeks old.
> 3. Should not be applied if the hair coat is wet. Bathing the animal 2 or more hours after treatment will not reduce the effectiveness.
> 4. Dogs should be tested for heartworm disease before initial treatment.

 INSECTICIDES

Pyrethrins

1. Extracted from pyrethrum or chrysanthemum flowers.
2. Generally considered safe for most mammals.
3. Have a quick-kill effect; low residual (stabilized or microencapsulated pyrethrins have increased residual).
4. Commonly found in pet sprays, dips, shampoos, dusts, foggers, premises sprays, and yard and kennel sprays.
5. Often used in conjunction with other insecticides.
6. Always used with synergists to maximize effects.

Synthetic Pyrethroids

1. Kirk (1986) identifies pyrethroids as "synthesized chemicals modeled on the chrysanthemate molecule of natural pyrethrins, with various substitutions and modifications."
2. Commonly used in pet sprays, dips, foggers, premises sprays, and yard and kennel sprays.
3. The following are common pyrethroids:
   a. D-trans allethrin (Duocide spray; Mycodex Pet Shampoo)
   b. Resmethrin (Durakyl pet spray and shampoo)
   c. Tetramethrin (Ectokyl IGR Pressurized Spray)
   d. D-Phenothrin (Duocide spray; Mycodex mini-fog)
   e. Permethrin (Defend EXspot; Permectrin spray; Ectokyl IGR Total Release Fogger)
4. Most have a quick-kill effect, and some have limited residual.
5. Safety is comparable to that of natural pyrethrins.
6. Synergists are not always needed with pyrethroids.

> **Technician's Notes**
> Read labels carefully; concentrations affect the use of certain products in some species (e.g., cats).

Chlorinated Hydrocarbons

1. Once common, most have been banned because of their instability (e.g., dichlorodiphenyl trichlorethane [DDT]).
2. They now have limited uses, and efforts are still being made to ban them completely.
3. The following are common chlorinated hydrocarbons:
   a. Lindane (Happy Jack Kennel Dip)
   b. Methoxychlor (Purina Cattle Dust, 2.5x Flea and Tick Powder)

Adverse Side Effects. These vary among products, but these products are considered very hazardous to humans and domestic animals. Read labels carefully before using.

> **Technician's Notes**
> Educate clients on the availability of safer products.

Carbamates

1. Act as cholinesterase inhibitors and should not be used with other cholinesterase inhibitors, phenothiazine derivatives, and succinylcholine.
2. Found in dusts, sprays, shampoos, flea and tick collars.
3. The following are common carbamates:
   a. Carbaryl. Mycodex Pet Shampoo with Carbaryl, Sevin Dust, Adams Flea and Tick Dust II (used on birds)
   b. Bendiocarb. Mainly large-animal products
   c. Propoxur. Mainly small-animal products

Adverse Side Effects. These include excessive salivation, vomiting, diarrhea, muscle tremors, and miosis.

> **Technician's Notes**
> 1. Read labels carefully.
> 2. Atropine and 2-PAM are antidotal.

Organophosphates

1. Act as cholinesterase inhibitors and should not be used with other organophosphates, carbamates, phenothiazine derivatives, and succinylcholine.
2. Found in dips, pet sprays, dusts, yard and kennel sprays, premises sprays, and systemics.
3. The following are common organophosphates:
   a. Chlorpyrifos (Adams Flea and Tick Dip, Yard & Kennel Spray)
   b. Dichlorvos (Vapona)
   c. Cythioate (Proban tablets and liquid—oral systemic flea control for dogs)
   d. Diazinon (Escort, Escort Plus, Terminator; used on snakes—Diazinon 25-E)
   e. Fenthion (Spotton)
   f. Phosmet (Paramite Dip for Dogs)

Adverse Side Effects. These include excessive salivation, vomiting, diarrhea, muscle tremors, and miosis.

> **Technician's Notes**
> 1. These products should not be used in dogs prone to seizure.
> 2. Read labels carefully for user and animal safety.
> 3. Atropine and 2-PAM are antidotal.

Formamidines

1. Amitraz is the most commonly used formamidine in veterinary medicine.
2. The following are products containing amitraz:
   a. Mitaban. Treatment for canine demodicosis
   b. Preventic Tick Collar for dogs
   c. Taktic. Large-animal insecticide
3. Amitraz is not an organophosphate.

Adverse Side Effects. These include transient sedation, lowered rectal temperature, increased blood glucose level, and seizures.

> **Technician's Notes**
> Read labels carefully.

Synergists

1. Increase efficacy of pyrethrins and some pyrethroids
2. The following are common synergists:
   a. Piperonyl butoxide
   b. *N*-octyl bicycloheptene dicarboximide

Adverse Side Effects. Piperonyl butoxide has shown evidence of toxicity to cats and a low incidence of chronic neurologic side effects (tremors, incoordination, lethargy) with sprays having levels equal to or greater than 1.5% (Kirk, 1986).

Repellents

1. Commonly used in human, equine, and companion animal products.
2. Most repel gnats, mosquitoes, and flies; when combined with pyrethrins and pyrethroids, they repel new fleas and ticks longer than the active ingredient alone.
3. The following are common repellents:
   a. 2,3,4,5-bis(2-butenylene)tetrahydro-2-furaldehyde (MGK 11)
   b. Di-*n*-propyl isocinchomeronate (MGK 326)
   c. Butoxypolypropylene glycol

Insect Growth Regulators ([IGRs], Insect Growth Hormones)

1. Maturation and pupation of flea larvae normally require a low level of natural IGRs.
2. Products containing IGRs mimic natural IGRs. They cause a high level of IGRs and interrupt the natural development of flea larvae.
3. The following are common IGRs:
   a. Methoprene
   b. Fenoxycarb
   c. Nylar
4. Found in pet sprays, flea collars, premises sprays.

Other Insecticides

1. Rotenone (Rotenone Shampoo, Ear Mite Lotion)
   a. Very toxic to fish and swine
   b. Commonly used in combination with other insecticides

2. Ivermectin (Ivomec 1% Injection for Cattle, Ivomec 1% Sterile Solution for Swine)
   a. Systemic injectable for the control of ectoparasites and some **helminths**
   b. Studies show efficacy against *Sarcoptes scabiei* and *Otodectes cynotis;* not approved for these uses in dogs or cats
3. D-Limonene (VIP Flea Dip, VIP Flea Control Shampoo)
   a. Extract of citrus peel
   b. Found in sprays, shampoos, and dips
   c. Provides a quick kill but is not residual
4. Benzyl benzoate. Effective against many ectoparasites and may be combined with other agents
5. Petroleum distillate. Usually added to products as the solvent for pyrethrin and pyrethroid products

REFERENCES

Kirk, R.W.: Current Veterinary IX: Small Animal Practice. W.B. Saunders Company, Philadelphia, 1986.

McCurnin, D.M.: Clinical Textbook for Veterinary Technicians, 3rd ed. W.B. Saunders Company, Philadelphia, 1994.

Plumb, Donald C.: Veterinary Drug Handbook, 3rd ed. Iowa State University Press, Ames, 1999.

Smith, P.: New Studies, Products Fuel Heartworm Debate. Veterinary Product News 11(4):34-36, 1999.

■ Review Questions

1. Why is the control of parasites such an important part of veterinary medicine?

   _____

2. What is the technician's role in the treatment of parasites? _____

3. What improvements have been made in today's common parasiticides versus older products?

   _____

4. What products have been approved for the prevention of heartworm disease in dogs? In cats?

   _____

5. How does an IGR improve a product's efficacy?

   _____

6. What should be done before using any products described in this section?

   _____

7. What products should never be used with organophosphates? _____

8. What are the signs of organophosphate toxicity?

   _____

9. What classes of endoparasites are commonly treated in clinical practice? _____

10. What are the common names of the endoparasites found in the classes described in question 9?

    _____

Chapter 14

Drugs Used to Relieve Pain and Inflammation

LEARNING OBJECTIVES

After studying this chapter, you should be able to:

1. Define terms related to the pharmacology of drugs used to relieve pain and inflammation
2. Develop an understanding of the anatomy and physiology associated with pain production and relief
3. Describe the mechanism of action of the category of drugs known as non-steroidal anti-inflammatory drugs (NSAIDs)
4. List indications for the use of NSAIDs
5. List potential adverse side effects of the NSAIDs
6. Describe the mechanism of action of the antihistamines
7. Differentiate between the action of H_1 and H_2 histamine receptors
8. List indications for muscle relaxants
9. List the two major categories of corticosteroids and the effects of each
10. Describe the hypothalamic-pituitary-adrenal axis, which controls the release of corticosteroids in the body
11. List indications for the use of corticosteroids
12. Describe potential adverse side effects of short-term and long-term corticosteroid use
13. Describe the mechanism of action of local anesthetic agents
14. List some indications for local anesthetic agents

KEY TERMS

Analgesia The absence of the sensation of pain.
Deep pain Pain arising from deep receptors in the periosteum, tendons, and joint structures.
Histamine A chemical mediator of the inflammatory response released from mast cells. Histamine may cause dilation and increased permeability of small blood vessels, constriction of small airways, increased secretion of mucus in airways, and pain.
Iatrogenic Caused by the physician (veterinarian).
Nerve block A loss of feeling or sensation produced by injecting an anesthetic agent around a nerve to interfere with its ability to conduct impulses.

Prostaglandin A substance synthesized by cells from arachidonic acid that serves as a mediator of inflammation and has other physiologic functions.
Regional anesthesia Loss of feeling or sensation in a large area (region) of the body by injecting an anesthetic agent into the spinal canal or around peripheral nerves.
Transdermal administration The use of a patch applied to the skin to deliver a drug through an intact cutaneous surface to the systemic circulation.

INTRODUCTION

Pain is a fundamental protective mechanism of the body that signals an underlying problem; it may occur alone or in combination with inflammation. Pain sensation arises in free nerve endings called *nociceptors,* located in the skin, joints, blood vessel walls, periosteum, hollow organs (e.g., stomach, intestines, bladder), and parietal surfaces of the thorax and abdomen. These free nerve endings may be activated through mechanical, thermal, and chemical stimulation. Chemical stimulation may be from an exogenous source or from those endogenous chemicals released in response to tissue damage.

Assessment of pain in animals can be very difficult because of the dependence on nonverbal communication in veterinary medicine. Signs indicating the presence of pain may include increased heart rate, increased respiratory rate, salivation, vocalization, changes in facial expression, guarding the painful site, restlessness, unresponsiveness, failure to groom, abnormal gait, abnormal stance, and rolling. A patient that is pain-free will be quiet and calm (Paddleford, 1999).

Drugs used to control pain (analgesics) include the NSAIDs and the narcotics (see Chapter 4). The body is able to produce its own opiate-like analgesic agents

called *endorphins* and *enkephalins;* efforts to synthesize these substances for commercial production have been unsuccessful.

Pain should be treated for humane reasons and to reduce the harmful side effects that accompany it. The treatment regimen may vary according to the assessment of the severity of the pain.

Inflammation is a basic process that occurs in the body in response to tissue injury from physical, chemical, or biologic trauma. The objectives of this process are to counteract the injury by removing or walling off the cause of the injury and to repair or replace the damaged tissue. The clinical manifestations (cardinal signs) of inflammation include *redness, heat, swelling,* and *pain.* Although the process is designed to be protective, it can continue to become a source of further injury or damage (e.g., allergy, shock, and "proud flesh").

Damage to cells from any source results in the release of several chemical mediators that may initiate or prolong the inflammatory response. These chemicals include **prostaglandins,** leukotrienes, **histamine,** cytokines, and other mediators. These substances cause helpful responses such as dilation and increased permeability of blood vessels, which result in increased blood flow to the injured tissue. The increased blood flow brings plasma to dilute the offending agent, fibrin to immobilize it, and phagocytic cells to remove it. The redness, heat, swelling, and to some extent the pain of inflammation are a result of the increased amount of blood in the damaged tissue. The chemical mediators serve other beneficial functions such as attracting phagocytic cells to the area of concern (chemotaxis) but also several potentially harmful ones such as initiation of bronchoconstriction (histamine), anaphylactic shock, pain (histamine), cell death, platelet aggregation, and intestinal spasm. The inflammatory process can be acute (anaphylaxis) or chronic (flea allergy, arthritis).

Drugs that are used to decrease the inflammatory process include the NSAIDs, the glucocorticosteroids, and several miscellaneous agents including dimethyl sulfoxide (DMSO).

Another process mediated by a chemical (or chemicals) released from damaged cells is fever. Fever is an increase in body temperature above normal; it is an important clinical indicator of disease. The purpose of fever may include destruction of invading microorganisms by heat inactivation and facilitation of biochemical reactions in the body (most chemical reactions are speeded up by increased heat).

Heat is generated by the metabolic activity of muscle and glands and is lost through radiation or conduction loss from the skin, sweat evaporation, and evaporation during panting. These mechanisms that control body temperature are regulated by a "thermostat" in the hypothalamus.

A substance that can initiate a fever is called a *pyrogen*. An exogenous pyrogen is a foreign substance (e.g., bacteria and viruses) that when introduced into the body causes the release of an endogenous pyrogen (a chemical mediator such as prostaglandin) from white blood cells, and this endogenous pyrogen causes a resetting of the hypothalamic thermostat. The hypothalamus then activates processes to generate or conserve body heat: shivering to generate more heat, constriction of blood vessels in the skin to prevent radiation and conduction loss, and decreased sweating or panting to reduce evaporation loss. Damaged cells in some instances may release endogenous pyrogens in the absence of exogenous pyrogens. The drugs used to control fever are primarily the NSAIDs.

ANATOMY AND PHYSIOLOGY

Pain sensation arises in nociceptors— "naked" nerve endings found in almost every tissue of the body. Pain impulses are carried to the central nervous system by two fiber systems: type C unmyelinated fibers are responsible for dull, poorly localized pain (in humans), and type A delta fibers are responsible for sharp, localized pain (Ganong, 1993). Both types carry impulses to the dorsal horn of the spinal cord (Figure 14-1), and the information is then relayed up the cord via the spinothalamic tract through the thalamus to the cerebral cortex, where it is interpreted as pain. If any part of this system is non-functional, pain sensation does not occur. Descending pathways can act to inhibit the activity of the sensory receptors.

When spinal cord lesions occur, superficial pain is inhibited before **deep pain** as lesion severity worsens. The absence of deep pain is often a poor prognostic sign.

NON-STEROIDAL ANTI-INFLAMMATORY AGENTS

The NSAIDs are thought to work by inhibiting an enzyme called *cyclooxygenase (cox)*. Two forms (cox-1 and cox-2) of cyclooxygenase exist. NSAIDs that selectively inhibit cox-2 are thought to produce fewer gastrointestinal side effects. This enzyme promotes the formation of prostaglandin from cell membrane arachidonic acid (Figure 14-2). The glucocorticoids exert their effect by blocking phospholipase, an enzyme necessary for the production of both the prostaglandins and the leukotrienes (intervention comes earlier in the sequence of the formation of the inflammatory mediators). Because the inflammatory reaction is blocked earlier by the glucocorticoids, they are more effective anti-inflammatory agents than the NSAIDs (Langston and Mercer, 1988). NSAIDs are often preferred, however, because they have fewer side effects and they promote **analgesia** and fever reduction. At this time, it is not known why the glucocorticoids do not induce the analgesic and antipyretic effects of the NSAIDs. It is also unknown why some NSAIDs provide relief of only mild pain (aspirin)

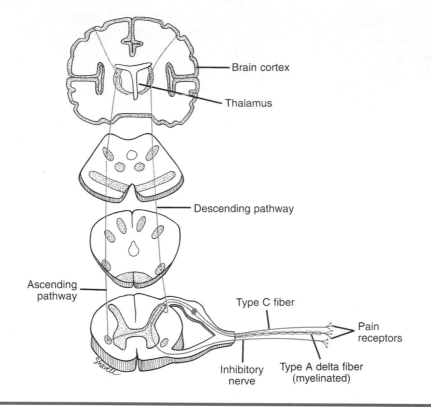

Brain cortex

Thalamus

Descending pathway

Ascending pathway

Type C fiber

Pain receptors

Inhibitory nerve

Type A delta fiber (myelinated)

Figure 14-1

Pain pathways.

and others provide relief of moderate to severe pain (flunixin).

The most common side effect of the NSAIDs is gastrointestinal ulceration and bleeding, which are probably a result of interference with the normal mucous coating of the stomach. Other side effects may include nephrotoxicity, inhibition of cartilage metabolism, bone marrow suppression, and bleeding tendencies (from reduced platelet aggregation).

Technician's Notes
1. NSAIDs should be used with caution in geriatric animals.
2. Combining NSAIDs or combining NSAIDs with corticosteroids should be used with great caution or avoided.

Salicylates

Aspirin, a salicylate, is also known as *acetylsalicylic acid*. Its actions include the following:

1. Relief of pain (analgesia)
2. Reduction of fever (antipyrexia)
3. Inhibition of inflammation (anti-inflammatory)
4. Reduction of platelet aggregation

These effects are thought to occur as a result of aspirin's ability to inhibit an enzyme (cyclooxygenase) that is responsible for the synthesis of prostaglandin. Prostaglandin is a chemical mediator of the processes that lead to pain, fever, inflammation, and platelet aggregation. Its inhibition results in a diminishing of each process.

Clinical Uses. Clinical uses of aspirin exist for most animal species and may include the following:

1. Relief of mild to moderate pain resulting from musculoskeletal conditions such as arthritis or hip dysplasia

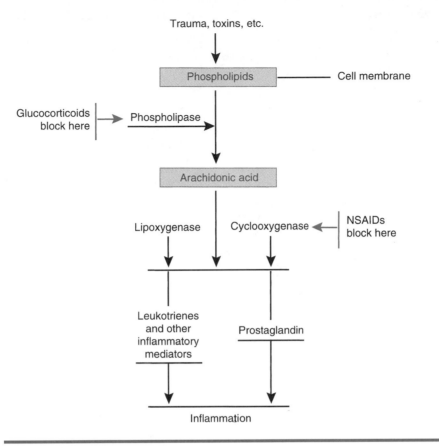

Trauma, toxins, etc.

Phospholipids — Cell membrane

Glucocorticoids block here → Phospholipase

Arachidonic acid

Lipoxygenase   Cyclooxygenase ← NSAIDs block here

Leukotrienes and other inflammatory mediators   Prostaglandin

Inflammation

Figure 14-2

Action of nonsteroidal anti-inflammatory drugs and the glucocorticoids to interrupt the inflammatory response.

2. Postadulticide treatment for heartworm disease
3. Analgesia/antipyrexia
4. Treatment of cardiomyopathy in cats
5. Treatment of endotoxic shock

Dosage Forms. These include plain uncoated tablets, buffered uncoated tablets, enteric coated forms, and boluses (large-animal applications). Many generic or brand names in many different strengths are available, including the following:

1. Aspirin bolus
2. Aspirin tablets
3. Cortaba (a combination of aspirin and methylprednisolone)

Adverse Side Effects. Adverse side effects of aspirin include gastric irritation, which can lead to ulceration and bleeding. *Cats are very susceptible to aspirin overdose because of their inability to metabolize it rapidly, and they should receive this drug only under the supervision of a veterinarian.*

Technician's Notes

1. Enteric coated aspirin such as Ecotrin may be used to prevent gastric irritation.
2. A 1-gr "baby" aspirin contains 65 mg; a 1.25-gr baby aspirin contains 81 mg.
3. There is no withdrawal time for aspirin in food animals.

Pyrazolone Derivatives

Phenylbutazone

Phenylbutazone, a pyrazolone derivative, is a commonly used NSAID in veterinary medicine. Its actions include the following:

1. Analgesia for mild to moderate pain
2. Anti-inflammatory action
3. Antipyrexia

Clinical Uses. These include relief of inflammatory conditions of the musculoskeletal system of horses and dogs. Phenylbutazone is used extensively in horses for the treatment of lameness and for the relief of pain associated with colic. It is sometimes used in dogs and cattle for its anti-inflammatory, analgesic, and antipyretic effects.

Dosage Forms. Dosage forms of phenylbutazone include a parenteral injection, tablets, boluses, an oral paste, an oral gel, and powder.

1. Butazolidin Tablets, Boluses, Paste, Injection
2. Phenylzone Paste
3. Butaron Gel
4. Equipalazone Powder
5. Equi-Phar Phenylbutazone Gel, Tablets
6. Phenylbutazone Tablets
7. Pro-Bute
8. Phenylbutazone Injection

Adverse Side Effects. These include gastrointestinal bleeding and bone marrow suppression.

Technician's Notes

1. Phenylbutazone injection should be administered by the intravenous route only. Subcutaneous and intramuscular injection may lead to sloughing of tissue.
2. Prolonged use or overdose can lead to bone marrow suppression in humans.
3. Prolonged use may also lead to ulcer formation.
4. Because of the possible bone marrow suppression and potential ulcer formation, animals that are receiving long-term treatment with phenylbutazone should be monitored carefully.

Flunixin Meglumine (Banamine)

Flunixin is an NSAID labeled for use in horses and cattle. It has extralabel uses in other species. Its actions are related to its ability to inhibit cyclooxygenase and include the following:

1. Analgesia
2. Antipyrexia
3. Anti-inflammatory

Clinical Uses. Clinical uses of flunixin in horses include alleviation of pain associated with musculoskeletal disorders and colic (flunixin apparently has great ability to inhibit visceral pain). Other uses in horses and other species include treatment of the following:

1. Disk disease
2. Endotoxic shock
3. Calf diarrhea
4. Parvovirus disease
5. Heatstroke
6. Ophthalmic conditions
7. Postsurgical pain

Dosage Forms. Dosage forms of flunixin include injectable, oral paste, and oral granule formulations.

1. Banamine Injection
2. Banamine Oral Paste
3. Banamine Oral Granules
4. Finadyne

Adverse Side Effects. These are limited in horses but may include swelling at the injection site and sweating. In dogs, vomiting, diarrhea, nephrotoxicity, and gastric ulceration may occur with long-term use.

Technician's Notes

1. Flunixin is labeled for intravenous and intramuscular use in horses.
2. Some equine clinicians believe that flunixin relieves abdominal pain so well in horses that it may cause a sense of false security about the condition of an animal with colic.
3. Small-animal patients receiving flunixin should be well-hydrated and should be receiving intravenous fluids and ulcer prophylaxis (Paddleford, 1999).

Dimethyl Sulfoxide

DMSO is a clear liquid that was originally developed as a commercial solvent. It is noted for its anti-inflammatory action as well as its ability to act as a carrier of other agents through the skin. Its anti-inflammatory actions may be related to its ability to trap products associated with the inflammatory response. DMSO causes vasodilation when applied topically.

Clinical Uses. Clinical uses of DMSO are varied; however, the only labeled use for DMSO is for topical application to reduce acute swelling resulting from trauma in dogs and horses. DMSO has reportedly been used as the following:

1. An adjunct to intestinal surgery (intravenously)
2. A treatment for cerebral edema or spinal cord injury (intravenously)
3. A treatment for perivascular injection of sodium caparsolate or other irritating substances (topical)
4. A carrier of drugs across the skin

Dosage Forms. Dosage forms of DMSO include a solution (90%) and a gel (90%).

1. DMSO Gel and Solution (90%)
2. Synotic (DMSO and a steroid)

Adverse Side Effects. Adverse side effects of DMSO are probably minimal with limited use or exposure but may include the following:

1. Garlic taste that occurs very shortly after the agent is applied to the skin
2. Skin irritation accompanied by a burning sensation
3. Induction of birth defects (teratogenic) in some species

Technician's Notes
1. Rubber gloves should be worn while applying DMSO.
2. Bandaging over an application of DMSO may cause skin irritation.
3. DMSO should be used carefully when cholinesterase inhibitors have been used.

Acetaminophen

Acetaminophen is an analgesic with limited antipyretic and anti-inflammatory activity.

Clinical Uses. Clinical uses of acetaminophen are limited in veterinary medicine, and its use should be discouraged because of the risk of potential toxicity and the availability of acceptable substitutes.

Dosage Forms. Dosage forms of acetaminophen include tablets, caplets, and liquid formulations. The following is a list of some of the human label brand names:

1. Tylenol
2. Datril
3. Tempra

Technician's Notes
1. Acetaminophen should never be given to cats.
2. Over-the-counter products should be checked carefully for the presence of acetaminophen before use in cats.

Adverse Side Effects. Adverse side effects of acetaminophen use in cats include the formation of methemoglobinemia, cyanosis, anemia, and liver damage. *Cats have a limited ability to biotransform acetaminophen and may succumb to a single dose.*

Propionic Acid Derivatives

Carprofen

Carprofen is a propionic acid derivative NSAID approved for oral use in dogs. Carprofen has been approved for oral and injectable use in dogs and cats in Europe. It has a half-life of 8 hours and is thought to work by inhibiting cyclooxygenase (cox).

Clinical Uses. Uses include the relief of pain associated with degenerative joint disease or postoperative pain resulting from soft tissue or orthopedic pain.

Dosage Form
1. Carporfen (Rimadyl)

Adverse Side Effects. Side effects such as gastrointestinal ulceration or bleeding are apparently rare with this agent.

Ketoprofen

Ketoprofen is a propionic acid derivative with analgesic, antipyretic, and anti-inflammatory activity. It is labeled for use in horses in the United States but has been used a great deal in dogs and cats in Europe and Canada.

Clinical Uses. In horses ketoprofen is used for treatment of pain and inflammation associated with musculoskeletal disorders. It has been used for postoperative and chronic pain in dogs and cats.

Dosage Forms

1. Ketofen (horses)
2. Orudis (human label)

Adverse Side Effects. Side effects may include gastrointestinal bleeding or ulceration, renal dysfunction, and generalized bleeding.

Naproxen

Naproxen is a propionic acid derivative similar to ketoprofen and ibuprofen. It is labeled for use in horses although it has been used in dogs.

Clinical Uses. Naproxen is labeled for the "relief of pain, inflammation, and lameness associated with myositis and other soft tissue diseases of the musculoskeletal system of horses."

Dosage Forms

1. Equiproxen (horses)
2. Naprosyn (human)

Adverse Side Effects. Few side effects are reported in the horse. GI ulceration has been reported in the dog.

Ibuprofen

Ibuprofen is reported to have potential for serious side effects in dogs and cats and is not recommended for use in these species.

OTHER NON-STEROIDAL ANTI-INFLAMMATORY DRUGS

Etodolac

Etodolac is an indole acetic acid derivative NSAID labeled for use in dogs.

Clinical Use. This drug is labeled for the management of pain and inflammation associated with osteoarthritis in dogs.

Dosage Form

1. EtoGesic

Adverse Side Effects. Side effects include anorexia, vomiting, diarrhea, and lethargy.

Other agents that are classified as NSAIDs or that have similar activity include the following:

Polysulfated Glycosaminoglycan (Adequan). Adequan is a semisynthetic mixture of glycosaminoglycans derived from bovine cartilage. This drug reduces degenerative changes induced by noninfectious or traumatic joint diseases and promotes activity of the synovial membrane. It is available in intra-articular and intramuscular forms and is labeled for use in horses and dogs.

Hyaluronate Sodium (Hyalovet). Hyalovet is a glycosaminoglycan that is labeled for intra-articular injection. It has activities similar to that of Adequan.

Legend. A solution of hyaluronate that may be given by intravenous or intra-articular injection for synovitis associated with osteoarthritis.

Meclofenamic Acid (Arquel Granules). This NSAID is labeled for oral treatment of acute or chronic inflammatory disease in horses.

Selenium and Vitamin E (Seletoc). Seletoc is labeled for relief of acute symptoms of arthritic conditions in dogs.

Ketorolac. Ketorolac is an NSAID with efficacy similar to that of morphine. It carries a human label and may cause serious side effects.

Orgotein (Palosein). Palosein is labeled for acute and chronic inflammatory conditions in horses and dogs.

Cosequin. Cosequin contains glucosamine, chondroitin sulfate, and manganese sulfate. It is a neutraceutical and has similar benefits on osteoarthritis as do the polysulfated glycosaminoglycans.

OPIOID ANALGESICS

The opioids and opioid receptors are discussed in a general fashion in Chapter 4. This section deals only with opioid use to control pain.

Opioids relieve pain by binding with specific receptor sites in the brain, spinal cord, and in peripheral tissues. By altering neurotransmitter release, they alter nerve impulse formation and transmission at many levels within the CNS. The ultimate effect is that the opioids block or inhibit pain impulses to the higher CNS centers responsible for the perception of pain.

Opioid Agonists

Opioid agonists remain one of the most effective drug classes in relieving moderate to severe pain (Paddleford, 1999). Opioid agonists are drugs that bind with all opioid receptor sites and produce opioid effects as well as respiratory depression, sedation, and addiction. The opioid agonists include alfentanil, carfentanil, codeine, etorphine, fentanyl, hydromorphine, meperidine, methodone, morphine, oxymorphone, and sufentanil. Even though some of these drugs are considered more potent than morphine, morphine is still considered to be one of the most effective of the opioids. All of the agonists are C-II controlled substances.

Clinical Uses. Opioid agonists are used to control moderate to severe pain in animals.

Selected Dosage Forms

1. Morphine sulfate (Infumorph, Astramorph PF) (human labels)
2. Oxymorphone (Numorphan)

3. Meperidine (Demerol)
4. Codeine (Codeine phosphate, codeine sulfate, Tylenol with codeine)
5. Fentanyl transdermal (Duragesic)

Adverse Side Effects. Side effects can include respiratory depression, sedation, excitement, and addiction. Cats are more sensitive to the excitatory effects of the opioid agonists than other species but do tolerate low doses well.

Transdermal Fentanyl Use

Transdermal application of fentanyl has been successfully used in humans for control of chronic pain for some time. This use has recently been adapted for the control of postoperative and chronic pain in dogs and cats (extralabel).

Care must be taken when using the transdermal patches to ensure that the animal does not eat or lick the patch (causing possible overdosage) or that accidental exposure to humans (especially children) does not occur. To apply the patch, gloves should be worn; the skin over the dorsum of the neck should be clipped, cleansed, and allowed to dry well; good skin contact with the patch should be achieved; and a snug bandage should be applied to hold the patch in place. The patch should never be cut because this interferes with the rate of release of the fentanyl. The patch should be carefully disposed of after use.

Opioid Agonists-Antagonists

The opioid agonist-antagonist drugs bind with opioid kappa receptors but antagonize opioid mu receptors. Opioid agonists-antagonists include butorphanol (C-IV), pentazocine (C-IV), and nalbuphine. These drugs are considered effective for mild to moderate pain and have few side effects.

Clinical Uses. The primary use is the relief of mild to moderate pain.

Dosage Forms

1. Butorphanol (Torbugesic, Torbutrol, Stadol)

2. Pentazocine (Talwin-V)
3. Nalbuphine (Nubain)

Adverse Side Effects. Side effects include sedation, ataxia, and salivation (pentazocine).

Opioid Partial Agonists

The opioid partial agonists bind with the mu receptors but only partially activate them. Buprenorphine is the primary drug in this category.

Clinical Uses. Uses include relief of mild to moderate pain in dogs and horses.

Dosage Form

1. Buprenex (human label)

Adverse Side Effects. Side effects include sedation and respiratory depression.

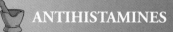

ANTIHISTAMINES

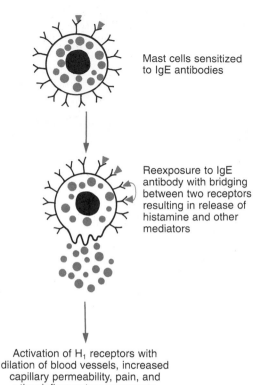

Mast cells sensitized to IgE antibodies

Reexposure to IgE antibody with bridging between two receptors resulting in release of histamine and other mediators

Activation of H_1 receptors with dilation of blood vessels, increased capillary permeability, pain, and other inflammatory responses

Figure 14-3

The release of histamine from mast cells when stimulated by IgE antibodies.

Antihistamines are drugs that are used to inhibit the effects or the spread of the inflammatory process. These drugs do not inhibit the formation of prostaglandins or other inflammatory mediators; they work by preventing histamine from combining with tissue receptors or by displacing histamine from receptor sites. Because histamine is a major chemical mediator of the allergic response, antihistamines may be useful in controlling allergic responses.

Histamine is a chemical that is released from mast cells when they are adequately stimulated by immunoglobulin E (IgE) antibodies to allergens (Figure 14-3). Histamine then combines with tissue receptors and causes dilation of small blood vessels, increased permeability of capillaries, smooth muscle spasm, and increased secretion of glands. Two types of antihistamine receptors have been identified: H_1 and H_2.

Antihistamines competitively block the binding of histamine to H_1 receptors, which may block the progression of the allergic response. Some antihistamines also block H_1 receptors that may contribute to motion sickness or nausea. Some antihistamines have a high affinity for H_1 receptors in the brain and cause a sedative effect.

Stimulation of H_2 receptors causes an increase in flow of hydrochloric acid by the gastric mucosa. H_2 blockers reduce secretion of hydrochloric acid and may be used to treat gastrointestinal irritation and ulceration.

Clinical Uses. Antihistamines are used to treat the following:

1. Pruritus
2. Urticaria and angioedema associated with acute allergic reactions
3. Laminitis in horses and cattle
4. "Downer" cow syndrome
5. Motion sickness

6. "Reverse sneeze" syndrome
7. Anaphylactic shock
8. Upper respiratory tract conditions

Dosage Forms. These include injectables, oral preparations, and topical agents. Many brand names are available under veterinary and human labels. A partial list of the formulations follows:

H_1 Blockers

1. Pyrilamine maleate (Antihistamine Injection)
2. Pyrilamine maleate injection
3. Pyrilamine maleate injection (Histavet-P)
4. Tripelennamine hydrochloride (Re-Covr Injection)
5. Pyrilamine maleate, phenylephrine hydrochloride with a decongestant and an expectorant (cough syrup)
6. Probahist Syrup (same ingredients as in No. 5)
7. Diphenhydramine HCl (Histacalm Shampoo, Spray)
8. Diphenhydramine (Benadryl)
9. Dimenhydrinate (Dramamine)
10. Meclizine (Bonine)
11. Promethazine (Phenergan)
12. Terfenadine (Seldane)
13. Hydroxyzine HCl (Atarax)
14. Chlorpheniramine maleate (Chlor-Trimeton)

H_2 Blockers

1. Cimetidine (Tagamet)
2. Ranitidine (Zantac)

Adverse Side Effects. Adverse side effects of the antihistamines include drowsiness, weakness, dry mucous membranes, urinary retention, and central nervous system stimulation on overdose.

> **Technician's Notes**
> Antihistamines are not as effective in controlling pruritus in animals as they are in humans.

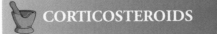

MUSCLE RELAXANTS

Skeletal muscle relaxants may be used as an aid in the treatment of acute inflammatory and traumatic conditions of muscle and the resulting spasms that may occur in these situations. They are thought to work by decreasing muscle hyperactivity without interfering with normal muscle tone. This action may be brought about by selective action on the internuncial neurons of the spinal cord.

Methocarbamol (Robaxin-V)

Robaxin-V is labeled for use in dogs, cats, and horses.
Clinical Uses. This product is used to treat the following:

1. Intervertebral disk syndrome
2. Strains and sprains
3. Myositis and bursitis
4. Muscle spasm
5. Tying up in horses

Dosage Forms. Dosage forms of Robaxin-V include tablets and an injectable.

Other Muscle Relaxants

1. Myotrol
2. Spasgesic

Adverse Side Effects. These include excessive salivation, emesis, muscle weakness, and ataxia when overdosed. The package insert states that adverse side effects are seldom encountered.

CORTICOSTEROIDS

Corticosteroid drugs are used in veterinary medicine to treat inflammatory, pruritic, and immune-mediated diseases. These drugs are also used to treat shock,

TABLE 14-1 Mineralocorticoid Versus Glucocorticoid Classification of Corticosteroids

Drug	Glucocorticoid Potency (Anti-Inflammatory Effect)	Mineralocorticoid Potency
Hydrocortisone	1	1
Cortisone	0.8	0.8
Prednisone	4	0.25
Prednisolone	4	0.25
Methylprednisolone	5	0
Triamcinolone	5	0
Paramethasone	10	0
Flumethasone	15	0
Dexamethasone	30	0
Betamethasone	35	0

TABLE 14-2 Duration of Action of Corticosteroids

Short Acting (<12 Hours)	Intermediate Acting (12-36 Hours)	Long Acting (>48 Hours)
Hydrocortisone	Prednisone	Betamethasone
Cortisone	Prednisolone	Dexamethasone
	Methylprednisolone	Flumethasone
	Triamcinolone	Paramethasone

laminitis, anorexia, adrenal insufficiency, and various other conditions. The technician should remember that corticosteroid therapy involves the treatment of the signs of disease; it is seldom, if ever, curative.

Natural corticosteroids are hormones that are produced by the adrenal cortex, whereas corticosteroids used clinically are synthetic reproductions (analogs) of the naturally occurring hormones. Corticosteroids are classified according to their activity as either mineralocorticoids or glucocorticoids (Table 14-1) and according to their duration of action (Table 14-2) as short, intermediate, or long acting. Mineralocorticoids, such as aldosterone, regulate electrolyte and water balance in the body. Glucocorticoids, such as cortisone, exert anti-inflammatory and immunosuppressive effects and influence the metabolism of carbohydrate, fat, and protein. No corticosteroid has complete glucocorticoid or mineralocorticoid activity, but each has a predominant

activity that determines its classification. Because mineralocorticoids are seldom used clinically, this discussion focuses on the glucocorticoids.

Control of the release of the naturally occurring corticosteroids (cortisol, corticosterone, and deoxycortisol) is complex and occurs through the hypothalamic-pituitary-adrenal axis (Figure 14-4). Control is exerted through this axis by two basic mechanisms. The first is a negative-feedback mechanism related to level of cortisol in the bloodstream: When the level of cortisol in the blood is lowered, the hypothalamus sends a chemical messenger called *corticotropin-releasing factor (CRF)* to the anterior pituitary gland, thus causing the pituitary to release a substance called *adrenocorticotropic hormone (ACTH)* into the bloodstream. ACTH is then carried by the blood to the adrenal cortex, where it stimulates this structure to release cortisol to raise the amount in the blood to appropriate levels. On the

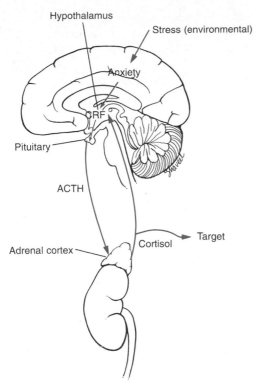

Hypothalamus

Stress (environmental)

Anxiety

CRF

Pituitary

ACTH

Adrenal cortex

Cortisol

Target

Figure 14-4

The release of corticosteroids is under the control of the hypothalamic-pituitary-adrenal (HPA) axis.

other hand, a high level of blood cortisol inhibits release of CRF by the hypothalamus, and the blood level is thus prevented from reaching excessive levels. It should be noted that the hypothalamus cannot distinguish between naturally occurring cortisol and the synthetic analogs administered by veterinarians.

The second mechanism for the control of the release of cortisol by the adrenal gland is through the stress response. External and internal stressors such as crowding, weaning, transporting, disease, surgery, trauma, pain, fear, anxiety, and many others can stimulate the hypothalamus, through impulses from the higher brain centers, to release CRF. The control mechanism then proceeds in a similar fashion as illustrated in Figure 14-4.

One of the major indications for the clinical use of corticosteroids is for their anti-inflammatory effects. These effects are brought about by their ability to block

the enzyme phospholipase, which promotes the reaction that results in the formation of prostaglandin—a primary mediator of the immune response. Corticosteroids also protect cells from inflammatory trauma by various mechanisms that include but are not limited to the following:

1. Stabilizing cell membranes to help prevent their breakdown
2. Stabilizing lysosomal membranes so that they do not release their harmful enzymes
3. Disrupting histamine synthesis
4. Inhibiting interleukin synthesis
5. Reducing exudative processes

Corticosteroids are also used clinically for their immunosuppressive effects. They are used to suppress the immune system in allergic conditions such as flea allergy dermatitis, atopy, autoimmune hemolytic anemia, rheumatoid arthritis, and uveitis. The immunosuppressive effect is a result of the ability of corticosteroids to do the following:

1. Inhibit antibody formation
2. Decrease the concentration of lymphocytes and eosinophils
3. Suppress the migration of neutrophils
4. Inhibit phagocytosis

Although the immunosuppressive qualities are very useful clinically, they can also mask the signs of serious infections that are simultaneously present.

Because corticosteroids are able to lyse lymphocytes, they may be useful in treating neoplasms of the lymphocyte cell lines (Chastain, 1989).

All steroid compounds are synthesized from a basic parent compound that has been described as resembling three rooms and a bath (Figure 14-5). Steroids are formed in three regions in the adrenal gland. Those regions and their respective products include the following:

1. Zona glomerulosa—mineralocorticoids
2. Zona fasciculata—glucocorticoids
3. Zona reticularis—sex hormones (androgen and estrogen)

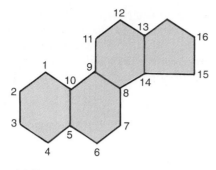

Figure 14-5 ━━━━━━━━━━

The configuration of the parent molecule of all steroid molecules including corticosteroids.

An increased number of double bonds in the parent compound, the addition of certain of side chains, or the addition of fluorine atoms to the parent molecule usually increase the anti-inflammatory effects of corticosteroids.

Clinical Uses. Corticosteroids are used for the treatment of the following conditions:

1. Allergic reactions/conditions
2. Inflammatory conditions of the musculoskeletal system
3. Shock/toxemia
4. Laminitis
5. Inflammatory ocular conditions such as conjunctivitis and uveitis
6. Addison's disease
7. Autoimmune disease such as autoimmune hemolytic anemia, lupus, and rheumatoid arthritis
8. Lymphocytic neoplasms

Dosage Forms. Corticosteroids are available in injectable, oral, and topical forms and in preparations containing antibiotics, antifungal, and corticosteroid products. These products may be applied to the skin or mucous membranes, injected into lesions, given orally, or administered parenterally. When emergency conditions call for administration of corticosteroids, the intravenous route is normally used with a water-soluble product in a water-soluble vehicle. Water-soluble products can be injected via the intramuscular or subcuta-

neous route when life-threatening conditions do not exist. The long-acting depot (repositol) products are prepared in a poorly soluble vehicle to prolong their effects. The justification for these long-acting products has been questioned by some clinicians.

A list of some of the many corticosteroid products available follows.

Injectables

1. Azium
2. Azium Sodium Phosphate
3. Betasone
4. Cortisate-20
5. Depo-Medrol
6. Dexamethasone Injection
7. Dexamethaxone Sodium Phosphate
8. Dex-A-Vet Injection
9. Dexasone
10. Flucort Solution
11. Meticorten
12. Predef
13. Solu-Delta-Cortef
14. Vetalog Parenteral

Oral

1. Azium Powder
2. Medrol
3. Methylprednisolone Tablets
4. Pet-Derm III
5. Temaril-P Tablets
6. Triamcinolone Tablets
7. Vetalog Oral Powder/Tablets
8. Prednisone generic tablets
9. Prednisolone generic tablets

Topical

1. Cort/Astrin Solution
2. CortiSpray
3. Hydro-Plus
4. Synalar Cream
5. Synalar Otic Solution
6. Vetalog Cream

Adverse Side Effects. Adverse side effects of the corticosteroids are numerous:

1. Polyuria and polydipsia
2. Thinning of the skin and muscle wasting resulting from the ability of corticosteroids to convert protein into glucose (seen with long-term administration)
3. Depressed healing
4. Polyphagia and resulting weight gain
5. **Iatrogenic** (caused by the veterinarian) hyper-adrenocorticism, iatrogenic Cushing's disease
6. Hypoadrenocorticism (iatrogenic) resulting from suppression of the hypothalamic-pituitary-adrenal axis by long-term administration of exogenous corticosteroids and then sudden cessation of the treatment (Addison's disease)
7. Gastric ulcers with or without bleeding
8. Osteoporosis (long-term)
9. Abnormal behavior

Because administration of corticosteroids is fraught with many potential side effects, clinicians must give careful consideration to their use. Much information has been written about the appropriate use of corticosteroids in veterinary medicine, and a selection of the principles of use follows:

1. Alternate-day dosing may help prevent iatrogenic hypoadrenocorticism.
2. Administration should never be stopped abruptly, but tapered off gradually.
3. Very large doses may be used in emergency situations.
4. Corticosteroids are generally not used for the treatment of corneal ulcers.
5. When corticosteroids are injected into joint spaces, extreme care should be given to aseptic technique.

LOCAL, REGIONAL, AND TOPICAL ANESTHETIC AGENTS

Many clinical situations call for the use of local or topical anesthesia to prevent or relieve pain. We have chosen to discuss these agents in this chapter on pain relief rather than in the traditional context of anesthesia.

In some situations, general anesthesia is not available or is too dangerous to a patient; in others, repair of a small laceration may not justify general anesthesia. In equine medicine, lameness may be diagnosed by administering a **nerve block** to an area and then observing abatement of the lameness. In bovine medicine, it may be useful to administer a regional nerve block to prevent straining in order to replace a prolapsed uterus. In cats, it may be useful to apply a local anesthetic to the larynx to facilitate placement of an endotracheal tube.

Local anesthetics work by preventing the generation and conduction of nerve impulses in peripheral nerves. These anesthetics are administered by the following routes:

1. Topically to the mucous membranes of the ear, eye, larynx, or other appropriate area
2. By infiltration in a localized area such as the margin of a wound to anesthetize nerve endings (Figure 14-6)
3. By injection into joint spaces
4. For intravenous regional nerve block—may be used for foot surgery in cattle by applying a tourniquet to the proximal area of a limb and then infusing a local anesthetic into the limb
5. Around nerve bodies
   a. Epidural anesthesia—injection of a local anesthetic into the epidural space (see Figure 14-6) of the spinal canal to provide anesthesia to the area around the anus and perineum for obstetric manipulations and to stop straining for the replacement of a prolapsed uterus
   b. Nerve block—local anesthetic deposited around a specific nerve (Figure 14-7) to facilitate minor procedures (e.g., lameness diagnosis, dehorning, lid or lip suturing)
   c. Paravertebral block—placement of a local anesthetic around a spinal nerve near where it leaves the intervertebral space; this procedure blocks a larger area and may be used for procedures such as cesarean sections and rumenotomies

Most of the local anesthetic agents provide anesthesia for approximately 5 to 30 minutes. The effects of local anesthetics can be prolonged by adding epineph-

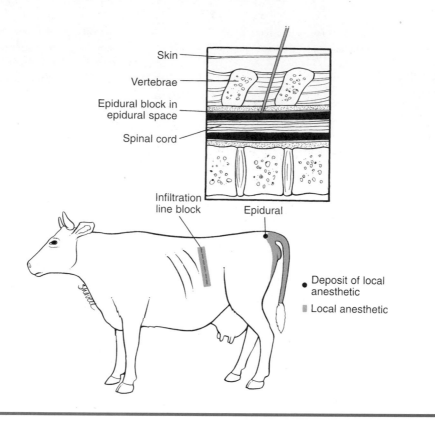

Skin

Vertebrae

Epidural block in epidural space

Spinal cord

Infiltration line block

Epidural

● Deposit of local anesthetic

▌ Local anesthetic

Figure 14-6

The use of local anesthetics to provide local and regional anesthesia.

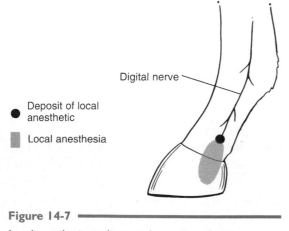

Digital nerve

● Deposit of local anesthetic

▌ Local anesthesia

Figure 14-7

Local anesthesia to diagnose lameness in horses.

rine, which causes vasoconstriction and therefore prolongs the absorption time owing to a reduced blood supply in the area. Using ethyl alcohol as a local anesthetic agent may considerably prolong the duration of the anesthesia. Some clinicians prefer to use xylazine or a narcotic agent for administering epidural anesthesia.

Clinical Uses. Local anesthetics are used for the following purposes:

1. Infiltration of local areas
2. Epidural anesthesia
3. Topical application in the eye, ear, larynx, and so forth
4. Nerve blocks
5. Their antiarrhythmic effects

Dosage Forms. Local anesthetic agents are available in injectable and topical forms. A partial list of these agents follows:

Injectable

1. Anthocaine Injection (lidocaine)
2. Carbocaine-V (mepivacaine)
3. Epidural Injection (procaine HCl)
4. Lidocaine hydrochloride injection
5. Other generic local anesthetics, including tetracaine and dibucaine

Topical

1. Ophthaine Solution Veterinary
2. Ophthetic

Adverse Side Effects. Local anesthetics can have adverse side effects if the total maximum dose for the species being treated is exceeded. The side effects may include restlessness, excitement, hypotension, and seizures.

Technician's Notes

Lidocaine with epinephrine should never be used if an antiarrhythmic is indicated.

REFERENCES

Chastain, C.B.: Use of corticosteroids. In Ettinger, S.J. (ed.): Textbook of Veterinary Internal Medicine. W.B. Saunders Company, Philadelphia, 1989.

Ganong, W.F.: Cutaneous and deep visceral pain. In Ganong, W.F. (ed.): Review of Medical Physiology. Appleton & Lange, East Norwalk, CT, 1993.

Langston, V.C., Mercer, H.D.: Non-steroidal anti-inflammatory drugs. In Proceedings of the 17th Seminar for Veterinary Technicians. The Western Veterinary Conference, Las Vegas, 1988.

Paddleford, R.R.: Analgesia and pain management. In Manual of Small Animal Anesthesia. W.B Saunders Company, Philadelphia, 1999.

■ Review Questions

1. Define the following terms:
   Analgesia _____
   Deep pain _____
   Histamine _____
   Inflammation _____
   Prostaglandin _____
   Pyrogen _____

2. Type _____ unmyelinated nerve fibers are responsible for dull pain, whereas type _____ are responsible for sharp pain.

3. Nerve impulses are interpreted as pain in the _____.

4. Describe how the NSAIDs relieve pain. _____

5. Acetaminophen should never be given to cats because _____.

6. List some of the potential adverse side effects of NSAID use. _____

7. How do the antihistamines exert their effects? _____

8. Where are histamine H_2 receptors found, and what activity do they control? _____

9. List two indications for the use of muscle relaxants in veterinary medicine. _____

10. What are the two major categories of corticosteroids? _____

11. Describe the mechanism that controls the release of naturally occurring corticosteroids.

12. Describe the side effects of short-term and long-term corticosteroid use. _____

13. What is the mechanism of action of the local anesthetic agents? _____

14. What are some indications for the use of local anesthetics? _____

Therapeutic Nutritional, Fluid, and Electrolyte Replacements

LEARNING OBJECTIVES

After studying this chapter, you should be able to:

1. Define terms related to fluid, electrolyte, and selected therapeutic nutritional preparations
2. Describe the distribution of water in the body
3. Describe the composition of body and therapeutic fluids
4. Define osmotic pressure and tonicity as they apply to fluids
5. Discuss the basic principles of fluid therapy
6. Describe fluid equipment and its use
7. Categorize and provide examples of the fluids used in fluid therapy
8. List and describe selected fluid additives
9. List and describe selected oral electrolyte preparations
10. List and describe selected parenteral vitamin/mineral products

KEY TERMS

Buffer A substance that decreases the change in pH when an acid or base is added.

Colloid A chemical system composed of a continuous medium throughout which small particles are distributed and do not settle out under the influence of gravity.

Dissociation The act of separating into ionic components (NaCl → Na+ and Cl−).

Electrolyte A substance that dissociates into ions when placed in solution, becoming capable of conducting electricity.

Empirical Based on observation and personal experience.

Hyperkalemia An excess of potassium in the blood.

Hypernatremia An excess of sodium in the blood.

Hypokalemia A deficiency of potassium in the blood.

Hyponatremia A deficiency of sodium in the blood.

Hypovolemia Decreased volume of circulating blood.

Metabolic acidosis Decreased body pH caused by excess hydrogen ions in the extracellular fluid.

Metabolic alkalosis Increased body pH caused by excess bicarbonate in the extracellular fluid (ECF).

Oncotic pressure The osmotic pressure generated by plasma proteins in the blood.

Solute A substance dissolved in a solvent to form a solution.

Transcellular fluid Cerebrospinal fluid, aqueous humor of the eye, synovial fluid, gastrointestinal fluid, lymph, bile, and glandular and respiratory secretions.

Turgor Degree of fullness or congestion; describes the degree of elasticity of the skin.

INTRODUCTION

Veterinary technicians often have an important role in fluid, electrolyte, and therapeutic nutritional therapy. They administer parenteral or oral fluid or nutritional products and monitor patients' responses under the direction of a veterinarian. Because the use of the products can be critically important to the outcome of a case, technicians should have a thorough knowledge of these products and their use.

ANATOMY, PHYSIOLOGY, AND CHEMISTRY

DISTRIBUTION OF BODY WATER AND ELECTROLYTES

Measurements of total body water (TBW) have shown that water represents 50% to 70% of the total body weight in adult animals; 60% is often used as the average figure. As much as 80% of a neonatal animal's

body weight may be water, a factor that makes fluid loss in young animals potentially very serious. An increase in body fat decreases the amount of TBW, and makes it important to estimate fluid needs based on lean body mass to avoid overhydration.

TBW is distributed in several compartments within the body (Figure 15-1). Sixty percent of the TBW is found within cells and is called *intracellular fluid (ICF)*. ICF makes up 40% of the total body weight. The other 40% of the TBW is found outside the cells and is called *extracellular fluid (ECF)*. The ECF accounts for 20% of the total body weight. The ECF (discounting the relatively small **transcellular** component) distributes itself between the interstitial fluid (15% of body weight) and the intravascular fluid or plasma (5% of body weight).

Body fluid compartments should be thought of as volumes of fluid and electrolytes in dynamic equilibrium, with fluids and electrolytes moving back and forth across semipermeable cell membranes. Changes in the quantity of fluid or electrolytes in one com-

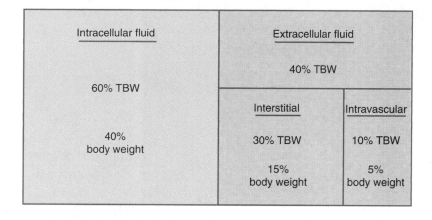

Figure 15-1

Body fluid compartments. *TBW,* total body water.

partment usually result in changes in the quantities in other compartments. Fluids administered intravenously to an animal first enter the intravascular space of the ECF, move into the interstitial space, and then enter the ICF (Figure 15-2). In most cases, the loss of fluids occurs first from the ECF and then from the other compartments as losses continue.

COMPOSITION OF BODY AND THERAPEUTIC FLUIDS

Body water contains an array of **solutes** varying in quantity from compartment to compartment. A solute is a substance that dissolves in a solvent; this solvent is usually water in biologic systems. The molecules of substances called **electrolytes** break down (dissociate) into charged particles called *ions.* Electrolytes are either positively charged (cations) or negatively charged (anions), and the number of cations always equals the number of anions in normal animals (Table 15-1). In the ECF, the most abundant cation is sodium and the most abundant anions are chloride and bicarbonate. In the ICF, the major cations are potassium and magnesium and the major anions are phosphates and proteins. Therapeutic fluids are described as balanced if they resemble ECF in composition and unbalanced if they do not. Lactated Ringer's solution is an example of a balanced solution, and saline is an example of an unbalanced solution. Table

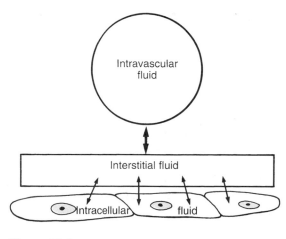

Figure 15-2

Schematic showing movement of fluid between compartments.

15–2 lists the composition of solutions used in fluid therapy.

It is important for readers to have a basic understanding of the way in which solute particles such as electrolytes are quantified in fluids. One of the oldest ways of measuring solute concentration is by describing the weight of the solute per 100 ml of solution (g%). A 0.9% sodium chloride (NaCl) solution (saline) would contain 0.9 g/100 ml or 900 mg/100 ml.

	Plasma	Interstitial Fluid
TABLE 15-1 Composition of Plasma and Interstitial Fluid		
Ion	Plasma (mEq/L)	Interstitial Fluid (mEq/L)
Cations		
Na^+	142	145.1
K^+	4.3	4.4
Ca^{2+}	2.5	2.4
Mg^{2+}	1.1	1.1
Total	**149.9**	**153.0**
Anions		
Cl^-	104	117.4
HCO_3^-	24	27.1
H_2PO_4	2	2.3
Protein	14	(none)
Other	5.9	6.2
Total	**149.9**	**153.0**

Other clinically significant ways of describing the quantity of solute particles include use of the concepts of (1) the milliequivalent, (2) osmolality, (3) osmolarity, and (4) tonicity.

The milliequivalent is the unit of measurement used to express the concentration of electrolytes such as sodium, potassium, and calcium in solutions. The concentration of these substances is usually expressed as milliequivalents per liter (mEq/L) in fluids and milliequivalents per milliliter in supplements. The milliequivalent describes the tendency of a particle to combine with another particle and is defined as 1:1000 of an equivalent. An *equivalent* is defined as the weight in grams of an element that will combine with 1 g of hydrogen ion. For all practical purposes, the equivalent weight of a compound is equal to the gram molecular weight of the substance divided by the total positive valence of the material in question (Blankenship and Campbell, 1976). For example, the equivalent weight of NaCl is 58.5/1 = 58.5, and 1 L of fluid containing 58.5 g of NaCl contains one equivalent weight or 1000 mEq of NaCl. The equivalent weight of sulfuric acid (H_2SO_4) is 98.1/2 = 49; therefore, 49 g of H_2SO_4 in 1 L of fluid contains one equivalent or 1000 mEq. The following formulas allow determination of milliequivalents of solute in a solution when the concentration in grams or milligrams is known:

$$mEq/L = \frac{\text{milligrams per liter}}{\text{molecular weight}} \times \text{valence}$$

or

$$mEq/L = \frac{\text{milligrams per deciliter} \times 10}{\text{molecular weight}} \times \text{valence}$$

OSMOTIC PRESSURE AND TONICITY OF FLUIDS

Body fluid compartments are usually separated by a semipermeable (cell) membrane that permits the passage of water and some solutes. Solutes that can cross the membrane tend to move from an area of higher to an area of lower concentration by the process called *diffusion*. Solutes that cannot cross the cell membrane tend to attract water toward them. This movement of water across a cell membrane is called *osmosis*, and the ability of particles to attract water is called *osmotic pressure*.

Osmolality is a determination of the osmotic pressure of a solution based on the relative number of solute particles in 1 kg of the solution. The greater the number of particles, the greater the pressure generated. The unit of measurement of osmolality is the osmol (osm), and 1 osm of any substance is equal to 1 g molecular weight divided by the number of particles formed by the **dissociation** of that substance. A substance that dissociates into two particles in solutions creates twice as much osmotic pressure as one that does not dissociate. Because the quantities being measured are very small in biologic systems, the milliosmole (mOsm) is used when describing fluids. One kilogram of a solution containing 29.25 g (58.5/2 particles) of NaCl would generate 1 osm/kg or 1000 mOsm/kg of osmotic pressure.

Osmolarity is also a measure of the osmotic pressure of a solution based on the number of solute particles in that solution. However, osmolarity refers to the number of particles per liter of solvent rather than per kilogram of solvent, as with osmolality. There is

TABLE 15-2 Composition of Solutions Used in Fluid Therapy

	Glucose* (g/L)	Na+ (mEq/L)	Cl− (mEq/L)	K+ (mEq/L)	Ca2+ (mEq/L)	Mg2+ (mEq/L)	Buffer† (mEq/L)	Osmolarity (mOsm/L)	kcal/L	pH
Dextrose Electrolyte Solution Composition										
5% dextrose	50	0	0	0	0	0	0	252	170	4.0
10% dextrose	100	0	0	0	0	0	0	505	340	4.0
2.5% dextrose in 0.45% NaCl	25	77	77	0	0	0	0	280	85	4.5
5% dextrose in 0.45% NaCl	50	77	77	0	0	0	0	406	170	4.0
5% dextrose and 0.9% NaCl	50	154	154	0	0	0	0	560	170	4.0
0.45% NaCl	0	77	77	0	0	0	0	154	0	5.0
0.85% NaCl (normal saline)	0	145	145	0	0	0	0	290	0	5.0
0.9% NaCl	0	154	154	0	0	0	0	308	0	5.0
3% NaCl	0	513	513	0	0	0	0	1026	0	5.0
Ringer's solution	0	147.5	156	4	4.5	0	0	310	0	5.5
Lactated Ringer's solution	0	130	109	4	3	0	23(L)	272	9	6.5
2.5% dextrose in lactated Ringer's solution	25	130	109	4	3	0	28(L)	398	94	5.0
5% dextrose in lactated Ringer's solution	50	130	109	4	3	0	28(L)	524	179	5.0
2.5% dextrose in half-strength lactated Ringer's solution	25	65.5	55	2	1.5	0	14(L)	263	89	5.0
Normosol-M in 5% dextrose‡	50	40	40	13	0	3	16(A)	364	175	5.5
Normosol-R‡	0	140	98	5	0	3	27(A) 23(G)	296	18	6.4
Plasma-Lyte§	0	140	103	10	5	3	47(A) 8(L)	312	17	5.5
Plasma-Lyte M in 5% dextrose‡	50	40	40	16	5	3	12(A) 12(L)	376	178	5.5
Plasma	1	145	105	5	5	3	24(B)	300	—	7.4
Additives and Solutions										
20% mannitol	200(M)	0	0	0	0	0	0	1099	—	
7.5% NaHCO₃	0	893(B)	0	0	0	0	893(B)	1786	0	
8.4% NaHCO₃	0	1000(B)	0	0	0	0	1000(B)	2000	0	
10% CaCl₂	0	0	2720	0	1360	0	0	4080	0	
14.9% KCl	0	0	2000	2000	0	0	0	4000	0	
50% dextrose	500	0	0	0	0	0	0	2780	1700	4.2

*All glucose, with one exception: M, mannitol.
†Buffers used: A, acetate; B, bicarbonate; G, gluconate; L, lactate.
‡CEVA Laboratories.
§Baxter Healthcare.
From Chew, D.J., DiBartola, S.P.: Manual of Small Animal Nephrology and Urology. W.B. Saunders Co., Philadelphia, 1986, pp. 308-309.

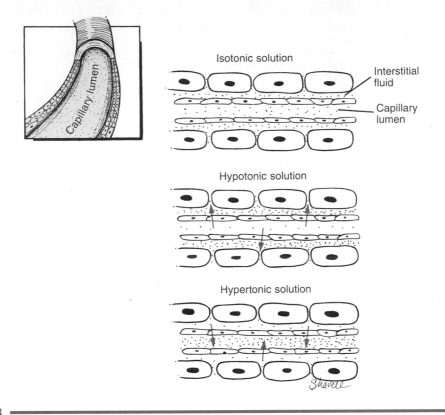

Figure 15-3

Schematic showing the osmotic effects of fluids.

very little difference, however, between osmolality and osmolarity of animals' fluids, and the terms are frequently used interchangeably. A 1 L solution containing a full gram molecular weight (58.5 g) of NaCl would generate 2 osm or 2000 mOsm/L of osmotic pressure.

Not all solutes contribute to osmotic activity (exert a "pull" on water molecules). Those particles that are capable of generating pressure are called *effective osmoles,* and those that are not are called *ineffective osmoles.* Sodium and glucose provide most of the effective osmoles in commercial fluid preparations (Chew, 1994). The total effective osmolarity/osmolality of a solution is called *tonicity.* The osmolarity of dog and cat serum is approximately 300 mOsm/L. Commercial fluids with an osmolarity of 300 mOsm/L are isotonic (e.g., Ringer's solution); those with an osmolar-

ity greater than 300 mOsm/L are hypertonic (e.g., 10% dextrose); and those with an osmolarity less than 300 mOsm/L are hypotonic (e.g., 0.45% saline). Tonicity can be an important consideration when choosing a fluid or its route of administration, because a hypotonic solution can shift fluid out of the intravascular space and a hypertonic solution can shift fluid into the intravascular space (Figure 15-3).

PRINCIPLES OF FLUID THERAPY

Fluid therapy is a critical but somewhat inexact component of veterinary medical care. It is critical because it is often lifesaving, but it is inexact because its application revolves around estimating the amount of fluid loss and consequently the amount of fluid that must be replaced. Fortunately, if the heart and kidneys and the processes that sense and control fluid balance are functioning normally, many errors of estimation are compensated for automatically.

INDICATIONS FOR FLUID THERAPY

A basic factor in the decision to administer fluids is the animal's hydration status. The hydration status is determined by evaluating the patient's history, physical examination status, and the results of basic laboratory tests. If it is determined that the animal has lost more water than it has taken in, it is said to be in a state of *dehydration,* and fluids must be administered to compensate. In addition, fluids are often administered to maintain normal hydration status in animals that are losing excessive fluid quantities, to replace electrolytes and nutrients, and to maintain an open intravenous line for administering medications.

FLUID BALANCE

In normal animals, the intake of fluid and electrolytes is adjusted to offset losses that occur. The sources of water intake include (1) water that is drunk, (2) water ingested in food, and (3) water that results from the metabolism of food (metabolic water). Normal routes of water loss include (1) urine, (2) fecal water, (3) sweat (horses), and (4) respiration. Respiratory loss can potentially be important in dogs because of panting, and sweating can be important in horses. Fluid losses are frequently characterized as sensible, or those that can be easily measured (e.g., urine), and insensible, or those that cannot be easily measured (e.g., fecal and respiratory losses).

Decreased fluid intake often accompanies anorexia, and increased fluid loss occurs in disease states that cause polyuria, vomiting, and diarrhea. Third-space shifts of body water may occasionally cause quantities to be taken out of circulation (e.g., intestinal obstruction, body cavity effusions, or hemorrhage). Extensive burns, uncommon in veterinary medicine, can also cause extensive fluid loss.

HISTORY, PHYSICAL EXAMINATION, AND LABORATORY FINDINGS

A patient's history provides important information about the route and extent of water intake and loss. Knowing the route of loss can aid a clinician in determining the type of fluid to use to correct dehydration and electrolyte imbalances. Table 15-3 lists various causes of dehydration and the fluid indicated for treating the condition. For example, acute vomiting leads to loss of potassium and chloride ions, whereas acute diarrhea causes primarily a potassium loss.

The physical examination provides important information about the extent of fluid loss. The skin **turgor** test, along with other physical findings, is used to determine the percentage of body weight that has been lost via fluid (Table 15-4). This skin turgor test is performed by pinching up a fold of skin over the thoracic or lumbar area and then determining how long it takes to return to a normal position. If the neck area is used in small animals, the extra skin may cause misleading results. The point of the shoulder should be used in horses, because the skin of the neck area can again be misleading. The longer the skin takes to return to normal, the greater the degree of dehydration. Animals with little body fat may appear to be more dehydrated than they really are (slow return to normal skin position) because of low body fat levels, whereas obese animals may appear to be well-hydrated when they are not because the increased fat increases skin elasticity. The presence of dry mucous membranes; an increased heart rate; weak, thready pulses; reduced jugular distention (especially in horses); and a reduced capillary refill time all may be indicators of dehydration. Because most of the evaluations mentioned earlier are subjective, simple laboratory tests may be performed to aid in assessing hydration status.

Simple laboratory tests that can aid in evaluating hydration status are the packed cell volume (PCV), total plasma protein (TPP) determination, and urine specific gravity. Dehydration generally results in an increase in the PCV, TPP, and urine specific gravity. Because anemia can make a dehydrated patient appear to be normally hydrated, the PCV should always be evaluated with the TPP. Readers should consult more

TABLE 15-3 Fluid and Electrolyte Disorders and Fluids Used in Their Correction

Abnormality	Type of Dehydration	Electrolyte Balance	Acid-Base Status	Fluid Therapy
Simple dehydration, stress, exercise	Hypertonic			Half-strength or balanced electrolyte solution; 5% dextrose solution
Heatstroke	Hypertonic	K^+ variable Na^+ variable	Metabolic acidosis	Half-strength electrolyte solution followed by balanced electrolyte solution
Anorexia	Isotonic	K^+ loss	Mild metabolic acidosis	Balanced electrolyte solution; KCl
Starvation	Isotonic	K^+ loss	Mild metabolic acidosis	Half-strength or balanced electrolyte solution; KCl; calories
Vomiting	Isotonic or hypertonic	Na^+, K^+, and Cl^- loss	Metabolic alkalosis; metabolic acidosis chronically	Ringer's solution; 0.9% saline with KCl supplementation
Diarrhea	Isotonic or hypertonic	Na^+ loss K^+ loss chronically	Metabolic acidosis	Balanced electrolyte solution; HCO_3^-; KCl (if chronic)
Diabetes mellitus	Hypertonic	K^+ loss	Metabolic acidosis	Balanced electrolyte solutions; KCl
Hyperadreno-corticism	Isotonic	K^+ loss	Occasionally mild metabolic alkalosis	Balanced electrolyte solutions; KCl
Hypoadreno-corticism	Isotonic or hypertonic	Na^+ loss K^+ retention	Metabolic acidosis	0.9% saline followed by balanced electrolyte solutions
Urethral obstruction	Isotonic or hypertonic	K^+ retention Na^+, Cl^- variable	Metabolic acidosis	0.9% saline followed by balanced electrolyte solution; KCl post-obstruction
Acute renal failure	Isotonic or hypertonic (with vomiting)	K^+ retention Na^+, Cl^- variable	Metabolic acidosis	Balanced electrolyte solutions
Chronic renal failure	Isotonic or hypertonic (with vomiting)	Na^+, K^+, Cl^- variable	Metabolic acidosis	Balanced electrolyte solutions
Congestive heart failure	Plethoric (Na^+, H_2O retention early); hypotonic chronically	Na^+ retention (but dilutional hyponatremia)	Metabolic acidosis (chronically)	5% dextrose solution
Hemorrhagic shock	Isotonic		Metabolic acidosis	Balanced electrolyte solutions; blood
Endotoxic shock	Isotonic		Metabolic acidosis	Balanced electrolyte solutions; 0.9% saline

From Muir W.W., DiBartola, S.P.: Fluid therapy. In Kirk, R.W. (ed.): Current Veterinary Therapy VIII: Small Animal Practice. W.B. Saunders Company, Philadelphia, 1983, p. 31.

TABLE 15-4 Clinical Signs of Dehydration	
Clinical Signs	**Percent Dehydration**
Not detectable	<5
Slight loss of skin elasticity	5-6
Noticeable delay in return of skin to normal position. Slight increase in capillary refill time. Dry mucous membranes.	6-8
Skin remains "tented." Continued increase in capillary refill time. Eyes sunken in orbits. Tachycardia and weak pulses.	10-12
Prominent signs of shock and/or death.	12-15

advanced references for interpretation of laboratory findings related to hydration status.

DETERMINING THE AMOUNT OF FLUID TO ADMINISTER

The three values that are calculated to determine the volume of fluid to administer are (1) the hydration deficit, (2) the maintenance requirement, and (3) the contemporary (ongoing) losses.

The hydration deficit is the amount of fluid that must be replaced to bring the animal back to a normal hydration status and is calculated by multiplying the percentage of dehydration by the patient's normal body weight. The percentage of dehydration is estimated from the history, physical examination, and laboratory findings. The saying "a pint is a pound the world around" can then be applied, because a pint is roughly equivalent to 500 ml. For example, if a 22 lb beagle is determined to be 5% dehydrated, the hydration deficit is calculated as follows:

22 lb × 0.05 (5%) = 1.1 lb of fluid loss

1.1 lb × 500 ml/lb = 550 ml replacement fluid needed

If an animal's weight is measured in kilograms, the calculations are made in a similar manner except that the weight of fluid loss (in kilograms) is multiplied times 1000 because 1 kg is roughly equivalent to 1 L (1000 ml). Using the same 22 lb (10 kg) beagle, the calculations are as follows:

10 kg × 0.05 (5%) = 0.5 kg of fluid loss

0.5 kg × 1000 ml/kg = 500 ml of replacement fluid

The second value needed to calculate the volume of fluids to administer is the maintenance value. Daily maintenance volumes are related to daily energy requirement and can be read from Figure 15-4. Many veterinarians calculate maintenance values by using thumb rules (20 to 30 ml/lb/day) established by Chew (1994), Muir and DiBartola (1983), DiBartola (1992), and others. Readers should consult these references if more precise calculations are required. Using the thumb rule, our 20 lb beagle would need:

22 lb × 25 ml/lb/day = 550 ml/day for maintenance

The final calculation to be made is that for ongoing losses. If we estimate that our beagle is losing 100 ml of fluid per day through vomiting, then we would need to add an additional 100 ml of fluid to our total calculated volume.

The total volume that our beagle would need to be given in 24 hours then, is

550 ml to correct the hydration deficit
550 ml for normal maintenance
100 ml for ongoing vomiting losses
1200 ml total

ROUTES OF FLUID ADMINISTRATION

The route by which fluids are administered depends on several factors, such as the nature of the condition being treated, its duration, and its severity. The routes that may be used are (1) intravenous, (2) subcutaneous, (3) oral, (4) intraperitoneal, and (5) intraosseous.

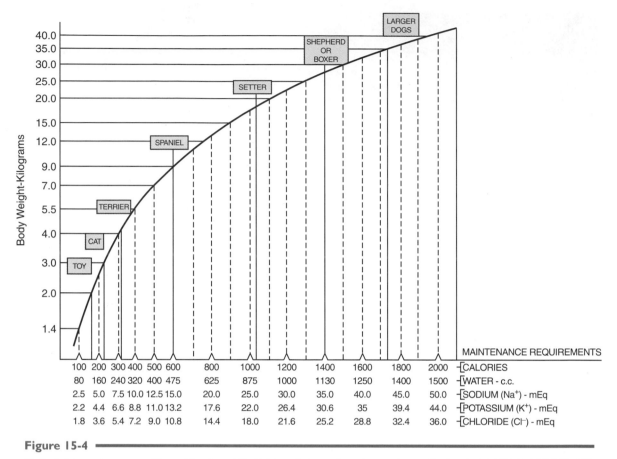

Figure 15-4

Daily fluid requirements. (From Harrison, J.B.: Fluid and electrolyte therapy in small animals. J.A.V.M.A. 137:637–645, 1960.)

The intravenous route is preferred when the loss has been great or the disorder is severe. The intravenous route allows quicker, more precise delivery of fluids than the other routes. This route does require placement of an intravenous catheter and closer monitoring because of potential complications such as obstruction or kinking of the catheter, septicemia, embolism, and phlebitis. Catheters should be flushed with heparinized saline (5 U/ml of 0.9% saline) every 6 to 12 hours and should be removed and replaced every 72 hours to minimize complications.

The subcutaneous route is useful when a patient's needs are not severe. The amount of fluid that can be administered subcutaneously depends on the size of the animal and the amount of loose skin that it has. Between 50 and 200 ml can generally be infused at a subcutaneous site. Great care should be taken not to administer enough fluid to dissect the skin loose from its blood supply, because this can cause sloughing of the skin over the site. Hypertonic or irritating fluids should not be given by the subcutaneous route.

The oral route is a practical means of administering fluids as long as an animal has no severe disorders of the gastrointestinal system. This route allows normal physiologic processes to control the amount of fluid and the amount and type of electrolytes absorbed. This route is not satisfactory when large volumes of fluid need to be given rapidly.

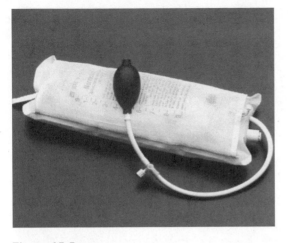

Figure 15-5

Pressure administration cuff. (Infusable Pressure Infuser is a registered trademark of Biomedical Dynamics. Sold by Sanofi Animal Health, Inc., Overland Park, KS.)

The intraperitoneal route allows for administration of large volumes of fluid, but the absorption is slow. Peritonitis is a potential complication, and this route is not commonly used.

The intraosseous (femur, ilium, or humerus) route is sometimes used in very small animals or in those with poor access to veins. This route allows rapid delivery of fluids and blood but does require more technical expertise for placing the delivery needle. Careful attention should be paid to sterile technique when this route is used to avoid causing osteomyelitis.

RATE OF ADMINISTRATION

Once the volume of fluid needed and the route of administration have been decided, the time frame for delivering the fluids must be established. Rapid losses of fluid usually call for rapid replacement. In veterinary practice, fluid flow rates are often determined **empirically**; however, some generalizations are helpful.

For treating shock, fluids should be administered rapidly (40 ml/lb/hour in dogs and 20 to 30 ml/lb/hour in cats). The use of a pressure administration cuff may allow more rapid infusion in these cases (Figure 15-5).

Fluids should ideally be infused continuously during a 24-hour period. One method of determining fluid flow rate is to calculate the hydration deficit, add maintenance and ongoing losses, and set the drip rate to administer the total during a 24-hour period. Some clinicians prefer to administer the hydration deficit during the first few hours and then give the remainder over a longer period. Some divide the total calculated volume into three equal parts and administer each in an 8-hour period. In many practices, fluid administration can be monitored for a part of the day only. In this case, the total 24-hour fluid volume can be administered during the period that the patient can be monitored (common sense and medical judgment must be exercised). Portions of the total volume may be administered subcutaneously when appropriate.

Fluids are administered from plastic bags or bottles or from glass bottles through intravenous administration sets (Figures 15-6 and 15-7). Two sizes of administration sets that are commonly used in veterinary medicine are the standard macrodrip set (15 drops/ml) and the minidrip/microdrip set (60 drops/ml). Other sizes (10 drops/ml and 20 drops/ml) are also available. The microdrip sets are suited for use in administering fluids to cats and small dogs. The size of the administration set must be known to calculate the drip or flow rate.

To calculate the drip rate, first divide the total number of milliliters to be administered by the total number of minutes for administration to determine the number of milliliters per minute to deliver. Then multiply the milliliters per minute by the drops per milliliter of the administration set you have chosen to use to arrive at the number of drops (gtt) per minute (gtt/min). For example, if we wish to give our beagle 1200 ml of fluid during a 24-hour period using a standard (15 gtt/ml) administration set:

$$\frac{\text{Volume of infusion (ml)}}{\text{Time of infusion (min)}} \times \text{drop factor (gtt/ml)} = \text{gtt/min}$$

$$\frac{1200 \text{ ml}}{24 \text{ hours} \times 60 \text{ min/hour}} = \frac{1200 \text{ ml}}{1440 \text{ min}}$$

$$= 0.83 \text{ ml/min} \times 15 \text{ gtt/ml} = 12.5 \text{ gtt/min}$$

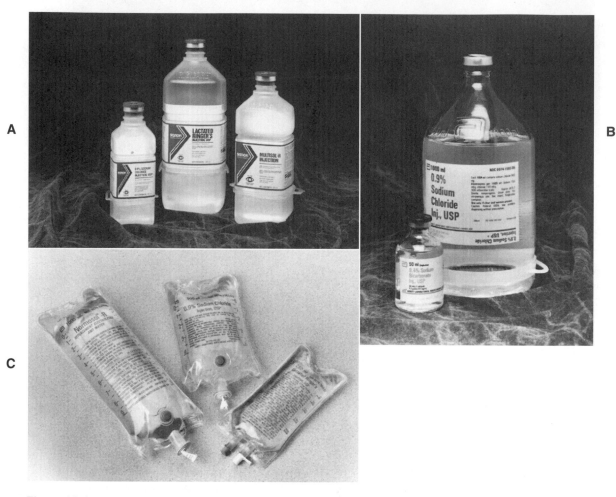

Figure 15-6

Types of fluid containers. **A,** RigiCare rigid plastic bottles. **B,** Glass bottles. **C,** LIFECARE flexible plastic bags. (Photo courtesy Sanofi Animal Health, Inc., Overland Park, KS; RigiCare is a registered trademark of Sanofi Animal Health, Inc., Overland Park, KS; LIFECARE is a registered trademark of Abbott Laboratories.)

A rate of 12.5 gtt/min can be thought of as 1 drop approximately every 5 seconds $\left(\frac{60}{12} = 5\right)$.

When standard gravity flow bags or bottles are used, drip rates are controlled by devices that are placed on the administration sets to adjust the diameter of the line (e.g., roller clamps, slide clamps, or screw clamps) (Figure 15-8). The flow rate is simply dialed in on the machine when fluid infusion pumps (ml/hour) or controllers (ml/min) are used.

MONITORING FLUID ADMINISTRATION

Fluids administered too rapidly or in too great a volume can be life threatening. Careful monitoring of the physical status of the animal is essential. Lung sounds, skin turgor, and the overall status of the animal should be monitored regularly, as well as the PCV and TPP. When a large volume of fluids is administered rapidly, it is prudent to insert a urinary catheter to monitor urine output and establish that the kidneys are functioning normally. Some clinicians also choose to in-

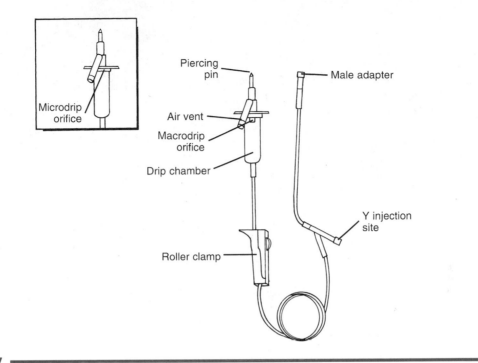

Figure 15-7

Intravenous administration set.

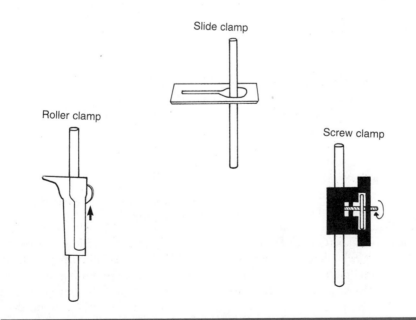

Figure 15-8

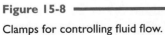

Clamps for controlling fluid flow.

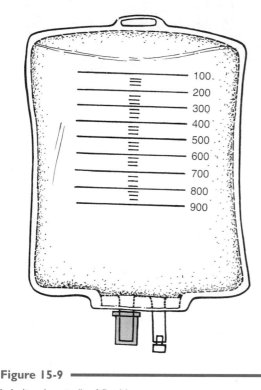

Figure 15-9

Labeling (vertical) of fluid bag.

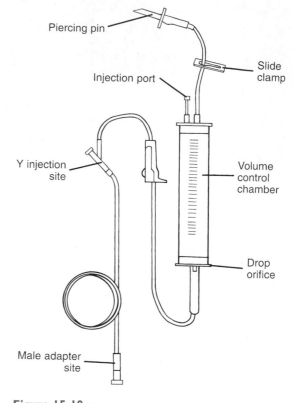

Figure 15-10

Volume control administration set.

sert a jugular catheter to monitor central venous pressure as a way of preventing fluid volume overload.

Signs of overhydration may include restlessness, serous nasal discharge, increased lung sounds (crackles), tachycardia, dyspnea, and others. Fluid infusion should be slowed or stopped and the veterinarian contacted at the first appearance of these signs.

Labeled adhesive tape should be placed vertically on fluid bottles or bags to allow monitoring of the volume delivered (Figure 15-9). Bottles or bags should also be labeled with all pertinent information, including the presence of any additives. It may be helpful to place a horizontal piece of tape across the fluid container to indicate when fluid delivery is to be stopped.

A volume control system or Buretrol device may

be used for administering small volumes of fluid (Figure 15-10). A clamp allows the volume control chamber to be filled with a predetermined amount of fluid from the bag or bottle. The line is then clamped off to prevent entry of additional fluid from the bag. The chamber can be refilled if desired.

PREPARING FLUID ADMINISTRATION EQUIPMENT

When preparing to administer intravenous fluids, you should follow a standard protocol. After gathering your supplies and preparing the injection site, check to see that you have the correct fluid type and that it is not out of date. Then determine that the container is not cracked or chipped and that the solution is clear.

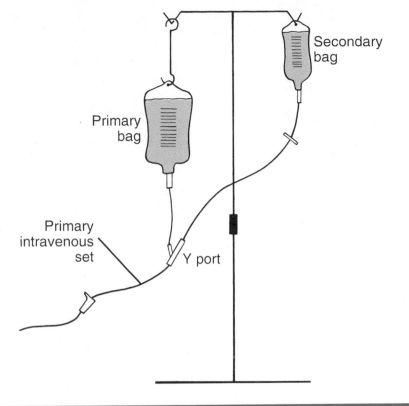

Figure 15-11

Piggyback setup of fluids.

Fluids should never contain precipitates or appear cloudy. After inspecting the container's cap to make sure that it is intact, remove the metal cap (bottle) or insertion port cover (bag), being careful not to contaminate the port. Close the flow clamp on the administration set and remove the cover from the administration set spike. Wipe the port with an alcohol swab and insert the administration set spike into the rubber stopper (bottle) or insertion port (bag). Hang the bottle or bag, and fill the administration set line by opening the flow clamp and allowing fluid to run through the line until all bubbles are cleared. Close the flow clamp and attach the adapter to the intravenous catheter using sterile technique. After the flow clamp is opened to determine that the catheter and the line are patent, the drip rate may be adjusted as required.

If at any time the flow rate slows or stops, check the following: (1) the catheter for correct placement and patency, (2) the position of the patient to determine whether limb position or flexion has occluded the flow, (3) the flow clamp to see whether it is in the open position, (4) the tubing to determine whether it is kinked or crimped, and (5) the fluid level in the bottle.

Two fluid solutions may be administered simultaneously by using a piggyback setup of the containers (Figure 15-11). The secondary bag is hung higher than the primary bag, and the secondary administration set line is connected to the Y port of the primary administration set.

It is useful for a technician to understand the use of a three-way valve. The three-way valve permits three-way connections to be made. Flow of fluid through the valve depends on the position at which the control handle is placed. The handle points toward the line

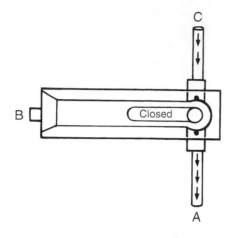

Figure 15-12

Operation of a three-way valve.

that is closed. Figure 15-12 illustrates the operation of a three-way valve.

TYPES OF SOLUTIONS USED IN FLUID THERAPY

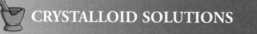

CRYSTALLOID SOLUTIONS

Crystalloids are solutions containing electrolyte and non-electrolyte substances that are capable of passing through cell membranes and can therefore enter all body fluid compartments. Administration of crystalloid solutions therefore results in rapid equilibration of fluid between the intravascular and the interstitial spaces. Crystalloid solutions are routinely used in veterinary medicine because of their versatility and relatively low cost. Crystalloid solutions can further be classified as replacement or maintenance solutions. Replacement solutions resemble ECF in content, whereas maintenance solutions contain less sodium and more potassium than replacement fluids.

Clinical Uses. Fluids are administered for correction of dehydration, treatment of shock, maintenance of normal hydration, replacement of electrolytes and nutrients, and as a vehicle for administration of intravenous drugs.

Dosage Forms. Dosage forms are numerous. Fluids are available in glass bottles, plastic bottles, and plastic bags that hold 250, 500, and 1000 ml. Containers that hold 3000 and 6000 ml are available for some solutions (see manufacturer product guides). The following section briefly describes the commonly used crystalloid solutions. For a listing of the composition and other characteristics of each, see Table 15-3.

Adverse Side Effects. Adverse side effects of fluid administration are primarily associated with overhydration. Signs of overhydration may include restlessness, shivering, serous nasal discharge, coughing, and pulmonary edema.

Physiologic Saline

Physiologic saline is a 0.9% solution of NaCl and is also called *normal saline*. It may also be called *isotonic saline* because it has an osmolarity of 308 mOsm/L. Saline is used to increase plasma volume or to correct a sodium deficiency (**hyponatremia**). It may also be used to bathe tissues during surgery to prevent them from drying out. Because of its high sodium content, saline should not be used in animals with known heart disease.

Lactated Ringer's Solution

Lactated Ringer's solution is one of the most versatile and commonly used fluids in veterinary medicine. It is a balanced electrolyte replacement solution and can be administered by any route that is available. It contains 28 mEq/L of lactate, which is converted by the liver to bicarbonate to act as a **buffer** against acidosis. Theoretically, lactated Ringer's solution should not be administered with blood because the calcium contents could cause clotting to occur.

Dextrose 5% in Water

Dextrose 5% in water (D5W) is a non-balanced solution that contains only dextrose (50 g/L) and water. Administering dextrose 5% is equivalent to administering pure water because the dextrose is metabolized to carbon dioxide and water. Dextrose 5% provides approximately 170 kcal/L (a quantity that cannot be relied on to meet the daily caloric needs of most small animals), although it may supplement other caloric sources. Dextrose 5% should not generally be given by the subcutaneous route because it may osmotically "draw" fluid from the vascular space. Dextrose in water should not be used as a maintenance solution because it may dilute out all electrolytes.

Ringer's Solution

Ringer's solution is a balanced replacement solution that contains more sodium, calcium, and chloride than lactated Ringer's solution. It contains no lactate, however, and can be used in cases of **metabolic alkalosis**.

2.5% Dextrose in Half-Strength (0.45%) Saline/Potassium Added

Half-strength (0.45%) saline in 2.5% dextrose with 5 mEq/L of potassium chloride is a maintenance solution that is appropriate for use in patients that have sodium restrictions.

Multisol-R/Normosol-R

Multisol-R is the veterinary trademark for Normosol-R. Both are balanced, multiple electrolyte solutions with a dual buffering system (acetate and gluconate). Acetate and gluconate are metabolized outside the liver, a factor that may have advantages in conditions such as liver disorders. Both Multisol-R and Normosol-R are calcium free and thus may help to prevent potential incompatibilities with transfused blood or added sodium bicarbonate.

Normosol-M in 5% Dextrose

Normosol-M in 5% dextrose is a balanced maintenance solution that has acetate as a buffer and contains 175 kcal/L.

Plasma-Lyte/Plasma-Lyte M in 5% Dextrose

Plasma-Lyte is a balanced replacement solution with 47 mEq/L of acetate and 8 mEq/L of lactate as buffers. Plasma-Lyte M in 5% dextrose is a maintenance solution with equal amounts of acetate and lactate (12 mEq/L) as buffers and 178 kcal/L.

Technician's Notes

1. Fluids containing preservatives such as benzyl alcohol should never be given to cats because of the likelihood of toxic reactions.
2. Some clinicians warn against administering fluids with preservatives to puppies and adult dogs.

COLLOID SOLUTIONS

Colloid solutions contain large–molecular-weight particles that are unable to cross cell membranes and are therefore confined to the vascular space. These confined particles are effective osmoles that are able to hold fluid in the vascular space and to draw fluid from the interstitial space into the vascular space (expand the plasma volume). They are especially useful when cerebral or pulmonary edema is a potential complication of fluid administration or when crystalloid therapy has not been successful.

Colloids include albumin, plasma, and the synthetic colloids (dextrans and hydroxyethyl starch). Only the commercially available synthetic products are discussed here.

Clinical Uses. Colloid solutions are used for expansion of the plasma volume in the treatment of **hypovolemic** or septic shock.

Dosage Forms

1. The dextrans. Dextran 40 and dextran 70 are large–molecular-weight polysaccharide solutions used in the treatment of shock. Dextran 40 is prepared as a 10% solution in 0.9% saline or in 5% dextrose. Dextran 70 (Macrodex) is supplied as a 6% solution in 0.9% saline and is the most commonly used form of the dextrans in veterinary medicine. The dextrans may cause allergic reactions or clotting deficits in some animals.
2. Hetastarch (Hespan). Hydroxyethyl starch (hetastarch) is a large-molecular–weight starch that is used in the treatment of hypovolemia and hypoproteinemia. Hetastarch expands the plasma volume longer and has fewer side effects than the

dextrans. It is prepared as a 6% solution in 0.9% saline. The primary disadvantage of hetastarch is its expense.

3. Oxypolygelatin (Plasm.ex). Oxypolygelatin is a hypo-osmolar 5.6% gelatin suspension in sodium chloride (Rudloff and Kirby, 1998). This product has no direct effects on coagulation proteins or platelets. Potential side effects include anaphylaxis.

Adverse Side Effects. Adverse side effects of colloid administration are usually related to clotting deficiencies or allergic reactions.

> **Technician's Notes**
>
> 1. Colloids are not intended for maintenance or long-term use.
> 2. References should be checked for determining the appropriate flow rate for colloid solutions.

HYPERTONIC SOLUTIONS

This discussion is confined to the use of hypertonic saline solutions. These solutions have been advocated by some clinicians in the treatment of hemorrhagic and endotoxic shock, as well as for patients undergoing major surgical procedures (e.g., gastric dilation or volvulus). Like the colloids, the hypertonic saline solutions also may be useful when brain or pulmonary edema is present or is a potential complication.

Clinical Uses. Hypertonic saline solutions are used for the treatment of shock associated with trauma, endotoxemia, burns, pancreatitis, and major surgical procedures.

Dosage Forms. Hypertonic saline solutions are available from commercial sources in 3%, 4%, 5%, 7%, and 23.4% preparations.

Adverse Side Effects. These may include phlebitis; tissue irritation; re-hemorrhage in traumatic shock; electrolyte imbalances; and, when the administration rate is too fast, hypotension, bronchoconstriction, and bradycardia.

> **Technician's Notes**
>
> 1. The rate of administration of the hypertonic saline solutions is a very important consideration because exceeding this rate may cause serious side effects.
> 2. These solutions should be infused through a well-secured intravenous catheter to prevent extravasation of the irritating fluids.

FLUID ADDITIVES

In some instances, special substances may be added to intravenous fluid solutions to enhance the solutions' therapeutic effects. These substances may be added to correct acid-base abnormalities and electrolyte imbalances, to supplement calories, and to provide supplemental vitamins to replace those washed out by fluid therapy.

Sodium Bicarbonate

Sodium bicarbonate (baking soda) is an alkalizing agent that may be added to correct **metabolic acidosis** and certain other conditions. Because lactate or acetate in fluid preparations often cannot correct severe metabolic acidosis, supplementation becomes necessary. Normal serum bicarbonate is 24 mEq/L. Required amounts for supplementation are calculated by measuring a patient's bicarbonate level (or carbon dioxide) and subtracting that value from 24 (normal). The difference is called the *bicarbonate deficit*. The bicarbonate deficit is multiplied by 0.6 and then by the animal's weight in kilograms to determine the number of milliequivalents of sodium bicarbonate to administer.

Bicarbonate supplementation (mEq) =
bicarbonate deficit × 0.6 × weight (kg)

When access to laboratory measurement of bicarbonate or carbon dioxide is not available, **empirical** estimations of supplementation levels are made based on clinical judgment.

TABLE 15-5 Potassium Supplementation Guide*			
Serum K+ (mEq/L)	mEq K+ (To Add to 250 ml Fluid)	mEq K+ (To Add to 1 L Fluid)	Maximum Infusion Rate of Intravenous Fluids (0.5 mEq/kg/hour)
<2.0	20	80	6
2.1-2.5	15	60	8
2.6-3.0	10	40	12
3.1-3.5	7	28	18
>3.5-<5.0	5	20	25

*For dogs or cats with hypokalemia or for those with potassium depletion and normal serum potassium levels. This regimen is designed to be infused in maintenance volume of fluids.

Bicarbonate concentration in commercial products is measured in milliequivalents per milliliter.

Clinical Uses. These include the treatment of metabolic acidosis and as an adjunctive therapy for the treatment of hypercalcemia or **hyperkalemia.**

Dosage Forms. Veterinary-approved forms include the following:

1. An 8% (1 mEq/ml) solution for injection that is available in 50-, 100-, and 500-ml vials
2. A 5% (0.6 mEq/ml) solution for injection

Adverse Side Effects. These may include metabolic alkalosis, hypokalemia, hypocalcemia, and **hypernatremia.**

Technician's Notes

1. Sodium bicarbonate is incompatible with several solutions and should be mixed only after consulting product inserts or appropriate references.
2. Some references indicate that sodium bicarbonate should not be added to solutions containing calcium because of potential for precipitates to form.
3. Replacement of the total number of milliequivalents should be made over several hours.

Potassium Chloride

Potassium chloride is a solution used to supplement potassium deficits (**hypokalemia**). Anorexia, diuresis, and diarrhea are some of the common causes of hypokalemia. Normal serum potassium levels are between 3.5 and 5.5 mEq/L. Table 15-5 provides a guide for potassium supplementation based on the measured serum level of potassium.

Clinical Uses. Potassium chloride is used for the treatment or prevention of potassium deficits.

Dosage Forms. Dosage forms for intravenous use include the following:

1. Potassium chloride for injection (2 mEq/ml) in 10- and 20-ml vials (veterinary approved)
2. Potassium chloride for injection (2 mEq/ml) in 5-, 10-, 20-, 30-, 100-, 200-, and 500-ml vials (human approved)

Adverse Side Effects. These may include hyperkalemia, which is manifested by muscle weakness, and cardiac conduction disturbances, which can be life threatening.

Technician's Notes

1. Potassium chloride solutions must be diluted before administering.
2. The rate of infusion of potassium is critical. Consult product inserts or other references for appropriate rates.

Calcium Supplements

Calcium gluconate and calcium chloride may be diluted (1:1 with saline) and given as an infusion to correct hypocalcemia. This is not a common procedure in practice, however. It is more common to inject the supplement, without diluting, for the treatment of emergency conditions such as eclampsia or milk fever.

Clinical Uses. Calcium supplements are used for the treatment of hypocalcemia that may result from various conditions, which may include parathyroid gland disorders, milk fever, eclampsia, and excessive sweating in horses. Calcium in combination with phosphorus, magnesium, potassium, and dextrose is used to treat conditions in cattle such as grass tetany, milk fever, and downer cow syndrome.

Dosage Forms

1. Calcium gluconate injection (generic and proprietary) 10%, in ampules, syringes, vials, and bottles (veterinary label)
2. Calcium gluconate (various proprietary names), 23%, in 100- and 500-ml bottles (veterinary label)
3. Calcium chloride injection (generic and proprietary), 10%, in ampules, vials, and syringes (human label)
4. Numerous combination products (CalDextro, Norcalciphos) containing calcium, phosphorus, magnesium, potassium, and dextrose

Adverse Side Effects. Adverse side effects that result from hypercalcemia may include hypotension, cardiac arrhythmias, and cardiac arrest. These effects are usually a result of too rapid an infusion of the calcium.

Technician's Notes

1. Any product containing calcium should be given by slow intravenous administration to prevent cardiac complications.
2. Products containing 23% calcium are labeled for large-animal use.

50% Dextrose

When caloric supplementation is indicated, 50% dextrose is often used as a stock solution to add to other fluids to provide a desired percent solution of dextrose. It is not usually possible to meet the total caloric needs of a small-animal patient through dextrose supplementation of intravenous fluids. Supplementation is often indicated, however, in patients that are hypoglycemic because of fever, sepsis, insulin overdose, insulinoma, liver disease, and others. Varying amounts of dextrose may be added in an attempt to keep the blood glucose level near the normal range (80 to 100 mg/dl).

Intravenous administration of 50% dextrose is used in ruminants as a treatment of uncomplicated ketosis.

To prepare a 2.5% solution of dextrose, add 50 ml (25 g) of 50% dextrose to 1 L of fluids. Fifty milliliters of the original fluid solution should be removed before adding the 50% dextrose to keep the dilution correct. To prepare a 5% solution, add 100 ml of 50% dextrose to 1 L of fluids. A formula that may be used to determine the quantity of a stock solution to use in preparing percent solutions follows:

$$\frac{\text{Desired strength}}{\text{Available strength}} = \frac{\text{how much you are going to use}}{\text{how much you are going to make}}$$

or

$$V_1 \times C_1 = V_2 \times C_2$$

For example, if you wish to make 250 ml of a 5% solution of dextrose using your stock supply of 50% dextrose, you would set up your formula in the following way:

$$\frac{5\%}{50\%} = \frac{X}{250}$$

Cross multiplying 50X = 1250

$$X = 25 \text{ ml}$$

Therefore, to prepare the 250 ml of 5% solution, draw up 25 ml of 50% dextrose and add 225 ml of a diluting fluid.

Clinical Uses. These include caloric supplementation in small-animal patients and treatment of ketosis in ruminants.

Dosage Forms. Various manufacturers supply 50% dextrose. The most common package is a 500-ml plastic bottle.

Adverse Side Effects. These are few if used according to directions.

> **Technician's Notes**
> A 50% solution of dextrose contains 500 mg/ml.

Vitamin Supplements

Patients that have been given large amounts of fluids undergo a diuresis that may cause a corresponding loss of the water-soluble vitamins (B complex and C), making fluid supplementation desirable. Animals with polyuria resulting from renal failure also lose water-soluble vitamins and benefit from supplementation of their parenteral fluids. Recommendations for supplementation vary from 0.5 to 2 ml/L of fluids.

Clinical Uses. Vitamin supplements are used for restoration of normal levels of the water-soluble vitamins.

Dosage Forms. Several manufacturers produce vitamin B complex. Care should be taken to ensure that the form selected may be given intravenously. Many are labeled for intramuscular or subcutaneous use only.

Adverse Side Effects. These include hypersensitivity reactions to the thiamine in the complex.

ORAL ELECTROLYTE PREPARATIONS

In severely dehydrated animals, fluids must be given by the intravenous route in order to be effective. In mild to moderate cases of dehydration, however, the oral route is a practical alternative to replenish water and electrolytes.

Oral electrolytes are packaged as powders that are mixed with water to form a solution that can be given free choice or by stomach tube. In some instances, oral pastes or fluids packaged for intravenous use may be given orally. The oral route of administration is especially useful for cases in which the veterinarian wishes to direct the pet or livestock owner in the home or farm treatment of the animal.

Diarrhea in young dairy calves, commonly called *calf scours,* is caused by bacteria, viruses, or nutritional factors and is a condition often treated with oral electrolyte solutions. The diarrhea is commonly a result

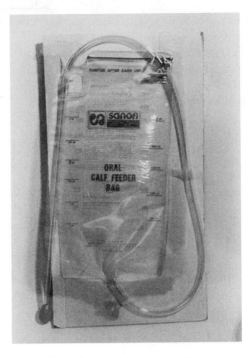

Figure 15-13
Esophageal feeder.

of the type or amount of milk replacer that the calf is being fed. A calf is treated by eliminating the milk replacer from its diet and by giving it an oral electrolyte solution with glucose or glycine for 24 to 48 hours. Glucose and glycine provide a source of calories and may enhance absorption of the electrolytes. The solution may be administered via an esophageal feeder—a device that has a plastic bag (for mixing the electrolyte solution) attached to a rigid delivery tube (Figure 15-13). The tube has a ball of sufficient diameter on the distal end to prevent introduction of the tube into the trachea.

Oral electrolyte solutions or pastes are often given to performance horses to replace the electrolytes lost through sweating. Horses participating in endurance races, 3-day events, and other athletically demanding events benefit from electrolyte replenishment.

Administration of oral electrolyte solutions may also be helpful as a follow-up to intravenous fluid therapy for dogs recovering from viral enteritis or other diseases causing prolonged vomiting or diarrhea.

Hypokalemia in dogs and cats may be treated with oral potassium products.

Clinical Uses. These include electrolyte and water replenishment.

Dosage Forms. Dosage forms are numerous, and the following is only a partial listing:

1. Avian Bluelite (powder)
2. Biolyte (powder)
3. Elpak-G Electrolyte Gel
4. Equine Bluelite (powder)
5. Entrolyte (powder)
6. Equi-Phar ElectrAmino Paste
7. Formula 911 (powder)
8. Ora-Lyte (powder)
9. Re-Sorb (powder)
10. Tumil-K (powder, gel, and tablets for dogs and cats)
11. Vedalyte 8X (powder)
12. Ritrol

Adverse Side Effects. These are rare if care is taken not to cause inadvertent administration into the respiratory system.

Technician's Notes

Some of the oral electrolyte products for farm animals also contain antibiotics.

PARENTERAL VITAMIN/MINERAL PRODUCTS

Parenteral vitamin/mineral products are used to prevent or treat various conditions in veterinary medicine. They are used as therapeutic agents in large-animal medicine more than in small-animal medicine. White muscle disease, "tying up," polyneuritis, pink eye, reproductive problems, bracken fern poisoning, and polioencephalomalacia are only a few of the conditions prevented or treated with vitamin products in large-animal practice. In small-animal practice, routine vitamin and mineral supplementation is not con-

sidered necessary if the animal receives a balanced diet. Many small-animal clinicians consider overuse of vitamin/mineral products a bigger problem than vitamin/mineral deficiencies. Warfarin poisoning (vitamin K) and certain dermatologic conditions (zinc) are exceptions.

Oral multiple vitamin/mineral products are numerous and are not listed here.

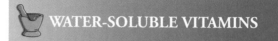

WATER-SOLUBLE VITAMINS

Vitamin B Complex

B complex vitamins are a group of water-soluble vitamins that include thiamine, riboflavin, niacinamide (niacin), *d*-panthenol (pantothenic acid), pyridoxine, cyanocobalamin (B_{12}), biotin, choline, and folic acid. B vitamins serve as co-enzymes for many metabolic reactions in the body. B complex is often added to intravenous fluids (discussed earlier) and may be given parenterally in an attempt to enhance the biochemical response of stressed or debilitated animals.

Clinical Uses. These vitamins are administered to replace or supplement a deficiency of B complex vitamins.

Dosage Forms

1. B Complex One-Fifty Injection
2. Vitamin B Complex
3. Vitamin B Complex Fortified
4. Vitamin B Complex Injectable

Adverse Side Effects. These can include allergic reactions and pain at the injection site.

Technician's Notes

1. Check the label before giving B complex intravenously.
2. Observe the animal for allergic reactions.
3. B complex injections may cause pain at the injection site.

Thiamine Hydrochloride (Vitamin B_1)

Thiamine is a water-soluble B complex vitamin that acts as a co-enzyme for biochemical reactions involved in carbohydrate metabolism. Deficiency of thiamine may occur as a consequence of decreased intake or synthesis or from increased destruction, which may result from bracken fern poisoning, thiamine-destroying factors in the rumen, or thiaminase in raw fish. Polioencephalomalacia of ruminants has also been associated with thiamine deficiency.

Clinical Uses. Thiamine is administered for the treatment of thiamine deficiency in all domestic species and as an aid in the treatment of lead poisoning in cattle.

Dosage Forms

1. Vita-Jec Thiamine HCl
2. Thiamine hydrochloride (generic)
3. Vitamin B_1 injection

Adverse Side Effects. These may include hypersensitivity reactions and muscle soreness at intramuscular injection sites.

Vitamin B_{12} (Cyanocobalamin)

Vitamin B_{12} is a B complex vitamin that contains cobalt and is thought to act as a co-enzyme in protein synthesis. Pernicious anemia is a condition that occurs in humans as a result of a failure to absorb B_{12} adequately. A deficiency in any case results in anemia because red blood cells fail to mature properly in the absence of B_{12}. B_{12} deficiencies are rare in veterinary medicine.

Clinical Uses. Vitamin B_{12} is administered for the management of B_{12} deficiencies.

Dosage Forms

1. Vita-Jec Vitamin B_{12}
2. Vitamin B_{12} injection

Adverse Side Effects. These may include allergic reactions to administration.

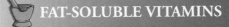 FAT-SOLUBLE VITAMINS

Vitamin A

Vitamin A is an organic alcohol that is converted from plant substances called *carotenoids* (e.g., beta carotene) in the intestine and liver and stored primarily in the liver. It is needed for proper growth and maintenance of surface epithelium, for proper bone growth, and for maintenance of visual pigments in the retina. A deficiency of vitamin A may be associated with many clinical signs, including poor growth and reproductive performance, susceptibility to infectious disease, and poor vision in dim light. Many of the commercial vitamin A products are combined with vitamin D or E.

Clinical Uses. Vitamin A is administered for the prevention or treatment of vitamin A deficiencies.

Dosage Forms

1. A-D Injection
2. Vitamin AD Injection
3. Vitamin AD_3
4. Vital E + A
5. AD = 5 (beta carotene for use in horses)

Adverse Side Effects. These are uncommon if label directions are followed.

Vitamin D

Vitamin D exists in two forms—D_2 and D_3. Vitamin D_2 is formed when a plant substance (ergosterol) is exposed to sunlight, and D_3 is formed when a provitamin precalciferol in the skin is converted by sunlight. A deficiency of vitamin D is characterized by the development of rickets in young animals or osteomalacia in adults. Vitamin D is often combined commercially with vitamin A or E.

Clinical Uses. Vitamin D is administered for the treatment or prevention of vitamin D deficiencies.

Dosage Forms. Refer to the dosage forms for vitamin A.

Adverse Side Effects. These are uncommon if label directions are followed.

Vitamin E

Vitamin E (alpha-tocopherol) is involved (with selenium) in the metabolism of sulfur and acts as an antioxidant. Vitamin E is used in the prevention or treatment of selenium/vitamin E deficiency syndromes such as white muscle disease (ewes, lambs, and calves), mulberry heart disease (sows and pigs), and myositis (horses).

Clinical Uses. Vitamin E is administered for the prevention and treatment of vitamin E deficiencies.

Dosage Forms

1. Bo-Se (selenium, vitamin E injection [approved for use in calves, swine, and sheep])
2. E-SE (selenium, vitamin E injection [approved for use in horses])
3. Mu-Se (selenium, vitamin E injection [approved for use in non-lactating dairy cattle and beef cattle])
4. L-Se (selenium, vitamin E injection [approved for use in lambs and baby pigs])
5. Seletoc (selenium, vitamin E injection [approved for use in dogs])
6. Velenium
7. Vital E-300 and Vital E-500 injectable tocopherol
8. Vital E + A

Adverse Side Effects. These include allergic reactions and soreness at injection sites.

Vitamin K

Vitamin K is a fat-soluble vitamin required for the formation of prothrombin and for this reason is very important to the clotting process. Vitamin K is discussed in Chapter 16.

REFERENCES

Blankenship, J., Campbell, J.B.: Solutions. In Blankenship, J., Campbell, J.B. (eds.): Laboratory Mathematics: Medical and Biological Applications. Mosby, St. Louis, 1976.

Chew, D.J.: Fluid therapy for dogs and cats. In Birchard, S., Sherding, R. (eds.): Saunders Manual of Small Animal Practice. W.B. Saunders Company, Philadelphia, 1994.

DiBartola, S.P.: Introduction to fluid therapy. In DiBartola, S.P. (ed.): Fluid Therapy in Small Animal Practice. W.B. Saunders Company, Philadelphia, 1992.

Muir, W.W., DiBartola, S.P.: Fluid therapy. In Kirk, R.W. (ed.): Current Veterinary Therapy VIII: Small Animal Practice. W.B. Saunders Company, Philadelphia, 1983.

Rudloff, E., Kirby, R.: Fluid therapy: crystalloids and colloids. In Boothe, D.M. (ed): The Veterinary Clinics of North America, Small Animal Practice. W.B. Saunders Company, Philadelphia, 1998.

■ Review Questions

1. Define hyperkalemia.

   _____

2. Intravascular fluid makes up approximately
   _____ body weight.
   a. 2%
   b. 5%
   c. 15%
   d. 40%

3. Explain the concept of a balanced solution for fluid
   therapy. _____

4. What are three units of measurement for quantifying
   electrolytes in fluids?

   _____

5. Therapeutic fluids with an osmolarity of approximately
   _____ mOsm/L are iso-
   tonic.
   a. 100
   b. 200
   c. 300
   d. 500

6. Give examples of sensible and insensible fluid losses.

   _____

7. Underestimation of the degree of dehydration is sometimes a problem in _____
   animals.

8. One pound of fluid is equivalent to
   _____ milliliters, and 1 kg
   is equivalent to _____
   milliliters.

9. The three volumes that are calculated to arrive at the
   total fluid volume are

   _____.

10. Calculate the fluid needed for a 44 lb dog that is 6%
    dehydrated and losing 100 ml of fluid daily through
    vomiting. _____

11. What drip rate should be used to deliver (over a 24-
    hour period) the fluid for the dog in question 10 (using
    a standard administration set)?

    _____

12. Describe how you would set up the first bag of fluids
    for the dog in question 10.

    _____

13. Tell how you would prepare 500 ml of 5% dextrose
    from a 50% stock solution.

    _____

14. What is the purpose of the lactate in lactated Ringer's
    solution? _____

15. Describe the use of an esophageal feeder.

    _____

16. What type of fluid (tonicity) should not be given sub-
    cutaneously? _____

Blood-Modifying, Antineoplastic, and Immunosuppressant Drugs

LEARNING OBJECTIVES

After studying this chapter, you should be able to:

1. Understand the role of erythropoietin in red blood cell formation
2. Understand the significance of iron in the hemoglobin molecule
3. List an example of iron deficiency anemia that occurs in veterinary medicine
4. Understand the potential indications for and limitations of hematinics and oxygen-carrying solutions
5. Describe the clotting mechanism in general terms
6. List four anticoagulants and their method of action
7. List examples of topical hemostatics
8. Name the antagonist for heparin overdose
9. List the indications for the use of vitamin K_1 and possible adverse side effects of its use
10. Define fibrinolysis and name a fibrinolytic agent
11. Describe the phases of the cell cycle
12. List six categories of antineoplastic drugs and give an example of each
13. Define biologic response modifier (BRM) and list two examples of BRMs
14. List indications for the use of immunosuppressive drugs and provide five examples
15. Discuss the safety precautions involved in the use of antineoplastic drugs

KEY TERMS

Alkylation Formation of a linkage between a substance and DNA that causes irreversible inhibition of the DNA molecule. Alkylating drugs are used in chemotherapy of cancer.

Cell cycle non-specific Capable of acting in several or all cell cycle phases.

Cell cycle specific Capable of acting during a particular cell phase only.

Cytostatic Capable of halting growth of cells.

Cytotoxic Capable of destroying cells.

Disseminated intravascular coagulation (DIC) Widespread formation of clots (thrombi) in the microscopic blood vessels of the circulatory system. DIC occurs as a complication of a wide variety of disorders and consumes clotting factors, with resultant bleeding.

Endothelial layer The smooth layer of epithelial cells that line blood vessels.

Erythropoietin A substance produced in the kidneys that stimulates the bone marrow to make red blood cells.

Fibrinolysis Fibrin (clot) breakdown through the action of the enzyme plasmin.

Hybridoma A cell culture consisting of a clone of a hybrid cell formed by fusing cells of different kinds, such as stimulated mouse plasma cells and myeloma cells.

Metastasis Generally refers to the transfer of cancer cells from one site to another.

Myeloma A malignant neoplasm of plasma cells (B-lymphocytes).

Thrombocytopenia A decreased number of platelets.

Thromboembolism The condition that occurs when thrombus material becomes dislodged and transported by the bloodstream to another site.

Thrombus A clot in the circulatory system.

Vesicant A substance that causes blister formation.

INTRODUCTION

The first section of this chapter deals with drugs or agents that influence blood formation or its processes (e.g., clotting, **fibrinolysis**). Hematinics, anticoagulants, anticoagulant antagonists/hemostatics, and fibrinolytic agents are discussed. Because the anticoagulants are used routinely in veterinary practice, veterinary technicians should have a complete working knowledge of their applications and their potential misuse.

The second section covers antineoplastic and immunosuppressant drugs. Antineoplastic drug categories include alkylating agents, antimetabolites, mitotic inhibitors (vinca alkaloids), antibiotics, hormones, and miscellaneous agents. Safe handling techniques for these potentially dangerous agents are listed. Selected immunosuppressant drugs, as well as their clinical applications, are discussed at the conclusion of this section.

Separate anatomy/physiology descriptions are used for each section listed earlier to provide continuity of the information.

BLOOD-MODIFYING DRUGS/AGENTS

HEMATINICS

Red blood cells are formed in the bone marrow in response to stimulation by **erythropoietin,** a chemical released by the kidneys when hypoxia is present in this organ (Pugh, 1991) (Figure 16-1). Their primary function is to carry oxygen to the tissues. This activity is greatly enhanced by the hemoglobin component of the red blood cells. Only a small portion of oxygen is carried in solution in the plasma.

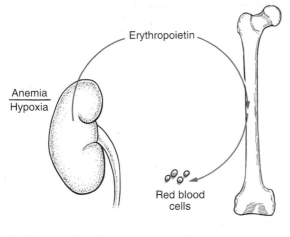

Figure 16-1

Erythropoietin stimulates the bone marrow to produce red blood cells.

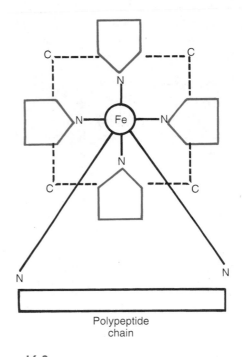

Polypeptide chain

Figure 16-2

The structure of hemoglobin.

Hemoglobin is made up of a protein and an iron-containing pigment (Figure 16-2). The iron in hemoglobin must be in the ferrous (Fe^{2+}) state in order to combine with oxygen in the most efficient way. If the iron in the hemoglobin is in the ferric (Fe^{3+}) state, hemoglobin cannot combine with oxygen and is called *methemoglobin*. Adequate amounts of iron, cobalt, copper, B vitamins, trace minerals, and protein are needed for normal hemoglobin and red blood cell formation.

Anemia can result from excessive loss of red blood cells, formation of inadequate numbers of red blood cells, or inadequate amounts of hemoglobin in the red blood cells. Iron deficiency anemia, a relatively common form in humans, is rare in animals that consume balanced diets. One exception, however, is baby pig anemia, a condition that results because of inadequate assimilation of iron from the placenta of the sow for future hemoglobin formation by the piglet. The piglet is born without adequate stores of iron for its rapid growth phase, and sow's milk is relatively low in this element. Baby pig anemia is a problem of pigs raised in confined environments (concrete or slatted floors), because those raised outdoors usually obtain adequate iron from the soil.

Hematinics are substances that tend to promote an increase in the oxygen-carrying capacity of the blood.

Hematinics are used to prevent or treat anemia, and the primary ingredient in most of these products is iron, a vital component of hemoglobin. Some also contain copper and B vitamins to enhance red blood cell formation. The response to hematinic administration is relatively slow, and this factor makes use of hematinics ancillary to whole blood transfusion in acute anemia.

Iron Compounds

Many injectable and oral iron preparations are available for veterinary use under generic and proprietary labels. The form of iron in these products may be iron dextran, ferrous sulfate, peptonized iron, gleptoferron, ferric hydroxide, and others, and the form apparently has little effect on utilization. Copper, B vitamins, liver fraction (an iron source), and palatability enhancers are often added to the oral products as well. The injectable forms are labeled for intramuscular injection and contain only iron. They may cause discoloration of muscle tissue at the site of injection.

Clinical Uses. Iron compounds are used for prevention or treatment of baby pig anemia or as a nutritional aid, depending on the form.

Dosage Forms

1. Injectable Iron 10%
2. Iron Dextran Complex Injection
3. Iron Hydrogenated Dextran Injection
4. Ferrodex 100
5. Iron-Gard 100
6. Purina Oral Pigemia
7. Lixotinic
8. Pet Tinic
9. Gleptosil

Adverse Side Effects. These are rare but may include muscle weakness, prostration, or muscle discoloration.

Technician's Notes

Pork quality assurance programs often recommend that iron injections be given in neck muscle rather than in the ham (a higher-quality cut) because of potential meat staining and subsequent condemnation.

Erythropoietin

Erythropoietin, a protein produced in the kidneys, stimulates the division and differentiation of committed erythroid precursors in the bone marrow. A synthetic product, Epogen, has the same properties of erythropoietin and is available commercially. It is approved for human use and is produced by recombinant DNA technology. It is labeled for the treatment of anemia related to chronic renal failure or for that associated with azidothymidine treatment in patients with human immunodeficiency virus infection. No veterinary approved product is available.

Clinical Uses. Erythropoietin is used in dogs and cats for the treatment of anemia associated with chronic renal failure or other causes.

Dosage Form

1. Epogen (Amagen)

Adverse Side Effects. In humans, adverse side effects may include hypertension, iron deficiency, polycythemia, and seizures. The use of human-coded proteins in dogs or cats could potentially cause allergic reactions.

Androgens

The treatment for anemia associated with chronic renal failure has traditionally been androgen therapy. The results of the use of androgens for chronic anemia have been inconsistent.

Clinical Uses. Androgens are used for the treatment of chronic (non-regenerative) anemia.

Dosage Forms

1. Winstrol-V
2. Equipoise
3. Deca-Durabolin (human approved)

Adverse Side Effects. These have included enlargement of the prostate, hepatic toxicity, and sodium and water retention.

Blood Substitutes

Researchers have looked for an oxygen-carrying substitute for red blood cells practically since it was learned that the hemoglobin in those cells was the transporting vehicle. Only recently has an acceptable substitute been developed.

The Biopure Corporation has prepared a polymerized bovine product with a hemoglobin concentration of 13 g/dl in a modified lactated Ringer's solution. This solution has obvious benefits over blood products that include availability, a long shelf life, universal compatibility, and freedom from disease-producing agents.

This hemoglobin solution picks up and distributes oxygen in a similar manner to red blood cells but the oxygen-carrying function is shifted to the plasma. Since the oxygen is carried in the plasma, diffusion of this gas across cell membranes occurs more efficiently than when carried by red blood cells because one fewer membrane must be crossed.

This product is stable for 2 years when unwrapped at room temperature or in the refrigerator (but it should not be frozen). Once the wrapper is removed, the product must be used within 24 hours. It is compatible with any other IV fluid, but other solutions should not be mixed in the same bag. A separate line should be used for these other solutions. No consideration needs to be made for blood typing or crossmatching when using this product.

Clinical Uses. This product is labeled for the treatment of anemia in dogs regardless of the cause. It has been used in cats but is not labeled for such use.

Dosage Form

1. Oxyglobin (hemoglobin glutamer-200)

Adverse Side Effects. Potential side effects include pulmonary edema, discolored urine, discolored membranes, ventricular arrhythmias, fever, and coagulopathy.

Technician's Notes
1. The recommended administration rate should not be exceeded.
2. Do not administer with other fluids or drugs through the same intravenous set.
3. Do not combine with other fluids in the same bag.

 ANTICOAGULANTS

Blood coagulation is an obviously essential process designed to inhibit the loss of vital blood constituents from the circulatory system. Two separate systems or pathways may initiate the clotting mechanism, the intrinsic (intravascular) and extrinsic (extravascular) systems.

The intrinsic pathway is activated by injury to the **endothelial layer** of a blood vessel, which disrupts blood flow and causes a chain of chemical reactions leading to a **thrombus,** or clot. This process helps to repair damage to blood vessel walls that occurs from routine wear as well as from pathologic processes.

The extrinsic pathway is activated by injury to tissues and vessels, releasing tissue thromboplastin. Thromboplastin stimulates the clotting mechanism. Vasoconstriction occurs in damaged blood vessels, causing a slowing of blood flow and facilitating clot formation. Platelet aggregation and adherence are also important steps in the clotting process.

The intrinsic and the extrinsic pathways converge into a common pathway in the final steps of clot formation (Figure 16-3, p. 299). At least 13 clotting factors participate in this series of reactions (called a *cascade*) in which the product of the preceding reaction promotes the next reaction (Table 16-1). The final step in the process is the conversion of fibrinogen to fibrin by thrombin. If any of the clotting factors in the cascade are deficient or missing, clotting does not occur.

A balance must be maintained in the body between clot formation and clot breakdown. Destruction of clots—fibrinolysis—occurs through the action of an enzyme called *plasmin.* Plasmin digests fibrin threads and other clotting products to cause clot lysis and the release of fibrin degradation products into the circulation.

Anticoagulants inhibit clot formation by tying up or inactivating one of the clotting factors to interrupt the cascade reaction. They are used clinically to prevent coagulation of blood (or other body fluid) samples that are collected for testing, to preserve blood for transfusions, to inhibit clotting in intravenous catheters, and to prevent or treat thromboembolic disorders (e.g., thromboembolic cardiomyopathy in cats).

Heparin is used paradoxically to treat the bleeding disorder **disseminated intravascular coagulation (DIC).**

Heparin

Heparin is an anticoagulant that is found in many tissues of the body and is thought to be stored in mast cells. It is obtained from pig intestinal mucosa, and its strength is expressed in terms of heparin units. Heparin acts as an anticoagulant by preventing the conversion of prothrombin (factor II) to thrombin. With-

TABLE 16-1 The Clotting Factors

Coagulation Factor	Synonym
I	Fibrinogen
II	Prothrombin
III	Tissue factor (thromboplastin)
IV	Calcium ions
V	Proaccelerin, labile factor, or accelerator globulin
VI	Activated factor V
VII	Serum prothrombin conversion-accelerator (SPCA), stable factor, or proconvertin
VIII	Antihemophilic factor (AHF), antihemophilic factor A, or antihemophilic globulin (AHG)
IX	Christmas factor, plasma thromboplastin component (PTC), or antihemophilic factor B
X	Stuart-Prower factor, thrombokinase
XI	Plasma thromboplastin antecedent (PTA) or antihemophilic factor C
XII	Hageman factor, glass factor, or contact factor
XIII	Fibrin-stabilizing factor (FSF) or fibrinase

out thrombin, fibrinogen is not converted to fibrin and a clot does not form. Heparin does not break down clots but can prevent clots from increasing in size. It is administered therapeutically by intravenous or subcutaneous injection.

Heparin has various uses in veterinary medicine. It is used in vitro as an anticoagulant to preserve blood samples for testing by heparinizing (drawing heparin into the syringe and then forcing all visible quantities out) a syringe before drawing the blood sample. It is also diluted in saline or sterile water for injection to form a flush solution for preventing clots in intravenous catheters. Heparin is sometimes used to preserve donated blood for transfusions when small quantities are needed (e.g., for cats, small dogs). It is used in vivo to aid in the treatment of DIC and **thromboembolism** and has been advocated for the treatment of laminitis in horses.

Clinical Uses. Clinical uses are listed in the previous paragraph.

Dosage Forms. Forms approved for use in humans are used in veterinary medicine:

1. Heparin sodium injection, 1000 U/ml
2. Heparin calcium
3. HepLock flush solution (10 or 100 U/ml)

Adverse Side Effects. These are usually bleeding or **thrombocytopenia.**

Technician's Notes

1. Heparin should not be used as an anticoagulant when collecting blood for performing a differential count because white blood cell morphology may be adversely affected.
2. A heparin flush solution may be prepared by diluting heparin in saline at a concentration of 5 U/ml (Crow and Walshaw, 1987).
3. Approximately 750 U of heparin should be drawn into a 60-ml syringe to act as an anticoagulant when collecting blood for transfusion (Norsworthy, 1992).
4. Heparin blood collection tubes have a green top.
5. Protamine sulfate is the antidote for heparin overdose.

Ethylenediamine Tetraacetic Acid (EDTA)

EDTA is an anticoagulant that prevents clotting by chelation of calcium (factor IV). With calcium ions tied up by the EDTA, clotting cannot occur. It is used in vitro to preserve blood samples and is the anticoagulant of choice when a differential count is needed (it preserves white cell morphology well). EDTA is prepared in lavender-topped collection tubes.

The calcium salt of EDTA (Calcium Disodium Versenate) is also used in vivo as a chelating agent to

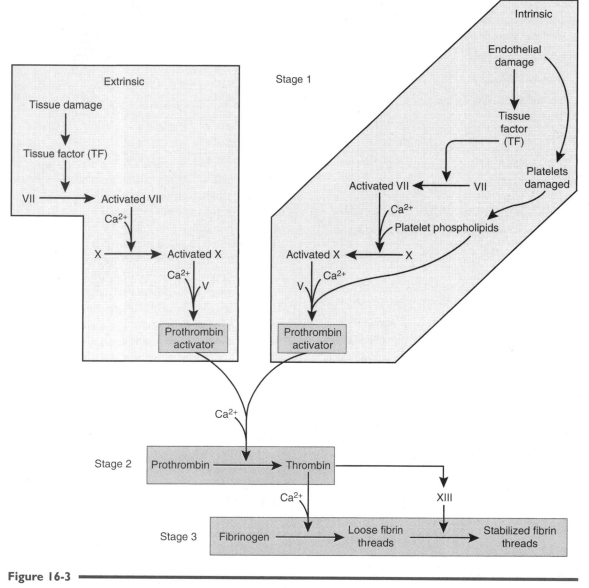

Figure 16-3

The clotting pathways.

treat lead poisoning. This function does not involve the clotting mechanism (see Chapter 18).

Coumarin Derivatives

Coumarin derivatives such as dicumarol and warfarin are oral anticoagulants that bind vitamin K and there-fore inhibit the synthesis of prothrombin (factor II) as well as factors VII, IX, and X. These compounds are indicated for long-term treatment of thromboembolic conditions. They are used clinically to a greater extent in human medicine than in veterinary medicine.

Dicumarol may be found in moldy sweet clover and has been associated with fatal hemorrhagic disease of cattle. Warfarin and related compounds are used in many rat poisoning products.

Clinical Uses. Coumarin derivatives are used for long-term management of thromboembolic conditions.

Dosage Forms

1. Coumadin tablets or injection
2. Panwarfin
3. Dicumarol tablets

Adverse Side Effects. Adverse side effects are related to hemorrhage.

> **Technician's Notes**
>
> Vitamin K_1 is the antidote for warfarin or dicumarol toxicity.

Acid Citrate Dextrose (ACD) Solution and Citrate Phosphate Dextrose Adenine (CPDA-1)

ACD solution contains dextrose, sodium citrate, and citric acid and prevents clotting by chelating calcium. It is prepared in bottles or plastic bags for blood collection under both veterinary and human labels. Bottles for collecting 250 and 500 ml of blood are available. ACD solution preserves blood for 3 to 4 weeks.

CPDA-1 solution is available in plastic bags for collection of 450 ml of blood. CPDA-1 also prevents clotting by chelating calcium and preserves blood for as long as 6 weeks.

Eight milliliters of ACD or CPDA-1 can be drawn into a syringe to collect 50 ml of blood when small quantities are needed (Norsworthy, 1992).

Antiplatelet Drugs

Antiplatelet drugs such as aspirin appear to impair clotting through inhibition of platelet stickiness and clumping. This activity is thought to be mediated through inhibition of the pro-aggregatory prostaglandin called *thromboxane* (Pugh, 1991).

Aspirin has been used to prevent thromboembolism associated with heartworm treatment in dogs and to treat cardiomyopathy in cats.

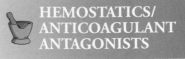

HEMOSTATICS/ ANTICOAGULANT ANTAGONISTS

Substances that promote blood clotting—hemostatics—may be divided into two categories: (1) those applied topically and (2) those given parenterally.

Topical Agents

Topical agents act by providing a framework in which a clot may form or by coagulating blood protein to initiate clot formation. Framework substances used in topical hemostatics include gelatins and collagens, whereas styptics, hemostatic powders, and solutions are substances that initiate clotting through coagulation. The framework substances are absorbed after clot formation. Topical hemostatics are used to control capillary bleeding or bleeding from other small vessels.

Clinical Uses. These include the control of capillary bleeding in surgical sites or superficial wounds.

Dosage Forms

1. Gelfoam absorbable gelatin sponge
2. Hemopad Absorbable Collagen Hemostat
3. Surgical Absorbable Hemostat
4. Hemostat Powder (ferrous sulfate powder)
5. Clotisol (ferric sulfate)
6. Silver nitrate sticks
7. Thrombogen topical thrombin solution

Adverse Side Effects. These are usually minimal but may include delayed wound healing.

Parenteral Agents

Parenterally administered hemostatic agents act as anticoagulant antagonists because they do not directly activate clotting. These substances either promote the synthesis of clotting factors that have been depleted through poisoning or disease or tie up (inactivate) anticoagulants that have been overdosed. These drugs are not used to control surgical or traumatic bleeding.

Protamine Sulfate

Protamine sulfate is a protein produced from the sperm or testes of salmon or related species (Plumb, 1999). Protamine has a strongly basic pH, and heparin has a strongly acidic pH. Protamine combines with heparin to form inactive complexes (salt).

Clinical Uses. Protamine sulfate is used for the treatment of heparin overdose. Slow intravenous administration is recommended.

Dosage Form

1. Protamine sulfate injection, USP

Adverse Side Effects. Hypotension and bradycardia can occur if given too rapidly.

Vitamin K$_1$ (Phytonadione)

Phytonadione is a synthetic substance that is identical to naturally occurring vitamin K$_1$. Vitamin K is necessary for the production (in the liver) of active prothrombin (factor II), proconvertin factor (factor VII), plasma thromboplastin component (factor IX), and Stuart factor (factor X). It is used clinically for treating cases in which vitamin K has been tied up or destroyed and in bleeding disorders associated with poor formation of vitamin K-dependent clotting factors. Immediate coagulant effect should not be expected after administration of vitamin K, because several hours may pass before synthesis of new clotting factors.

Clinical Uses. In veterinary medicine, vitamin K$_1$ is used for the treatment of rodenticide toxicity, for bleeding disorders related to faulty synthesis of vitamin K-dependent clotting factors, and for unknown anticoagulant toxicity.

Dosage Forms. Human forms of vitamin K$_1$ are used:

1. AquaMEPHYTON, phytonadione injection
2. Konakion, phytonadione injection
3. Mephyton, phytonadione tablets

Adverse Side Effects. These include anaphylactoid reactions (intravenous use) and bleeding at the injection site.

Technician's Notes

Because of the possibility of anaphylactoid reactions, many consider intravenous administration of phytonadione to be contraindicated.

FIBRINOLYTIC (THROMBOLYTIC) DRUGS

Thrombolytic drugs are used to break down or dissolve thrombi. Occlusion of an artery by a thromboembolus can cause necrosis of tissue distal to the blockage if the obstruction is not removed quickly. In humans, damage to heart muscle that occurs when a coronary artery is occluded in a heart attack is a classic example of this process. Pulmonary thromboemboli sometimes occur in dogs after heartworm treatment and may accompany cardiomyopathy in cats.

Thrombolytic agents may help to remove or reduce the size of the occluding thromboembolus and minimize tissue damage. This action is brought about by stimulating conversion of plasminogen to the enzyme plasmin, which lyses the clots. The sooner the therapy is initiated after thromboembolism has occurred, the better the chances of success. Thrombolytic activity of one of the products (alteplase) is activated by the presence of fibrin so that recent clots are targeted.

The expense of these drugs often precludes their use in veterinary medicine.

Clinical Uses

1. Treatment of pulmonary embolism
2. Treatment of arterial thrombosis and emboli
3. Treatment of coronary thrombosis
4. Intravenous catheter clearance

Dosage Forms

1. Streptase, streptokinase
2. Abbokinase, urokinase
3. Activase, alteplase

Adverse Side Effects. These are related to bleeding episodes, especially if anticoagulants have also been used.

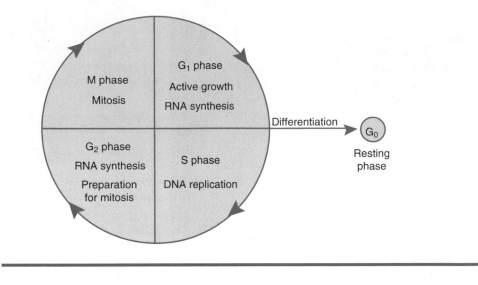

Figure 16-4

The cell cycle.

ANTINEOPLASTIC DRUGS

Antineoplastic drugs are administered to animal patients to cure or lessen the effects of neoplasms. Anticancer chemotherapy may be used alone or in combination with other treatment methods such as surgery, radiation, or immune modulation. Chemotherapy can reduce tumor size, relieve pain, destroy microscopic **metastases,** and in some instances prolong periods of remission and survival time (MacEwen and Rosenthal, 1989). The goal of cancer therapy is to kill all of the neoplastic cells, but this is seldom a reality.

Carcinogenesis has been associated with many factors, including (1) aging (improved health care has led to an increasing population of older animals), (2) oncogenes, (3) stress, (4) viruses, (5) chemicals, (6) nutritional factors, and (7) irritation. No matter what the cause, all cancers are characterized by populations of cells with defective growth control: they multiply rapidly, form large growths, and may spread to other sites.

The cytotoxic drugs used in chemotherapy have been developed to interfere with activities such as DNA/RNA synthesis, mitotic spindle formation, or other processes involved with cell division. These effects are not limited to cancer cells. All rapidly dividing cells such as those of the bone marrow, gastrointestinal tract, reproductive organs, and hair follicles are affected by antineoplastic drugs.

All cells go through a series of cell cycle phases to replicate themselves (Figure 16-4). These phases are described as G_0, the resting or nonproliferative phase; G_1, presynthesis preparation; S, DNA synthesis; G_2, RNA production; and M, mitosis (Jenkins, 1991). The cytotoxic activity of antineoplastic drugs often targets activity of one or more of these phases to interfere with synthesis of products or with division processes. In general, antineoplastic drugs are divided into two groups: (1) the **cell cycle non-specific** drugs, which act at all stages of the cycle except the resting phase (G_0), and (2) the **cell cycle specific** drugs, which act selectively at a certain phase of the cycle (usually S or M). Cell cycle specific drugs are most effective against rapidly growing neoplasms. Malignant cells in the resting phase may be difficult to destroy because they are not very susceptible to chemotherapeutic drugs. This is one reason why prolonged use of antineoplastic drugs may be needed.

Many potential adverse side effects are associated with the use of antineoplastic drugs. These may include anaphylactic reactions, immunosuppression,

Box 16-1 **Recommendations for Safe Handling of Antineoplastic Agents**

1. Designate a specific hospital location for drug handling (reconstitution, preparation, disposal, etc.).
2. Use an absorbent, disposable, plastic-backed sheet to cover the work surface; change regularly.
3. Wear latex nonpermeable gloves when handling all cytotoxic agents.
4. Reduce exposed skin surfaces by wearing laboratory coats, gowns, etc. Wear particulate respiratory filtration masks to prevent inhalation of aerosolized drug particles.
5. Reconstitute all materials carefully and safely, avoiding potential contamination of materials or aerosolization.
6. Clean reconstituted material of any contamination and properly mark and date it.
7. Dispose of contaminated materials in leak-proof, puncture-resistant containers. Proper disposal by health regulatory officials is necessary.
8. Wash hands thoroughly after removing gloves.

TABLE 16-2 Conversion of Body Weight in Kilograms to Body Surface Area in Meters for Dogs

kg	m²	kg	m²
0.5	0.06	26.0	0.88
1.0	0.10	27.0	0.90
2.0	0.15	28.0	0.92
3.0	0.20	29.0	0.94
4.0	0.25	30.0	0.96
5.0	0.29	31.0	0.99
6.0	0.33	32.0	1.01
7.0	0.36	33.0	1.03
8.0	0.40	34.0	1.05
9.0	0.43	35.0	1.07
10.0	0.46	36.0	1.09
11.0	0.49	37.0	1.11
12.0	0.52	38.0	1.13
13.0	0.55	39.0	1.15
14.0	0.58	40.0	1.17
15.0	0.60	41.0	1.19
16.0	0.63	42.0	1.21
17.0	0.66	43.0	1.23
18.0	0.69	44.0	1.25
19.0	0.71	45.0	1.26
20.0	0.74	46.0	1.28
21.0	0.76	47.0	1.30
22.0	0.78	48.0	1.32
23.0	0.81	49.0	1.34
24.0	0.83	50.0	1.36
25.0	0.85		

The conversion table is based on the following formula:

$$\frac{kg^{0.67}}{10} = m_2$$

From Ettinger, S.J.: Textbook of Veterinary Internal Medicine, Vol. I. W.B. Saunders Company, Philadelphia, 1975.

vomiting, diarrhea, hair loss, cystitis, pain associated with administration, and tissue damage resulting from drug extravasation. Several of the drugs that are administered intravenously (e.g., doxorubicin, vinblastine, and vincristine) are severe **vesicants,** and great care should be taken to avoid extravasation.

Great care should be taken, as well, to avoid accidental exposure to these drugs by technicians, veterinarians, and other employees because of their ability to directly irritate the skin and because of their potential to cause cancer on exposed skin or mucous membranes (Madewell and Simonson, 1989). Box 16-1 provides a list of recommendations for safe handling of antineoplastic agents.

Dosage of most antineoplastic agents is based on body surface area as measured in square meters (Page, 1992). Body surface area can be converted from body weight into kilograms (Table 16-2).

The antineoplastic drugs have been divided into six major categories: alkylating agents, antimetabolites, plant alkaloids, antibiotics, hormonal agents, and miscellaneous agents (Thompson, 1989). Table 16-3 lists the commonly used antineoplastic agents and the indications for their use in veterinary medicine.

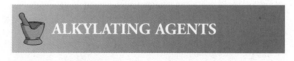

ALKYLATING AGENTS

Alkylating agents are cell cycle non-specific drugs that are able to cross-link strands of DNA to inhibit its replication. This brings protein synthesis and cell division to a halt; cell death often follows.

TABLE 16-3 Common Antineoplastic Drugs and Indications for Their Use

Drugs	Indication	Recommended Dosages	Toxicity
Alkylating Agents			
Cyclophosphamide (Cytoxan; Mead-Johnson)	Lymphoproliferative disorders, mast cell tumors, hemangio-sarcoma, miscellaneous carcinomas	50 mg/m²/PO every 48 hours 50 mg/m² PO every 24 hours for 4 days weekly 100-300 mg/m² IV every 3 weeks	BM, GI, hemorrhagic cystitis
Chlorambucil (Leukeran; Burroughs-Wellcome)	Lymphoproliferative disease, macroglo-bulinemia	2-4 mg/m² every 24-48 hours	BM
Melphalan (Alkeran; Burroughs-Wellcome)	Multiple myeloma	2-4 mg/m² PO every 24-48 hours	BM
Cisplatin (Platinol; Bristol)	Osteosarcoma, transitional cell carcinoma, squamous cell carcinoma	50-70 mg/m² IV every 3 weeks (vigorous hydration)	BM, GI, renal; do not use in cats
Carboplatin (Paraplatin; Bristol)	Similar to cisplatin	250-300 mg/m² IV every 3 weeks	BM, GI
Antimetabolites			
Methotrexate (Lederle)	Lymphoproliferative disorders	2.5 mg/m² PO every 24 hours 15-20 mg/m² IV every 3 weeks	BM, GI, renal
5-Fluorouracil (Roche)	GI and hepatic carcinoma	150-200 mg/m² IV every 7 days	BM, GI, CNS; do not use in cats

m^2, body surface area in square meters; *PO*, per os; *IV*, intravenously; *IM*, intramuscularly; *SC*, subcutaneously; *IP*, intraperitoneal; *BM*, bone marrow; *GI*, gastrointestinal; *CNS*, central nervous system.
From Birchard, S., Sherding, R. (eds.): Saunders Manual of Small Animal Practice. W.B. Saunders Company, Philadelphia, 1994, p. 189.

Clinical Uses

1. Treatment of various neoplastic disorders including lymphoproliferative neoplasms, osteosarcoma, hemangiosarcoma, and squamous cell carcinoma
2. Treatment of certain immune-mediated diseases (immune suppression)

Dosage Forms

1. Cytoxan, cyclophosphamide injection
2. Platinol, cisplatin for injection
3. Leukeran, chlorambucil tablets
4. Alkeran, melphalan tablets
5. Paraplatin, carboplatin injection

Adverse Side Effects. Adverse side effects of the alkylating agents may include leukopenia, nephrotoxicity, thrombocytopenia, vomiting, and hemorrhagic cystitis.

Technician's Notes

1. Cisplatin use is contraindicated in cats because of adverse side effects (pulmonary edema and dyspnea)
2. Cyclophosphamide is also used as an immunosuppressant.

TABLE 16-3 Common Antineoplastic Drugs and Indications for Their Use—cont'd

Drugs	Indication	Recommended Dosages	Toxicity
Antimetabolites—cont'd			
Cytosine arabinoside (Cytosar-U; Upjohn)	Lymphoproliferative disorders, myeloproliferative disorders	100 mg/m² IV or SC for 4 days every 3-4 weeks	BM, GI
Plant Alkaloids			
Vincristine (Oncovin; Eli Lilly)	Lymphoproliferative disorders, mast cell tumors, sarcomas, carcinomas	0.5-0.7 mg/m² IV every 7 days	GI, peripheral neuropathy; vesicant
Antibiotics			
Doxorubicin (Adriamycin; Adria Labs)	Lymphoproliferative disorders, soft tissue sarcoma, carcinomas	30 mg/m² IV every 3 weeks (maximum cumulative dose = 180-240 mg/m²)	BM, GI, cardiac, severe vesicant, urticaria, alopecia
Mitoxantrone (Novantrone; Lederle)	Lymphoproliferative disorders	5-6 mg/m² every 3 weeks	BM
Hormones			
Prednisone	Lymphoproliferative disorders, mast cell tumors, brain tumors	20-50 mg/m² every 24-48 hours as needed	Iatrogenic Cushing's syndrome, GI
Miscellaneous			
L-Asparaginase (Elspar; Merck, Sharp & Dohme)	Lymphoproliferative disorders	10,000-30,000 IU/m² IM, SC, or IP as needed (pretreat with antihistamines, steroids)	Anaphylaxis, pancreatitis, coagulopathy

 ## ANTIMETABOLITES

The antimetabolites are cell cycle specific drugs that affect the S phase (DNA synthesis) of the cycle. These drugs are analogs of purines and pyrimidines—naturally occurring bases in DNA—and may be incorporated into the DNA molecule to inhibit protein and enzyme synthesis. Cellular functions needed for normal activity are thus blocked.

Clinical Uses

1. Treatment of lymphoproliferative neoplasms
2. Treatment of gastrointestinal and hepatic neoplasms
3. Treatment of central nervous system lymphoma

Dosage Forms

1. Methotrexate, oral tablet or injection
2. Cytosar-U, cytosine arabinoside injection
3. Fluorouracil injection

Adverse Side Effects. These may include anorexia, nausea, vomiting, diarrhea, bone marrow suppression, hepatotoxicity, and neurotoxicity.

Technician's Notes
Fluorouracil is contraindicated in cats because of adverse side effects.

PLANT ALKALOIDS

The plant alkaloids are cell cycle specific for the M phase, inhibiting mitosis and causing cell death. They are thought to bind microtubular proteins and inhibit formation of the mitotic spindle, thus suspending mitosis in metaphase.

The two drugs in this category—vincristine and vinblastine—are natural alkaloids derived from the periwinkle plant (*Vinca rosea,* Linn). Protective clothing should be worn when administering these drugs to prevent possible skin contact irritation.

Clinical Uses

1. Treatment of lymphoproliferative neoplasms
2. Treatment of carcinomas
3. Treatment of mast cell tumors
4. Treatment of splenic tumors

Dosage Forms

1. Oncovin, vincristine sulfate injection
2. Alkaban-AQ, vinblastine sulfate for injection

Adverse Side Effects. These may include gastroenteritis, bone marrow suppression, stomatitis, alopecia, and peripheral neuropathy.

Technician's Notes

1. Extravasation of plant alkaloids may cause tissue necrosis.
2. Skin contact causes irritation.

ANTIBIOTIC ANTINEOPLASTIC AGENTS

The antibiotic antineoplastic agents are derived from soil fungi of the *Streptomyces* genus. They are cell cycle non-specific and exert their effects by binding with DNA and thus inhibiting mitotic activity. Doxorubicin is the most commonly used drug in this class in veterinary medicine; it is widely used for various neoplastic conditions.

Clinical Uses. These agents are used for the treatment of lymphoproliferative neoplasms and various carcinomas and sarcomas.

Dosage Form

1. Adriamycin, doxorubicin hydrochloride for injection

Adverse Side Effects. These include bone marrow suppression, cardiotoxicity (cardiomyopathy), gastroenteritis, and anaphylaxis.

Technician's Notes

1. Some clinicians use antihistamines to premedicate animals to be treated with doxorubicin to suppress allergic reactions.
2. Doxorubicin is a strong vesicant. Tissue sloughing can follow extravasation, and skin irritation can result from contact with the drug.
3. Doxorubicin is commonly used in combination with other antineoplastic agents.

HORMONAL ANTINEOPLASTIC AGENTS

The glucocorticoids prednisone and prednisolone are the most commonly used hormonal agents for the treatment of neoplastic disorders. They are cell cycle non-specific. Corticosteroids have a lympholytic action that makes them useful for treating lymphoid neoplasms. They are also helpful in the management of secondary complications of neoplastic diseases such as hypercalcemia and immune-mediated (thrombocytopenia) problems. In addition, they can increase appetite and the overall feeling of well-being in patients being treated for neoplasm. They are usually used in combination protocols with other antineoplastic drugs.

MISCELLANEOUS ANTINEOPLASTIC AGENTS

Asparaginase

Asparaginase is the most commonly used miscellaneous agent. It is a cell cycle specific (G1) enzyme extracted from *Escherichia coli* bacteria. Asparaginase acts as a catalyst in the breakdown of asparagine, an amino acid required by cancer cells. Deprived of a needed amino acid, the cancer cells die. Asparaginase has no effect on normal cells, and it is usually used in combination protocols.

Clinical Uses. Asparaginase is used for the treatment of lymphoproliferative neoplasms.

Dosage Form

1. Elspar, asparaginase for injection

Adverse Side Effects. The adverse side effects of this drug include immediate hypersensitivity and gastrointestinal disturbances.

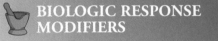

BIOLOGIC RESPONSE MODIFIERS

Biologic response modifiers (BRMs) are agents that alter the relationship between the tumor and the host animal in a way that improves the host's ability to mount an antitumor response (Grant and Shelton, 1989). BRMs are used as an adjunct to conventional chemotherapy protocols, not as the sole agent of treatment.

Many animals develop cancer because of an immunosuppressed state, and chemotherapy exacerbates the immunosuppression. The BRMs may be used to stimulate or restore the compromised immune response of the host.

Examples of BRMs include bacterial agents, chemical agents, interferons, thymosins, cytokines/lymphokines, and monoclonal antibodies.

Monoclonal Antibodies

Monoclonal antibodies are identical immunoglobulin molecules formed by a single clone of plasma cells. They are produced by a **hybridoma,** a fusion of a specific antibody-producing B cell with **myeloma** cells (Figure 16-5). Hybridomas secrete large quantities of a very specific (for the tumor) antibody. Monoclonal antibodies may have direct cytotoxic effects on tumor cells, or they may be attached (conjugated) to chemotherapeutic agents such as

radioisotopes, BRMs, or other agents to deliver them directly to the tumor cells. In this way, they become a "magic bullet" directed at the cancer cells (Figure 16-6).

Clinical Uses. Clinical use of monoclonal antibodies in practice is primarily confined to the treatment of canine lymphoma.

Dosage Form

1. Canine Lymphoma Monoclonal Antibody 231 (CL/MAb 231)

Adverse Side Effects. Adverse side effects of the sequential intravenous infusions may include pruritus, facial edema, vomiting, diarrhea, or anxious behavior. Reactions are usually a result of infusing the agent too rapidly.

Interferon

Interferons are chemicals produced by leukocytes, fibroblasts, and epithelial cells. Interferons can exert antitumor, antiviral, and immunoregulatory effects. Several categories of interferons have been identified. The products that are available are approved for use in humans and have been used in humans to treat hairy cell leukemia, Kaposi's sarcoma, genital warts, and certain granulomatous diseases. In veterinary medicine, they have been used to attempt to prevent the development of fatal disease in feline leukemia virus (FeLV)-infected cats and to attempt to extend the survival time of cats infected with feline infectious peritonitis (FIP).

Clinical Uses. These may include the amelioration of FeLV- and FIP-related conditions.

Dosage Forms

1. Roferon-A injection, recombinant interferon alfa-2a
2. Intron A, recombinant interferon alfa-2b for injection
3. Alferon N injection, human leukocyte–derived interferon alfa-N3
4. Actimmune injection, recombinant interferon gamma-1b

Adverse Side Effects. Adverse side effects in humans have included fever and flulike symptoms.

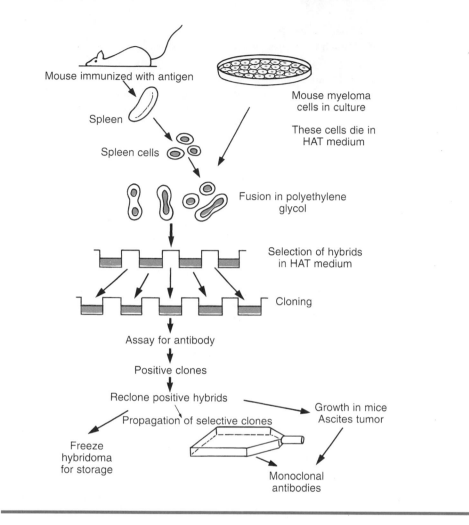

Figure 16-5

Production of monoclonal antibodies. *HAT,* hypoxanthine-aminopterin-thymidine. (From Tizard, I.: Veterinary Immunology: An Introduction, 3rd ed. W.B. Saunders, Philadelphia, 1987, p. 75.)

Other Biologic Response Modifiers

1. Acemannan. This product is licensed for the treatment of fibrosarcoma in dogs and cats.
2. Interleukins. There are 17 identified interleukins; their functions include various activities in the immune system, such as cell enhancement or suppression, hematopoietic growth, or regulation of leukocyte function.
   a. Interleukin 2. This substance's primary function is

the promotion of the clonal expansion of antigen-specific T cells and may be useful in treating certain canine and feline neoplasias (Kruth, 1998).

3. G-CSF and GM-CSF. These growth factors affect specific myeloid cell lines and may have some use in the treatment of neutropenia associated with the chemotherapy of canine or feline neoplasia or in the management of feline panleukopenia.

Direct destruction

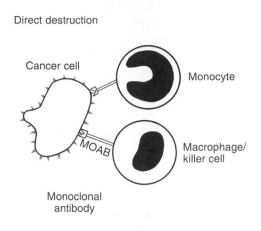

Delivery of cytotoxic drugs to cancer cells

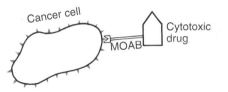

Figure 16-6

Antitumor mechanisms of monoclonal antibodies. *MOAB,* monoclonal antibody.

IMMUNOSUPPRESSIVE DRUGS

The immunosuppressive drugs are used in veterinary medicine to treat various immune-mediated disorders. Some of the diseases related to an overactive or improperly responding immune system include lupus erythematosus, lymphocytic-plasmacytic enteritis, rheumatoid arthritis, immune-mediated skin disease, and hemolytic anemia. Many of the immunosuppressive drugs work by interfering with one of the stages of the cell cycle or by affecting cellular messengers.

Azathioprine

Azathioprine is an antimetabolite that affects cells in the S phase of the cell cycle. It inhibits both T- and B-lymphocytes to bring about immunosuppression. It has fewer side effects than cyclophosphamide and some of the other immunosuppressants. It is often used in combination with prednisone or prednisolone. Because cats are more likely to be affected by the side effects of this drug, it should not be used in this species.

Clinical Uses. Azathioprine is primarily used for the treatment of immune-mediated disease in dogs.

Dosage Forms
1. Imuran tablets, azathioprine (50 mg)
2. Imuran, azathioprine injection

Adverse Side Effects. Adverse side effects are related to bone marrow suppression. Long-term use may predispose to infection.

Cyclosporine

Cyclosporine is a substance isolated from a fungus that inhibits proliferation of T-lymphocytes (Gregory, 1989). It was approved for use in humans for prevention of organ transplant rejection; however, it has also been used to treat several immune-mediated diseases (e.g., uveitis, Graves' disease, psoriasis, and pemphigus). It has been used in veterinary medicine for the prevention of organ transplant rejection, for treating immune-mediated skin disorders, and for the management of keratoconjunctivitis sicca (KCS) in dogs.

Clinical Uses. Clinical use of cyclosporine in practice is limited mainly to ophthalmic application for treatment of KCS in dogs.

Dosage Forms
1. Optimmune ointment
2. Sandimmune, cyclosporine gelatin capsules
3. Sandimmune, cyclosporine oral solution
4. Sandimmune, cyclosporine for injection

Adverse Side Effects. In humans, these may include nephrotoxicity, hepatotoxicity, nausea, vomiting, anaphylaxis (intravenous form), and others.

> **Technician's Notes**
> Monitor the eyes for irritation or infection if cyclosporine is being used for KCS.

> **Technician's Notes**
> Clients must be warned about the potential severe side effects of this drug.

Metronidazole

Metronidazole is a substance that has antibacterial, antiprotozoal, and immunosuppressive activities. It may be used in conjunction with corticosteroids to enhance its immunosuppressive effects.

Clinical Uses

1. Treatment of lymphocytic-plasmacytic enteritis in dogs
2. Treatment of giardiasis
3. Treatment of anaerobic bacterial infections

Dosage Forms

1. Flagyl, metronidazole tablets
2. Flagyl, metronidazole powder for injection
3. Flagyl IV, injectable

Adverse Side Effects. These may include gastrointestinal upset, neurologic disturbances, and lethargy.

Cyclophosphamide

Cyclophosphamide is an alkylating agent that is used as an antineoplastic agent as well as an immunosuppressant (see the earlier section on antineoplastic agents). Cyclophosphamide may be accompanied by serious side effects (e.g., hemorrhagic cystitis, bone marrow suppression, and gastroenteritis). It is an injectable agent sold under the trade name Cytoxan.

Clinical Uses. Cyclophosphamide is used primarily as an immunosuppressant.

Dosage Form

1. Cytoxan

Adverse Side Effects. These include bone marrow suppression, gastrointestinal signs, alopecia, and hemorrhagic cystitis.

Corticosteroids

Corticosteroids exert anti-inflammatory and immunosuppressive effects through their inhibitory influence on neutrophils, T-lymphocytes, blood vessels (decreased permeability), and cellular messengers (e.g., prostaglandin). They are generally considered to be anti-inflammatory at lower doses and immunosuppressive at higher doses. Corticosteroids are often used in combination with other immunosuppressant/antineoplastic agents.

REFERENCES

Crow, S.E., Walshaw, S.O.: Placement and care of intravenous catheters. In Crow, S.E., Walshaw, S.O. (eds.): Manual of Clinical Procedures in the Dog and Cat. J.B. Lippincott Company, Philadelphia, 1987.

Grant, C.K., Shelton, G.H.: Biological response modifiers. In Kirk, R.W., Bonagura, J.D. (eds.): Current Veterinary Therapy X: Small Animal Practice. W.B. Saunders Company, Philadelphia, 1989.

Gregory, C.: Cyclosporine. In Kirk, R.W., Bonagura, J.D. (eds.): Current Veterinary Therapy X: Small Animal Practice. W.B. Saunders Company, Philadelphia, 1989.

Jenkins, W.L.: Chemotherapeutic agents affecting host cellular functions: Antineoplastics and immunomodulators. In Brander, G.C., Pugh, D.M., Bywater, R.J., et al. (eds.): Veterinary Applied Pharmacology and Therapeutics, 5th ed. Bailliere Tindall, London, 1991.

Kruth, S.A.: Biologic response modifiers: Interferons, interleukins, recombinant products, liposomal products. In Boothe, D.M. (ed): The Veterinary Clinics of North America, Small Animal Practice. W.B. Saunders Company, Philadelphia, 1998.

MacEwen, E.G., Rosenthal, R.C.: Approach to treatment of cancer patients. In Ettinger, S.J., (ed.): Textbook of Veterinary Internal Medicine, 3rd ed. W.B. Saunders Company, Philadelphia, 1989.

Madewell, B.R., Simonson, E.R.: Special considerations in drug preparation and administration. In Kirk, R.W., Bonagura, J.D. (eds.): Current Veterinary Therapy X: Small Animal Practice. W.B. Saunders Company, Philadelphia, 1989.

Norsworthy, G.D.: Clinical aspects of feline blood transfusions. Comp. Cont. Educ. Pract. Vet. 14:470, 1992.

Page, R.L.: Chemotherapy: Pharmacologic and toxicologic considerations. In Kirk, R.W., Bonagura, J.D. (eds.): Current Veterinary Therapy XI: Small Animal Practice. W.B. Saunders Company, Philadelphia, 1992.

Plumb, D.C.: Veterinary Drug Handbook. Iowa State University Press, Ames, 1999.

Pugh, D.M.: Blood formation, coagulation, and volume. In Brander, G.C., Pugh, D.M., Bywater, R.J., et al. (eds.): Veterinary Applied Pharmacology and Therapeutics, 5th ed. Bailliere Tindall, London, 1991.

Thompson, J.P.: Antineoplastic agents in cancer therapy. In Kirk, R.W., Bonagura, J.D. (eds.): Current Veterinary Therapy X: Small Animal Practice. W.B. Saunders Company, Philadelphia, 1989.

■ Review Questions

1. Anemia in baby pigs can be treated by the administration of _____.

2. A 10-year-old cocker spaniel is presented to the veterinary clinic with polyuria/polydipsia and mild anemia. What is a potential cause of these signs, and what may be used to treat the anemia?

   _____

3. Why are hematinics not indicated for cases of acute blood loss? _____

4. What is the anticoagulant of choice for collecting blood for hematologic studies?

   _____

5. How can you explain the fact that clots may form in the vascular system with no external trauma to blood vessels? _____

6. You have accidentally cut the quick of a rottweiler puppy's nail. What would you use to stop the bleeding, and how does this agent work?

   _____

7. A 3-month-old chow is presented to the pet emergency clinic because it has eaten a box of rat poison. What drug would the veterinarian use to treat this condition, and by what route would it be administered?

   _____

8. An 8-year-old male Persian cat is presented to the veterinary clinic with an acute onset of apparent rear leg paralysis and tachycardia. What agent may be used to treat this condition? _____

9. Briefly describe the phases of the cell cycle.

   _____

10. List the six categories of the antineoplastic drugs, and give an example of each.

    _____

11. A 12-year-old Labrador retriever has been through a treatment protocol for lymphoma, and the owner has opted for the use of a BRM. What agent could be used in this case? _____

12. List four indications for the use of immunosuppressive agents. _____

13. Why should you be very careful to avoid extravasation of antineoplastic drugs?

    _____

14. List eight precautions that should be taken when handling antineoplastic drugs.

    _____

Immunologic Drugs

LEARNING OBJECTIVES

After studying this chapter, you should be able to:

1. Understand the principles associated with vaccination
2. Understand the differences between vaccine types
3. Be familiar with the advantages and disadvantages of the different types of vaccines
4. Know common diseases that have available vaccines
5. Understand the different routes of administration of vaccines
6. Be familiar with drugs used in immunotherapy

KEY TERMS

Active immunity Immunity that occurs by an animal's own immune response after exposure to foreign antigen.

Adjuvant A substance given with an antigen to enhance the immune response to the antigen. Adjuvants may form a localized granuloma at the injection site or produce systemic hypersensitivity. Adjuvants have received much attention as a result of a possible (but not proven) link with the increased incidence of fibrosarcomas in vaccinated cats. Examples of adjuvants are aluminum hydroxide, aluminum phosphate, aluminum potassium sulfate, water in oil, saponin, and diethylaminoethyl (DEAE) dextran.

Anaphylaxis A systemic, severe allergic reaction.

Antibody An immunoglobulin molecule that combines with the specific antigen that induced its formation.

Antigen Any substance that can induce a specific immune response, such as toxins, foreign proteins, bacteria, and viruses.

Avirulent The inability of an infectious agent to produce pathologic effects.

Bacterin A killed bacterial vaccine.

Monovalent A vaccine, antiserum, or antitoxin developed specifically for a single antigen or organism.

Passive immunity Immunity that occurs by administration of antibody produced in another individual.

Polyvalent A vaccine, antiserum, or antitoxin active against multiple antigens or organisms; mixed vaccine.

Preservative A substance such as an antibiotic, anti-infective, or fungistat added to a product to destroy or inhibit multiplication of microorganisms.

Recombinant DNA technology A process that removes a gene from one organism or pathogen and inserts it into the DNA of another; this may also be referred to as gene splicing.

Virulence The ability of an infectious agent to produce pathologic effects.

PRINCIPLES OF VACCINATION

Vaccinations are an important part of the preventive health care program for companion animals and food animals alike. Vaccines are given to lessen the chance for a particular disease to occur. A patient's response is determined by several factors such as (1) the health and age of the patient, (2) the type of vaccine given, (3) the route of administration, (4) concurrent incubation of infectious disease, (5) exposure to an infectious disease before complete immunity is reached, and (6) drug therapy. The ideal vaccine would be safe, effective on challenge, and have no undesirable side effects. Immunology is a very complex field of study. This chapter outlines only the basics of common vaccines and immunostimulants. Reference to an immunology textbook may be helpful if further information is desired.

The future of vaccination is looking to the development of protocols that individualize vaccine schedules instead of having every animal vaccinated for every disease. There is also research that will hopefully provide optimal revaccination intervals. Some studies have suggested that with some vaccines, protective immunity may last for years and annual revaccination may not be necessary. With new information and technology, the 21st century will see many changes in vaccines.

COMMON VACCINE TYPES THAT PRODUCE ACTIVE IMMUNITY

INACTIVATED

In the manufacture of inactivated vaccines, organisms are treated most commonly by chemicals to kill the organisms, but very little change occurs in the **antigens** that stimulate protective immunity. Inactivated vaccines are also referred to as *killed,* or *dead, vaccines.*

Advantages
1. Inactivated vaccines are usually very safe.
2. They are stable in storage.
3. They are unlikely to cause disease through residual virulence.

Disadvantages
1. Inactivated vaccines require repeated doses to achieve adequate protection.
2. **Adjuvants** may cause severe local reactions.
3. Because of the need to repeat doses, costs may be higher.
4. Inactivated vaccines contain **preservatives** such as penicillin, streptomycin, and fungistats.

Examples
Leukocell 2: Feline leukemia virus
Duramune Cv-K: Rabies virus
Vibo-5/Somnugen: *Campylobacter fetus,* leptospirosis, *Haemophilus somnus,* **bacterin**

LIVE

A live vaccine is prepared from live micro-organisms or viruses. These organisms may be fully **virulent** or **avirulent.** Few vaccines of this origin are in use, with the exception of several poultry vaccines.

Advantages
1. Live vaccines necessitate fewer doses to achieve an immune response.
2. Adjuvants are unnecessary, but the vaccine may contain preservatives.
3. Live vaccines pose less risk of allergic responses.
4. They are inexpensive.

Disadvantages
1. Live vaccines may be contaminated with unwanted organisms.
2. They require careful handling. For example, accidental injection, ingestion, or exposure through a cut or the mucous membranes of brucellosis vaccine can cause undulant fever in humans.
3. They do not store as well as inactivated vaccines.
4. They may possess residual virulence.

Examples
Brucella Abortus Vaccine: *Brucella abortus* strain RB-51
Ovine Ecthyma Vaccine: Ovine ecthyma virus or sore mouth infection
Chick Ark Bronc: Infectious bronchitis (Massachusetts and Arkansas types)
Protex-Bb: *Bordetella bronchiseptica*

MODIFIED LIVE

In modified live vaccines, organisms undergo a process (attenuation) to lose their virulence so that when introduced to the body via inoculation they cause an immune response instead of disease.

Advantages
1. Effective vaccines for many viruses can be developed through attenuation of the causative virus.
2. Immunity is comparable in response and longevity to that with killed products.

Disadvantages
1. Modified live vaccines may cause abortion when given to pregnant animals.

2. Some vaccines can cause mild immunosuppression.
3. Residual virulence can cause a mild form of the disease.
4. These vaccines contain preservatives such as penicillin, gentamicin, thimerosal, or a fungistat.

Examples

Eclipse 3: Feline rhinotracheitis, calicivirus, and panleukopenia
BoviShield 4: Infectious bovine rhinotracheitis (IBR) virus, bovine virus diarrhea (BVD), parainfluenza3 (PI3) virus, bovine respiratory syncytial virus

RECOMBINANT

In the past few years, vaccines produced by **recombinant DNA technology** have become available for veterinary medicine. These vaccines are recognized as being safe, highly specific, potent, pure, and efficacious. These attributes cause recombinant vaccines to be more desirable than any other vaccine type. Recombinant vaccines are divided into three categories:

Type I recombinant (subunit) vaccines—These vaccines are derived by inserting a foreign gene from a specific pathogen into a recombinant organism (e.g. yeast, bacterium, or a virus). The recombinant organism multiplies, and the product of the gene is extracted, purified, and prepared for administration as a vaccine.
Type II recombinant (gene-deleted) vaccines—The manufacturing of these vaccines involves deletion of specific genes from a pathogenic organism. This manipulation produces a vaccine that has a low risk of producing disease but can still stimulate a protective immune response.
Type III recombinant (vectored) vaccines—These vaccines are derived from the insertion of specific pathogenic genetic material into a nonpathogenic or gene-deleted organism (e.g. poxvirus). This altered organism is then propagated in vitro and used to manufacture the vaccine (Van Kampen, 1998).

Advantages

1. These vaccines produce fewer adverse effects.
2. They provide effective immunity.
3. Type I and Type III vaccines cannot revert to virulence because of the way they are manufactured.
4. Some of these vaccines can be administered orally.

Disadvantages

1. Currently there are not many recombinant vaccines available.
2. New technology often brings with it a higher cost.

Examples

Type I
RM Recombitek Lyme: *Borrelia burgdorferi*
Type III
RM Recombitek C4: Canine distemper, adenovirus type 2, parainfluenza, and parvovirus
Raboral V-RG: oral vaccine for rabies virus (used in baiting devices for wildlife)
Newcastle Disease-Fowl Pox Vaccine (Recombinant): Newcastle disease and fowl pox
Trovac-AIV H5: Avian influenza subtype H5 and fowl pox

TOXOID

A toxoid is a vaccine for producing immunity to a toxin rather than a bacterium or a virus. The toxin is treated by heat or chemicals to destroy its damaging properties without destroying its ability to stimulate **antibody** production.

An anaculture combines toxoid and killed bacteria in a single dose prepared from highly toxigenic cultures and culture filtrates.

Characteristics

1. Toxoids and anacultures provide protection for up to 1 year.
2. Toxoids may contain adjuvants.
3. Many contain preservatives such as phenol, thimerosal, and formaldehyde solution.

Examples

Tetanus toxoid: *Clostridium tetani*

Tetnogen: *C. tetani*

Fermicon CD/T: *Clostridium perfringens* types C and D and *C. tetani*

COMMON VACCINE TYPES THAT PRODUCE PASSIVE IMMUNITY

 ANTITOXIN

An antitoxin is a specific antiserum aimed against a toxin that contains a concentration of antibodies extracted from the blood serum or plasma of a hyperimmunized, healthy animal (usually a horse).

Characteristics

1. An antitoxin neutralizes toxins produced by microorganisms.
2. It may contain preservatives such as thimerosal, phenol, or oxytetracycline.
3. Antitoxins produce immediate **passive immunity.**
4. Immunity is short lived (about 7 to 14 days).
5. Biologic products of equine origin may be associated with the development of equine serum hepatitis (Theiler's disease). This link has not been proven, but clients should be made aware of this possible risk before these products are administered.

Examples

Clostratox BCD: *C. perfringens* types C and D

Tetanus antitoxin: *C. tetani*

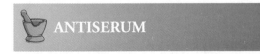 **ANTISERUM**

An antiserum is a serum containing specific antibodies extracted from a hyperimmunized animal (usually a horse) or an animal that has been infected with microorganisms containing antigen.

Characteristics

1. An antiserum kills living, infectious antigens.
2. It may contain preservatives such as phenol, thimerosal, or oxytetracycline.
3. An antiserum produces immediate passive immunity.
4. Do not vaccinate within 21 days after giving antiserum. For example, if a calf is treated with a *Corynebacterium–Escherichia Coli–Pasteurella–Salmonella* antiserum, then that calf should not be vaccinated with BVD, IBR, PI₃, *H. somnus,* or *Pasteurella haemolytica* within 21 days after receiving the antiserum.
5. Immunity is short lived.

Examples

Erysipelothrix Rhusiopathiae Serum Antibodies: *Erysipelothrix rhusiopathiae*

E.-Colicin-B: *E. coli*

Septi-Serum: *Salmonella typhimurium*

OTHER TYPES OF VACCINES

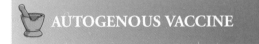 **AUTOGENOUS VACCINE**

An autogenous vaccine contains organisms isolated from an infected animal on a farm where a disease problem is occurring. This carefully prepared vaccine contains antigens needed for protection at that particular location.

MIXED VACCINE

A mixed vaccine contains a mixture of different antigens. It is also referred to as a **polyvalent** vaccine (Figure 17-1). Each component of a mixed vaccine is required to achieve an immune response comparable to that of a vaccine containing a single antigen (**monovalent** vaccine).

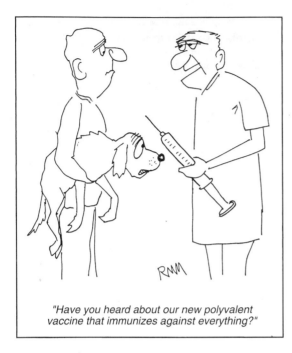

"Have you heard about our new polyvalent vaccine that immunizes against everything?"

Figure 17-1

From Vet. Forum, January 1994, p. 16.

ADMINISTRATION OF VACCINES

The intramuscular and subcutaneous routes are by far the most common methods for vaccine administration. These routes are easily accessible and provide systemic immunity, which is important in many diseases. Some diseases also respond well to local immunity. Vaccines against feline rhinotracheitis and calicivirus, canine infectious tracheobronchitis, and infectious bovine rhinotracheitis are examples of vaccines that may be administered intranasally, or in some cases, intraocular administration may be used to provide local immunity. After administration of these vaccines, the animal may experience slight watery eyes and occasional sneezing for a few days.

All of the previously mentioned routes of vaccine administration require that each animal be handled individually. When a large number of animals require vaccination, these routes may not be feasible. Some vaccines may be mixed with the drinking water or the feed. Others can be aerosolized and inhaled by the animals. For example, on mink ranches, vaccine for canine distemper and mink enteritis may be administered in this manner, or poultry houses may vaccinate for Newcastle disease by aerosolization. There is a greater margin for incomplete vaccination when aerosolization or mixing with feed or water is used. Some animals may not drink or eat enough to provide adequate protection, or the aerosolized vaccine may not distribute equally throughout the room. Vaccine failure may be implicated if these animals contract the disease, whereas in reality the animal did not receive enough vaccine to provide adequate immunity.

When using conventional measures for vaccination, it is very important to carefully read the insert provided with the vaccine. Some vaccines may be administered intramuscularly or subcutaneously, but others may be administered by only one route. For example, some rabies vaccines require an intramuscular route to be most effective. If a vaccine requires reconstitution, it should be done with the diluent provided by the manufacturer, and the vaccine should not be reconstituted until just before it is to be administered (see Chapter 2 for proper reconstitution procedure). The full recommended dose should be given. Splitting a vaccine dose may cause an animal to fail to develop an adequate immune response and may lower its protection.

Mixing different vaccines so that an animal does not have to receive so many injections is not recommended. This procedure can cause antigen blocking, resulting in one component's interfering with the action of another so that the animal does not receive adequate antigen to promote an effective immune response. Mixing different vaccines may also cause an increased chance of an allergic response. When administering different types of vaccines, give each vaccine in a separate site. It is also advisable to note the locations of administration and vaccine lot numbers on the patient's medical record. If a reaction or problem develops later, a reference will be available for checking.

When vaccinating food animals, several things must be considered. Almost all vaccines warn not to vaccinate within 21 days of slaughter. Vaccines such as those for *B. abortus* are under federal limitations and regulations, and complete records are maintained on the administration of these vaccines. Brucellosis vaccines are restricted to use by or under the direction of a licensed veterinarian. Carcass destruction is also a factor concerning food animal producers. Injection site lesions may cause damage to muscle tissue, requiring that area to be trimmed and discarded. If a vaccine may be administered either intramuscularly or subcutaneously, the subcutaneous route would produce less tissue reaction and eliminate muscle damage. This is important when dealing with animals used for meat consumption.

BIOLOGIC CARE AND VACCINE FAILURE

Biologics (especially modified live and live vaccines) are sensitive to inactivation by heat or sunlight. Clients purchasing vaccines should be provided with a cold pack if needed and should be warned against leaving such biologics in vehicles or in sunlight, where they may become warm and inactivated. The performance of even killed products can be altered if proper handling and storage measures are not practiced. When these vaccines are shipped from the manufacturer, cold packs are put in the box to provide some refrigeration during shipment. In some areas, it may be advisable to anticipate how much vaccine may be needed during the hot summer months and to stock up on that amount during early spring to prevent shipments from overheating during summer transportation. Once a shipment is received, it should be quickly unpacked and placed under refrigeration. Vaccines should never be frozen because cells may rupture, releasing toxins that can damage tissue or cause tissue death.

Inappropriate care of vaccines may lead to inactivation of the vaccine and may be perceived as a vaccine failure. Actual vaccine failure is relatively uncommon. If vaccines are purchased from a reputable manufacturer, one can be fairly sure that a good vaccine has been provided. Failure usually occurs because of improper handling, storage, or administration.

Live vaccines, especially, are affected by concurrent antibiotic therapy. Live and modified live vaccines can

be inactivated by chemicals used to clean or sterilize syringes and by use of excessive alcohol or other disinfectants to swab the skin before injection. As mentioned earlier, the route of administration may affect the ability of an animal to achieve an adequate immune response. Immunosuppressed, parasitized, stressed, or malnourished animals or those incubating disease are not able to mount an adequate immune response to prevent disease. Clients should always be advised that such problems can occur. In most cases, an adequate immune response is not achieved before 10 to 14 days. An 8-week-old puppy may not develop a strong enough immune response to protect against an infectious disease if challenged because of maternal antibodies. Because it is not feasible to check immune titers to determine whether maternal antibodies are still present and to determine when they disappear, it is recommended that puppies receive boosters every few weeks until about 4 to 5 months of age. Boosters allow vaccines to produce an optimum immune response. Clients often find it difficult to understand why they need to bring their pet in for boosters. If the reasons are explained and if clients are advised about why they should isolate their pet from animals with questionable vaccination histories, many cases of infectious diseases among young animals would be prevented. Clients often perceive one vaccine to be enough or do not understand that their animal is not protected immediately after an injection. Technicians should add this information to their education of clients on animal/pet care.

ADVERSE VACCINATION RESPONSES

The most significant risks involving vaccination include residual virulence and toxicity, allergic reactions resulting from hypersensitivity, disease in immunosuppressed animals, possible effects on a fetus, or abortion. The veterinarian assesses these risks before a vaccine is administered. In most cases, the benefits of vaccination far outweigh the risks, but it may occasionally be necessary to omit or delay vaccination because of some of the factors mentioned.

One of the most common reactions noticed with vaccine administration is the sting felt by the animal after injection. This is most often a result of inactivating agents used in manufacturing the vaccine. Manufacturers are constantly researching ways to decrease these undesirable effects and still produce a quality product. This stinging reaction is short lived and does not usually cause a problem unless the animal reacts violently. Other common but not usually serious reactions include a slight fever, lethargy, and soreness at the injection site. These usually subside within 1 day. Hypersensitivity may be caused by several factors, including the immunizing antigens, antigens acquired during the vaccine manufacturing, and reactions to adjuvants used in the vaccine. Some animals may have an anaphylactic shock reaction after receiving a vaccine, although this is uncommon. Clinical signs of **anaphylaxis** include vomiting, salivation, dyspnea, and incoordination. Epinephrine is usually the antidote of choice in cases of anaphylactic shock. Other adverse side effects that are possible include vaccine-associated fibrosarcoma in cats and immune-mediated hemolytic anemia in dogs (Ford, 1998). The possible etiologies for these effects are under investigation.

VACCINATIONS FOR PREVENTIVE HEALTH PROGRAMS

CANINE

As stated earlier, vaccination is an important part of any preventive health program. Many vaccines may be available as a monovalent or polyvalent product. For dogs, a common polyvalent vaccine includes canine distemper (D), respiratory diseases caused by adenovirus type 2 (A_2), canine parainfluenza (P), leptospirosis (L), and canine parvovirus (P). This vaccine may be referred to as *DA₂PLP.* Many different combinations are available, as well as many different product names. Most veterinarians choose a particular manufacturer from whom to buy vaccine products. This helps to lessen the confusion caused by different names used to designate the manufacturers' products. Other canine vaccines available include those for canine infectious bronchitis *(Bordetella bronchiseptica),* canine

coronavirus, rabies, and Lyme disease *(B. burgdorferi).* Manufacturer recommendations regarding age, route of administration, and follow-up boosters needed for each individual vaccine should be followed. Table 17-1 provides an example of a vaccination program for dogs.

EQUINE

Many horse vaccines are available, including those for tetanus, equine encephalomyelitis (may include Eastern, Western and/or Venezuelan strains), equine rhinopneumonitis, equine influenza, *Streptococcus* (strangles), equine viral arteritis, equine monocytic ehrlichiosis (Potomac horse fever), anthrax spore, and rabies vaccine. Tetanus antitoxin is used in wounded horses with no history of recent tetanus toxoid vaccination. It provides immediate immunity that lasts for about 2 weeks. Tetanus toxoid may be given to a horse to boost its immunity and provide longer protection. Manufacturer recommendations regarding age, route of administration, and follow-up boosters needed for each individual vaccine should be followed. Table 17-2 provides an example of a general preventive health program for horses.

FELINE

A common polyvalent vaccine for cats is for the prevention of feline viral rhinotracheitis (FVR), feline calicivirus (C), and feline panleukopenia (P). This combination may be referred to as *FVRCP.* Other vaccines available include those for feline chlamydiosis, feline leukemia, feline infectious peritonitis, bordetella, and rabies. Manufacturer recommendations regarding age, route of administration, and follow-up boosters needed for each vaccine should be followed. Table 17-3 provides an example of a vaccination program for cats.

BOVINE

Many vaccines in many different combinations are available for cattle. Vaccine schedules for cattle vary

TABLE 17-1 General Vaccination Program for Dogs

I. First office visit—usually at 6-8 weeks of age
Perform physical examination
Check for external parasites, and begin appropriate treatment
Do fecal examination, and begin appropriate treatment
Initiate heartworm preventative program
Vaccinate with DA₂PL-PvC*; also with kennel cough vaccine if indicated
Provide client education on pet care, and answer questions

II. Second office visit—usually at 9-12 weeks of age
Perform physical examination
Check for external parasites, and begin appropriate treatment
Do fecal examination, and begin appropriate treatment
Increase dosage of heartworm preventative according to weight increase
Vaccinate with DA₂PL-PvC*; also with kennel cough and Lyme disease vaccines if indicated
Provide client education on pet care, and answer questions

III. Third office visit—usually at 12-15 weeks of age
Perform physical examination
Check for external parasites, and begin appropriate treatment
Do fecal examination, and begin appropriate treatment
Increase dosage of heartworm preventative according to weight increase
Vaccinate with DA₂PL-PvC*; also with kennel cough and Lyme disease vaccines if indicated
Provide client education on pet care, and answer questions

IV. Fourth office visit—usually at 15-18 weeks of age
Perform physical examination
Check for external parasites, and begin appropriate treatment
Do fecal examination, and begin appropriate treatment
Increase dosage of heartworm preventative according to weight increase; for large breeds it may be necessary to weigh before the annual visit to ensure that the correct dose is being administered
Vaccinate with DA₂PL-PvC* and rabies vaccine; also with kennel cough and Lyme disease vaccines if indicated
Discuss recommendations for spaying or neutering
Provide client education on pet care, and answer questions

V. Annual office visit
Perform physical examination
Check for external parasites, and begin appropriate treatment
Do fecal examination, and begin appropriate treatment
Increase dosage of heartworm preventative according to weight increase
Vaccinate with DA₂PL-PvC* and rabies vaccine; also with kennel cough and Lyme disease vaccines if indicated
Provide client education on pet care, and answer questions

*This refers to the use of a vaccine to protect against: D-canine distemper, A₂-canine adenovirus type 2 (infectious canine hepatitis), P-canine parainfluenza, L-leptospira, Pv-canine parvovirus, and C-canine coronavirus.

depending on the type of cattle-raising operation, and a veterinarian can best decide what program an individual operation needs. Examples of common vaccines used include leptospirosis, vibriosis, clostridial combinations, respiratory tract disease vaccines, and enteric disease vaccines. As with all vaccines, manufacturer recommendations should be carefully followed for the best results. Tables 17-4 and 17-5 provide examples of preventive health programs for beef and dairy cattle.

TABLE 17-2 General Outline of a Preventive Health Program for Horses

First Quarter: January-March

All Horses

Deworm—minimum of every 8 weeks. Exercise care in choice of anthelmintics for mares in the third trimester. Begin deworming foals at 2 months of age.

Trim feet—every 6 weeks. More frequently in foals requiring limb correction.

Dentistry—check adults twice yearly and float teeth as needed. Remove wolf teeth in 2-year-olds and retained caps in 2-, 3- and 4-year-olds. Immunize for respiratory disease: influenza, strangles, and rhinopneumonitis.

Stallions

Perform complete breeding examination. Maintain stallions under lights if being used for early breeding.

Pregnant Mares

Immunize with tetanus toxoid, and open sutured mares 30 days prepartum. Develop a colostrum bank. Ninth-day breeding only for mares with normal foaling history and normal reproductive tract. Wash udders of foaling mares.

Open Mares

Maintain under lights if being used for early breeding. Perform daily teasing. Perform reproductive tract examination during estrus. Mares should not be too fat but in gaining condition during breeding season.

Newborn Foals

Dip navel in disinfectant. Carefully, give a cleansing enema at birth. Administer tetanus prophylaxis if indicated by history.

Second Quarter: April-June

All Horses

Deworm—minimum of every 8 weeks.

Trim feet–every 6 weeks. Don't forget the foals and yearlings.

Dentistry—check teeth and remove or float teeth as needed.

Immunize for equine encephalomyelitis. Administer appropriate vaccine boosters.

Stallions

Maintain an exercise program. Monitor the semen quality.

Broodmares

Palpate at 21, 42, and 60 days after successful breeding.

Foals

Creep-feed the foals and provide free-choice minerals. Immunize at 3 months of age. Group the foals by sex and size when weaned.

Third Quarter: July-September

All Horses

Deworm—minimum of every 8 weeks. Clip and sweep the pastures.

Trim feet—every 6 weeks. Continue corrective trimming on foals.

Dentistry—check teeth and remove or float teeth as needed.

Stallions

Maintain an exercise program.

Broodmares

Administer rhinopneumonitis boosters to pregnant mares according to manufacturer's labeled directions. Administer appropriate vaccine boosters to foals and yearlings. Check condition of mare's udder at weaning and reduce the amount of feed given until milk flow is reduced.

Foals

Administer all appropriate immunizations. Provide free-choice minerals. Maintain a protein supplement in creep feeders.

Fourth Quarter: October-December

All Horses

Deworm—minimum every 8 weeks. Select anthelmintics appropriate for season.

Trim feet—every 6 weeks. Continuous corrective trimming on foals.

Dentistry—check teeth and remove or float teeth as needed.

Stallions

Continue the exercise program. Check immunizations. Perform breeding examination.

Broodmares

Confirm pregnancy. Begin treating the open mares. Check immunizations.

From McCurnin, D.M.: Clinical Textbook for Veterinary Technicians, 4th ed. W.B. Saunders Company, Philadelphia, 1998.

TABLE 17-3 General Vaccination Program for Cats

I. First office visit—usually at 8-10 weeks of age
    Perform physical examination
    Check for external parasites, and begin appropriate treatment
    Do fecal examination, and begin appropriate treatment
    Vaccinate with FVRCP-C and FeLV; possibly test for FeLV/FIP before initial FeLV vaccine*; if indicated, recommend bordetella vaccine
    Provide client education on pet care, and answer questions

II. Second office visit—usually at 12-14 weeks of age
    Perform physical examination
    Check for external parasites, and begin appropriate treatment
    Do fecal examination and begin appropriate treatment
    Vaccinate with FVRCP-C and FeLV and rabies*
    If indicated, recommend FIP and ringworm vaccines be given at 16 weeks of age (boosters will be necessary)
    Discuss recommendations for spaying and neutering
    Provide client education on pet care, and answer questions

III. Annual office visit
    Perform physical examination
    Check for external parasites, and begin appropriate treatment
    Do fecal examination, and begin appropriate treatment
    Vaccinate with FVRCP-C and FeLV and rabies; also with FIP and ringworm vaccines if indicated*
    Provide client education on pet care, and answer questions

*This refers to the use of a vaccine to protect against: FVR-feline viral rhinotracheitis, C-feline calicivirus, P-feline panleukopenia, C-feline chlamydiosis (Chlamydia psittaci), FeLV-feline leukemia virus, FIP-feline infectious peritonitis.

TABLE 17-4 General Outline of a Preventive Health Program for Beef Cattle

Cow-Calf Herd Recommendation*

At Birth

Ingestion of colostrum within the first few hours after birth is an important factor in baby calf survival.
    Immunize with oral bovine rotavirus and coronavirus enteric disease vaccine if a calf diarrhea problem exists in the herd.

1- to 3-Month-Old Calves

Immunize with a seven-way clostridial diseases product. Deworm with commercial product that is safe for calves.

Preweaning Calves

Deworm with broad-spectrum commercial dewormer and immunize as follows:

IMMUNIZING VACCINE	AGE FOR VACCINE ADMINISTRATION
Brucella abortus, strain 19 (calfhood vaccination—replacement heifers only)	5-6 months of age (dependent upon federal and state regulations)
Clostridial diseases *Clostridium perfringens* types C and D, *C. chauvoei, C. novyi, C. septicum,* and *C. sordelli*	5-6 months of age

*Other optional vaccines that may be incorporated into the immunization program, depending on individual herd needs and diseases endemic to the area, include anthrax and anaplasmosis.

Continued

Cow-Calf Herd Recommendation*—cont'd

Preweaning Calves—cont'd

IMMUNIZING VACCINE—CONT'D	AGE FOR VACCINE ADMINISTRATION—CONT'D
Infectious bovine rhinotracheitis (IBR) and parainfluenza-3 (PI-3) respiratory diseases (inactivated vaccines only)	5-6 months of age, booster at 12-13 months of age
Bovine virus diarrhea (BVD) (inactivated vaccines only)	5-6 months of age, booster at 12-13 months of age

Weaning Calves

Deworm with broad-spectrum commercial dewormer and treat for lice and grubs. Castrate the bull calves. Immunize with *Pasteurella* (optional) and *Haemophilus* (optional) vaccines.

Prebreeding Replacement Heifers

Deworm with broad-spectrum commercial dewormer and treat for lice. Immunize as follows:

IMMUNIZING VACCINE	TIME OF VACCINE ADMINISTRATION
Infectious bovine rhinotracheitis (IBR) and parainfluenza-3 (PI-3) respiratory diseases	10-12 months of age
Clostridial diseases	10-12 months of age
C. perfringens types C and D, *C. novyi*, *C. septicum*, *C. sordelli*, and *C. chauvoei*	
Bovine virus diarrhea (BVD)	10-12 months of age
Leptospirosis	10-12 months of age
Campylobacteriosis	10-12 months of age

Prebreeding Cows

Deworm with broad-spectrum dewormer and treat for lice. Immunize for leptospirosis and campylobacteriosis.

Precalving Cows

Immunize as follows:

IMMUNIZING VACCINE	TIME OF VACCINE ADMINISTRATION
Infectious bovine rhinotracheitis (IBR) and parainfluenza-3 (PI-3) respiratory diseases (inactivated vaccines only)	Prior to calving
Bovine virus diarrhea (BVD) (inactivated vaccines only)	Prior to calving
Bovine rotavirus and coronavirus enteric diseases	Prior to calving
Escherichia coli enteric disease	Prior to calving
Clostridial diseases	Prior to calving
C. perfringens types C and D, *C. chauvoei*, *C. novyi*, *C. septicum*, and *C. sordelli*	

Bulls

Deworm annually with broad-spectrum dewormer and treat for lice and grubs. Immunize as recommended for prebreeding replacement heifers annually (see the above section).

Feedlot Recommendations†

On Arrival into the Feedlot

Deworm with a broad-spectrum dewormer and immunize for infectious bovine rhinotracheitis (IBR), parainfluenza-3 (PI-3), bovine virus diarrhea (BVD), and clostridial diseases (use seven-way vaccine). Inactivated infectious bovine rhinotracheitis, parainfluenza-3, and bovine virus diarrhea vaccines are the safest.

3-4 Weeks After Arrival into the Feedlot

Implant a commercial implant product. Treat for lice and grubs. Administer booster immunizations if necessary. Abort the heifers if necessary. Castrate and dehorn if necessary.

†Other optional vaccines that may be incorporated into the immunization program, depending on individual herd needs and diseases endemic to the area, include *Haemophilus somnus, Pasteurella* spp., respiratory syncytial virus, leptospirosis, and anthrax.

TABLE 17-5   General Outline of a Preventive Health Program for Dairy Cattle*

Calves

At Birth

Immunize with bovine rotavirus and coronavirus enteric disease vaccine† and administer orally *Escherichia coli* enteric disease vaccine. *Weaning Age (about 2 months of age) to Breeding Age (about 15 months of age)*

Immunizing Vaccine	*Age for Vaccine Administration*
Brucella abortus, strain 19 (calfhood vaccination—replacement heifers only)	4-8 months of age optimal time (dependent upon federal and state regulations)
Clostridial diseases	2-4 months of age
Clostridium perfringens types C and D, *C. chauvoei, C. novyi, C. septicum,* and *C. sordelli*	
Infectious bovine rhinotracheitis (IBR) and parainfluenza-3 (PI-3) respiratory diseases	4-6 months of age, booster at 12-13 months of age
Bovine virus diarrhea (BVD)	6-8 months of age, booster at 12-13 months of age
Leptospirosis	4-6 months of age, booster in 2 weeks
Campylobacteriosis (if natural breeding)	4-6 months of age, booster at 12-13 months of age

Fresh Cows and Heifers

Immunizing Vaccine	*Time of Vaccine Administration*
Infectious bovine rhinotracheitis (IBR) and parainfluenza-3 respiratory diseases (inactivated vaccines only)	30 days post partum
Bovine virus diarrhea (BVD) (inactivated vaccines only)	30 days post partum
Leptospirosis	30 days post partum
Campylobacteriosis	30 days post partum

Dry Cows and Bred Heifers

The goal of dry cow immunization is to provide for optimal protection for the newborn calf.

Immunizing Vaccine	*Time of Vaccine Administration*
Leptospirosis	At time of dry-off
Bovine rotavirus and coronavirus enteric diseases†	At time of dry-off, booster in 2-3 weeks
Escherichia coli enteric disease†	At time of dry-off, booster in 2-3 weeks
Clostridial diseases	At time of dry-off, booster in 2-3 weeks
C. perfringens types C and D, *C. chauvoei, C. novyi, C. septicum,* and *C. sordelli*	

*Other vaccines may be incorporated into the vaccination program, depending on individual herd needs and diseases endemic to the area, including *Haemophilus somnus, Pasteurella* spp., *Salmonella* spp., *Clostridium haemolyticum,* anthrax, and anaplasmosis.
†Use if problem of neonatal calf diarrhea exists on the farm.
From McCurnin, D.M.: Clinical Textbook for Veterinary Technicians, 4th ed. W.B. Saunders Company, Philadelphia, 1998.

OTHERS

Vaccines are also available for sheep, poultry, and swine. These animals may be raised in large numbers on farms, and as for cattle-raising operations, vaccination schedules may vary according to the type of conditions and location. Ferrets have become common household pets and should be vaccinated for canine distemper according to the schedule used for dogs. Some rabies vaccines are approved for use in ferrets. Public health authorities can require a rabies-vaccinated ferret that bites a human to be euthanized and tested for rabies virus.

IMMUNOTHERAPEUTIC DRUGS

It may often be desirable to use drugs to stimulate the body's immunologic response. Immunotherapy involves using drugs to stimulate or suppress the body's immunologic response to diseases or conditions caused by agents such as bacteria, viruses, or cancer cells. Immunostimulants are agents that stimulate the immune response. Immunomodulators are agents used to adjust the immune response to a desired level. Table 17-6 lists some of the drugs commonly used in immunotherapy.

Immunotherapy involves using drugs to stimulate or suppress the body's immunologic response to diseases or conditions caused by agents such as bacteria, viruses, or cancer cells. Immunostimulants are used to stimulate the body's immunologic response. They may do this by stimulating macrophage activity, producing lymphokine, increasing natural killer cell activity, and enhancing cell-mediated immunity. These drugs may be used in the treatment of chronic pyoderma in dogs, equine sarcoids, and bovine ocular squamous cell carcinoma. They may also be used as adjunctive therapy for some other types of cancers such as canine malignant lymphoma, fibrosarcoma, and feline retrovirus infections. Some immunostimulants may be used to help reduce the clinical signs and mortality associated with some infections such as *E. coli* diarrhea in calves. Many other immunostimulants such as interferons, interleukin-1, and interleukin-2 are being investigated for potential use in veterinary medicine. Immunosuppressive drugs are used to suppress the body's immunologic response. They are used in veterinary medicine to treat various immune-mediated disorders. Further information on immunosuppressive drugs may be found in Chapter 16.

IMMUNOSTIMULANTS

Complex Carbohydrates

Acemannan: This is a complex carbohydrate derived from aloe vera.

Clinical Uses. Acemannan is used as an aid in the treatment of fibrosarcoma in cats and dogs. It has also been used for stimulating wound healing and in treatment of FeLV- and FIV-infected cats.

TABLE 17-6 Immunotherapeutic Drugs and Indications for Their Use

Product Name and Manufacturer	Product Type	Product Indications
Acemannan Immunostimulant (Carrington)	A complex carbohydrate derived from aloe vera; stimulates macrophage activity	An aid in the treatment of fibrosarcoma in cats and dogs and feline leukemia; also for stimulating wound healing (Tizard, 1992)
Staphage Lysate (SPL) (Delmont)	*Staphylococcus aureus* phage lysate	Treatment for canine pyoderma and related skin infections with a staphylococcal component
Rubeola Virus Immunomodulator (Eudaemonic)	Inactivated rubeola virus with histamine phosphate	Treatment of equine chronic myofascial inflammation
Nomagen (Fort Dodge)	A mycobacterial cell-wall fraction immunostimulant	Treatment of equine sarcoids and bovine ocular squamous cell carcinoma
Immunoregulin (ImmunoVet)	*Propionibacterium acnes* immunostimulant	Chronic recurrent pyoderma in dogs
CL/MAb 231 (Synbiotics)	Canine lymphoma monoclonal antibody	Adjunctive therapy for dogs with lymphoma

Dosage Form

1. Acemannan Immunostimulant

Adverse Side Effects. None.

Immunomodulatory Bacterins

***Staphylococcus* Phage Lysate (SPL):** This is prepared by lysing *Staphylococcus aureus* with a polyvalent bacteriophage.

Clinical Uses. SPL is used in the treatment of canine pyoderma and related skin infections with a staphylococcal component.

Dosage Form

1. Staphage Lysate (SPL)

Adverse Side Effects. These include malaise, fever, chills, and injection site irritation.

Propionibacterium Acnes Bacterin: This is prepared from killed *Propionibacterium acnes.*

Clinical Uses. *P. acnes* is used in the treatment of chronic recurrent pyoderma and as an adjunct therapy in the treatment for equine respiratory disease complex. It has also been used as an adjunctive therapy in the treatment of feline retrovirus infections.

Dosage Forms

1. Immunoregulin
2. Eqstim

Adverse Side Effects. These include malaise, fever, and chills.

Mycobacterial Cell Wall Fraction: This is an emulsion of cell wall fractions that are modified to reduce their toxicity and allergic effects.

Clinical Uses. These include the treatment of equine sarcoids and bovine ocular squamous cell carcinoma. It is also used in the treatment of mixed mammary tumors and mammary adenocarcinoma in dogs.

Dosage Forms

1. Regressin-V
2. Nomagen

Adverse Side Effects. These include malaise, fever, and decreased appetite.

Technician's Notes
The effects of immunotherapy may be decreased with the administration of immunosuppressive drugs.

REFERENCES

Ford, Richard B.: Vaccines and Vaccinations. Issues for the 21st Century. Suppl. Compend. Contin. Educ. Pract. Vet. 20(8C):19-24, 1998.
Tizard, I.: Veterinary Immunology: An Introduction, 4th ed. W.B. Saunders Company, Philadelphia, 1992.

■   Review Questions

1. What factors affect an animal's response to a vaccine?
   _____

2. Describe the differences between inactivated, live, and modified live vaccines.
   _____

3. Why must live vaccines be handled carefully during administration? _____

4. Describe the main difference between an antiserum and an antitoxin. _____

5. What are some common routes for vaccine administration? _____

6. Why should different vaccines not be mixed?
   _____

7. What factors may lead to vaccine failure?
   _____

8. What antidote is usually recommended for anaphylactic shock due to a vaccine?
   _____

Miscellaneous Therapeutic Agents

LEARNING OBJECTIVES

After studying this chapter, you should be able to:

1. Develop a knowledge of glycosaminoglycans and how they act as chondroprotectives
2. Develop a general knowledge about the uses and adverse side effects of common antidotes
3. Understand the use of naloxone and yohimbine HCl as reversal agents
4. Be familiar with the names of common lubricants

KEY TERMS

Chelating agent An agent used in the chemotherapy of metal poisoning.
Methemoglobinemia The presence of methemoglobin in the blood; caused by injury or toxic agents that convert a larger-than-normal proportion of hemoglobin into

methemoglobin, which does not function as an oxygen carrier.
Nutraceutical Any nontoxic food component that has scientifically proven health benefits.

ALTERNATIVE MEDICINES

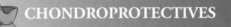 **CHONDROPROTECTIVES**

Glycosaminoglycans

Chondroprotectives contain glycosaminoglycans (GAGs), which occur naturally in the articular cartilage and connective tissue. When used in degenerative joint conditions, these GAGs stimulate synovial fluid secretion, increase viscosity, and inhibit enzymes that damage proteoglycans and collagen within joints. GAGs also promote the synthesis of proteoglycans, collagen, and hyaluronic acid. Although some controversy exists about the efficacy of these agents, research continues to provide promise for their use in veterinary medicine. Polysulfated glycosaminoglycan (PSGAG) contains glycosamine and hexuronic acid, which studies have shown to "inhibit catabolism of collagen and proteoglycan in chick embryonic and human articular cartilages, as well as to stimulate their synthesis in tissue culture systems" (Altman et al, 1989). It is used in veterinary medicine as a chondroprotective agent.

Adverse Side Effects. Adverse side effects are minimal with use of this product.

Clinical Uses. PSGAG is used in the treatment of noninfectious degenerative or traumatic joint dysfunction and associated lameness of the carpal joints in horses. It has also been used to treat degenerative joint disorders in dogs and lameness in swine.

Dosage Forms

1. Adequan I.A., for intra-articular injection
2. Adequan I.M., for intramuscular injection
3. Adequan Canine
4. Legend

Technician's Notes

1. Amikacin may be used concurrently with intra-articular use to prevent infection resulting from possible contamination.
2. PSGAG should not be used in horses intended for food.
3. Safety in breeding animals is undetermined.

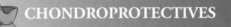 **NUTRACEUTICALS**

A **nutraceutical** has been defined as any nontoxic food component that has scientifically proven health benefits, including disease treatment and prevention. The popularity of these products that may have characteristics of nutrients and pharmaceuticals has seen tremendous growth in use by people in recent years, and the medical community has acknowledged that some of them may have treatment or preventive effects (Boothe, 1997). Products such as niacin, beta carotene, calcium, fiber, and antioxidants have widespread use for therapeutic purposes or prevention of selected medical conditions in people.

As people have become more aware of alternative medical options for themselves, they have come to expect similar options for their pets. Veterinarians and their clients can be expected to use nutraceuticals as treatment options to complement traditional medicine or when traditional treatment options have been exhausted.

The North American Veterinary Nutraceutical Council has defined a veterinary nutraceutical as "a nondrug substance that is produced in a purified or extracted form and administered orally to provide agents required for normal body structure and function with the intent of improving the health and well-being of animals." Even though the definitions listed for nutraceutical and veterinary nutraceutical seem straightforward, a great deal of confusion exists over what is actually a nutraceutical. It has been stated that the term nutraceutical was developed to refer to a product marketed under the premise of being a dietary supplement, but with the real intent of preventing or treating a disease (Fascetti, 1998).

The question often asked about these products is "is it a food (nutrient) or a drug?" If it is a food, then it is not subject to FDA approval, and if it is a drug, it must go through the FDA approval process at a great deal of expense to the manufacturer. A product is usually determined to be a drug if its label has a claim that indicates a therapeutic or preventive intent. If a product is determined to be a food, it is usually determined to be "generally regarded as safe (GRAS)" by the FDA.

The Dietary Supplement Health and Education Act (DSHEA) of 1994 listed dietary supplements as vitamins, minerals, amino acids, herbal products, and substances that supplement the diet by increasing total dietary intake. This action made these products "food" and excluded them from FDA regulation. The act does require, however, that the manufacturer show a disclaimer on the label after the product claim that says "this statement has not been evaluated by the Food and Drug Administration. This product is not intended to diagnose, treat, cure, or prevent any disease." Because of concerns about potential residues and the potential differences in response across species, the Center for Veterinary Medicine (CVM) of the FDA has stated that the DSHEA does not apply to animals or animal feeds.

Since nutraceuticals have not been through an extensive evaluation process to validate their safety and efficacy, it is up to the veterinarian to evaluate the suitability of particular products for use in companion animals and to promote their use in the context of a valid veterinarian-client-patient relationship. Some questions that should be answered when evaluating a nutraceutical product include the following:

1. What controlled studies have been done to determine whether the product does what it claims to do and who performed the studies?
2. Does the product contain what it says it does, and is that product bioavailable?
3. Is the label easily understandable with all ingredients listed in the same units?
4. Is the dosage appropriate?

A partial list of the substances marketed as nutraceuticals is included in the following.

Glucosamine and Chondrotin Sulfate

Glucosamine is an aminosaccharide manufactured from glucose and used by the body in the synthesis of glycoproteins and glycosaminoglycans, whereas chondrotin sulfate is a mucopolysaccharide found in the cartilaginous tissue of mammals. The mechanisms of action of these substances are believed to be a positive effect on cartilage metabolism and an inhibition of cartilage breakdown. They have been used extensively in the treatment of osteoarthritis in dogs and horses. A common veterinary product containing these substances is called Cosequin, which is comprised of glycosaminoglycan derived from the chitin of crab shell and condrotin sulfate from bovine trachea. Glyco-Flex and Syno-Flex derive their glycosaminoglycan from the Perna canaliculus mussel.

Echinacea

Echinacea is a commonly used remedy for colds and flu in people in the United States and Europe where research has been done demonstrating that it is an immunostimulant. It is derived primarily from the American cone flower. No major side effects have been reported other than the occasional allergic reaction (Fascetti, 1998).

Garlic

Garlic is a perennial bulb in the lily family that is related to the onion. This plant has been used for centuries for its reported medicinal value. People have claimed that it produces disinfectant, diuretic, and/or expectorant effects. There is some evidence that it does lower cholesterol values in people. There is no evidence, however, that garlic has any value in the treatment of parasites in animals. Garlic can produce a Heinz body anemia in cats and possibly in dogs at high dosages.

Ginseng

Ginseng is made from the dried roots of several species of plants from the Panax family. The Chinese believe that ginseng increase vitality and overall strength possibly by improving aerobic metabolism. Side effects may include hypertension, nervousness, and excitement.

Fatty Acids

The omega-6 and omega-3 fatty acids are the ones most often found in commercial veterinary fatty acid supplements. Omega-6 fatty acids have double bond 6 carbons from the methyl end, whereas omega-3 fatty acids have double bond 3 carbons from the methyl end. Fatty acid supplementation has been shown to be useful in treating certain dermatologic conditions in dogs and cats because of their anti-inflammatory effects. They also may be helpful in treating cancer, autoimmune disease, and rheumatoid arthritis in people. The proper ratio of omega-6 to omega-3 fatty acids in a product has apparently not been determined and is often debated. Fish oil and plant oils are common sources of these fatty acids. Side effects may include increased bleeding times and possible decreased immune function.

Brewer's Yeast

The claim has been made that brewer's yeast given to a pet will cause fleas to be repelled. No controlled studies have shown this effect to be true. Brewer's yeast is a good source of the B vitamins.

Probiotics

Probiotics are substances that competitively inhibit enteropathogens. They have been used to treat inflammatory bowel disease, food allergy, chronic antibiotic use, and diarrhea.

Bioflavonoids

Bioflavonoids are plant chemicals (phytochemicals) also called bioflavins or vitamin P. They are found in citrus pulp and a variety of other plants. They are known for their potential antioxidant activity.

Fiber

Soluble fiber from fruits and insoluble fiber from vegetables and whole grains are known for their ability to soften stool. Fiber is used to treat constipation and diabetes mellitus.

Ginkgo

Ginkgo biloba is thought to increase circulation to the brain and extremities and has been reported to improve memory and symptoms of senile dementia in people.

St. John's Wort

St. John's Wort is a plant that has reported (anecdotal) anti-anxiety and anti-depression effects in people.

Saw Palmetto

Saw palmetto plant extract may be of value in treating benign prostatic hyperplasia because of its possible ability to reduce testosterone formation.

Superoxide Dismutase

Superoxide dismutase from protein sources is an oxygen radical scavenger that has been used as an anti-inflammatory agent for musculoskeletal problems.

Coenzyme Q

This substance is an enzyme co-factor of mitochondrial membranes that is important in electron transport and ATP formation. It is used in the treatment of cardiovascular problems.

Aloe Vera

The aloe vera plant is known to contain substances with immunomodulator activity.

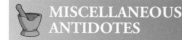
MISCELLANEOUS ANTIDOTES

Activated Charcoal

Activated charcoal is a fine, black, odorless, tasteless powder used to adsorb certain drugs or toxins to prevent or reduce their systemic absorption from the upper gastrointestinal tract.

Clinical Uses. These include oral administration to prevent or reduce the systemic absorption of certain drugs or toxins.

Dosage Forms
1. Toxiban Suspension
2. Toxiban Granules
3. Activated charcoal powder (generic) (for reconstitution with water)

Adverse Side Effects. These include vomiting after very rapid administration of activated charcoal. Activated charcoal can also cause either constipation or diarrhea, and the stool is black.

> **Technician's Notes**
> 1. Activated charcoal is not considered effective against heavy metals (e.g., lead, mercury, and inorganic arsenic), mineral acids, caustic alkalies, nitrates, sodium, chloride/chlorate, ferrous sulfate, or petroleum distillates.
> 2. Other oral therapeutic agents should not be administered within 3 hours after activated charcoal therapy.
> 3. Dairy products and mineral oil reduce activated charcoal's adsorptive properties.

Calcium EDTA

Calcium EDTA (CaEDTA) is a heavy metal **chelating agent** available commercially (human) as an injection. It may also be referred to as edetate calcium disodium, calcium disodium edetate, calcium edetate, calcium disodium ethylenediaminetetra-acetate, and sodium calcium edetate.

Clinical Uses. In veterinary medicine, calcium EDTA is used for the treatment of lead poisoning.

Dosage Forms
1. Calcium Disodium Versenate injection (human label)
2. Meta-Dote

Adverse Side Effects. These include renal toxicity, depression (dogs), and vomiting/diarrhea (dogs). Zinc deficiency may occur from chronic therapy.

> **Technician's Notes**
> 1. Calcium EDTA should not be used in anuric patients, and caution should be exercised when used in patients with renal insufficiency.
> 2. Calcium EDTA should not be administered orally.
> 3. Do not confuse with edetate disodium, which may cause severe hypocalcemia.
> 4. Magnesium sulfate (Epsom salt) or sodium sulfate may be used orally to prevent further intestinal absorption of lead.

Methylene Blue

Methylene blue is a thiazine dye that occurs as dark green crystals or crystalline powder with a bronze-like luster. It is an oxidating agent that helps to convert methemoglobin (a compound formed from hemoglobin by oxidation of the iron atom) from the ferrous (Fe^{2+}) to the ferric (Fe^{3+}) state. It does not function as an oxygen carrier to hemoglobin.

Clinical Uses. Methylene blue is used for treatment of **methemoglobinemia** resulting from oxidative agents (e.g., nitrites, nitrates, and chlorates) in ruminants. It may be used for cyanide toxicity in ruminants. It can be used in dogs to intraoperatively stain pancreatic islet cell tumors preferentially and for treatment of acetaminophen poisoning.

Dosage Forms

1. Methylene blue injection (generic) (human label)
2. Methylene blue tablets (generic)
3. Methylene blue powder (generic)

Adverse Side Effects. These include the development of Heinz body anemia or morphologic changes in red blood cells, as well as decreased red blood cell life span. Methemoglobinemia may occur but is usually dose- and species-dependent. Tissue necrosis may occur with subcutaneous administration or extravasation during intravenous injection.

Technician's Notes

1. Methylene blue is usually contraindicated in cats.
2. Dogs and horses may show greater occurrence of side effects than ruminants.
3. Methylene blue should not be used in patients with renal insufficiency.
4. Safety during pregnancy is unknown.

Acetylcysteine

Acetylcysteine is a white crystalline powder that is soluble in water or alcohol. It may also be referred to as *N*-acetylcysteine or *N*-acetyl-L-cysteine.

Clinical Uses. These include oral therapy for acetaminophen poisoning in dogs and cats. It may also be used as a mucolytic agent for pulmonary (via nebulization) or ophthalmic (via topical application) conditions.

Dosage Forms

1. Mucomyst (human label)
2. Mucosil (human label)
3. Acetylcysteine (human label)

Adverse Side Effects. These include nausea, vomiting, and occasionally urticaria (hives) when administered orally. Chest tightness, bronchoconstriction, bronchial or tracheal irritation, and acetylcysteine hypersensitivity are rare but possible side effects when administered into the pulmonary tract. Acetylcysteine may cause bronchospasm in some patients receiving treatment via the pulmonary tract.

Technician's Notes

1. Acetylcysteine is incompatible with amphotericin B, chlortetracycline hydrochloride, erythromycin lactobionate, oxytetracycline hydrochloride, ampicillin sodium, tetracycline hydrochloride, iodized oil, hydrogen peroxide, chymotrypsin, and trypsin.
2. Activated charcoal may adsorb acetylcysteine, reducing its effectiveness in treating acetaminophen toxicity.
3. Carefully monitor patients that have bronchospastic diseases and that receive pulmonary treatment.
4. Oral solution has a bad taste, and a masking agent (e.g., colas, juices) may be used.
5. Open vials should be refrigerated and discarded after 96 hours.

Dimercaprol

Dimercaprol is a dithiol chelating agent that occurs as a colorless or nearly colorless viscous liquid with a disagreeable odor. The commercial solution may be cloudy or may contain small amounts of flaky material or sediment. This is normal and does not indicate deterioration of the product. It may also be referred to as BAL, British antilewisite, dimercaptopropranol, or dithioglycerol.

Clinical Uses. Dimercaprol is primarily used for the treatment of toxicity resulting from arsenic compounds but may be used for lead, mercury, or gold toxicity.

Dosage Forms

1. Dimercaprol injection 100 mg/ml (human label)
2. BAL in oil (human label)

Adverse Side Effects. Intramuscular injections are painful. Vomiting and seizures may occur with high doses. It is potentially nephrotoxic. Most side effects subside quickly because of rapid elimination of the drug.

Pralidoxime Chloride

Pralidoxime chloride is a quaternary ammonium oxime cholinesterase reactivator. It reverses the action of cholinesterase inhibitors such as certain organophosphates.

It may also be referred to as a 2-PAM chloride or 2-pyridine aldoxime methylchloride.

Clinical Uses. Pralidoxime chloride is used for oral treatment of organophosphate poisoning. It may be used in conjunction with atropine and supportive therapy.

Dosage Form

1. Protopam injection (human label)

Adverse Side Effects. These are uncommon, but rapid intravenous injection may cause tachycardia, muscle rigidity, transient neuromuscular blockade, and laryngospasm.

Technician's Notes

1. Pralidoxime, like other anticholinesterases, may potentiate the action of barbiturates.
2. Patients with impaired renal function require a lower dose and careful monitoring.

Penicillamine

Penicillamine is a chelating agent of metals such as copper, lead, iron, and mercury. It is a degradation product of penicillins but does not have antimicrobial activity. It may also be referred to as D-penicillamine, *B, B*-dimethylcysteine, or D,3-mercaptovaline.

Clinical Uses. Penicillamine is used for copper-associated hepatopathy and for long-term oral treatment of lead poisoning and cystine urolithiasis.

Dosage Forms

1. Depen Titratabs, tablets (human label)
2. Cuprimine capsules (human label)

Adverse Side Effects. These include nausea and vomiting. Other rare side effects include fever, lymphadenopathy, skin hypersensitivity reactions, or immune-complex glomerulonephropathy.

Technician's Notes

Absorption of penicillamine may be reduced by concurrent administration of food, antacids, or iron salts.

Sodium Thiosulfate

Sodium thiosulfate uses the enzyme rhodanese to convert cyanide to a non-toxic thiocyanate ion that is excreted in the urine.

Clinical Uses. Sodium thiosulfate is used in the treatment of cyanide poisoning in horses and ruminants. It may be used in combination with sodium molybdate for the treatment of copper poisoning in ruminants. It has also been used for treatment of arsenic poisoning. When applied topically, sodium thiosulfate has antifungal properties.

Dosage Forms

1. Cya-dote Injection
2. Sodium Thiosulfate for Injection 25% (human label)

Adverse Side Effects. These are uncommon.

Technician's Notes

When administering sodium thiosulfate intravenously, it should be given slowly.

Ethanol

Ethanol is an alcohol that is a competitive inhibitor of ethylene glycol metabolism. It may also be referred to as pure grain alcohol, grain alcohol, or ethyl alcohol.

Clinical Uses. Ethanol is used to treat ethylene glycol (antifreeze) poisoning.

Dosage Form

1. Ethanol

Adverse Side Effects. Ethanol reduces body temperature and can be fatal if overdosed.

Technician's Notes

1. A 20% to 50% solution of pure ethanol is administered intravenously until the animal is comatose and does not respond to a toe pinch. Administration is repeated as needed to maintain a comatose state for 3 days.
2. Sodium bicarbonate is usually administered to control metabolic acidosis.

Fomepizole

Fomepizole is competitive inhibitor of alcohol dehydrogenase. Its action prevents the conversion of ethylene glycol into glycoaldehyde and other toxic metabolites. This allows ethylene glycol to be excreted primarily unchanged. It may also be referred to as 4-methylpyrazole (4-MP).

Clinical Uses. Fomepizole is used to treat ethylene glycol (antifreeze) poisoning in dogs.

Adverse Side Effects. Clinical signs of possible anaphylaxis include tachypnea, gagging, excessive salivation, and trembling.

Dosage Form

1. Antizol-Vet

Technician's Notes

1. Fomepizole must be diluted with 0.9% NaCl before intravenous injection.
2. Dogs treated within 8 hours of ingestion have a better prognosis (Plumb, 1999).

REVERSAL AGENTS

Atipamezole HCl

Atipamezole acts as a reversal agent for alpha$_2$-adrenergic agonists by competitively inhibiting alpha$_2$-adrenergic receptors.

Clinical Uses. Atipamezole HCl is used for the reversal of medetomidine (Domitor). It has also been used in the treatment of amitraz toxicity.

Dosage Form

1. Antisedan

Adverse Side Effects. These include vomiting, diarrhea, hypersalivation, tremors, and apprehension.

Technician's Notes

1. Pain perception returns after administration of atipamezole.

Flumazenil

Flumazenil acts as a benzodiazepine antagonist by acting as a competitive blocker of benzodiazepines at benzodiazepine receptors.

Clinical Uses. Flumazenil is used for the reversal of benzodiazepines.

Dosage Form

1. Romazicon (human label)

Adverse Side Effects. Seizures may occur.

Naloxone HCl

Naloxone is a narcotic antagonist. It is structurally related to oxymorphone and may be referred to as *N*-allylnoroxymorphone HCl.

Clinical Uses. Naloxone is used for the treatment, prevention, or control of narcotic depression.

Dosage Forms

1. P/M Naloxone HCl injection
2. Narcan (human label)

Adverse Side Effects. These are uncommon.

Technician's Notes

1. Intravenous injection provides the quickest response.
2. A repeat dose may be necessary if the action of the narcotic outlasts the action of naloxone.
3. Naloxone also reverses the effects of butorphanol (Torbugesic), pentazocine (Talwin-V), and nalbuphine (Nubain).

Tolazoline HCl

Tolazoline is a competitive alpha$_1$ and alpha$_2$-adrenergic receptor blocking agent that reverses the effects of alpha$_2$-adrenergic agonists.

Clinical Uses. Tolazoline HCl is used in horses for the reversal of xylazine (Rompun).

Dosage Form

1. Tolazine

Adverse Side Effects. These include transient tachycardia, peripheral vasodilation, licking lips, piloerection, clear lacrimal and nasal discharge, muscle fasciculations, and apprehension.

> **Technician's Notes**
>
> 1. Tolazoline is not approved for use in food-producing animals.
> 2. Tolazoline has a short duration and may require repeated doses.

Yohimbine HCl

Yohimbine is an alpha$_2$-adrenergic receptor antagonist that reverses the effects of alpha$_2$-adrenergic agonists.

Clinical Uses. Yohimbine is used to reverse the effects of xylazine (Rompun). This action usually occurs within 1 to 3 minutes. It is approved for use in dogs and deer but is also effective in other species.

Dosage Forms

1. Yobine
2. Antagonil (approved for deer)

> **Technician's Notes**
>
> 1. Normal pain perception remains after administration of yohimbine.
> 2. Caution should be exercised when using in epileptic or seizure-prone patients.
> 3. Yohimbine should not be used in food-producing animals.
> 4. Safety in pregnant or breeding animals is unknown.

LUBRICANTS

Lubricants are used to lubricate hands, arms, or instruments before gynecologic and rectal examinations.

Dosage Forms

1. K-Y Jelly
2. Lube Jelly
3. Lubiseptol (may cause local irritation if excess is not rinsed off patient)
4. Lubri-Nert
5. Lubrivet

Adverse Side Effects. Adverse side effects are uncommon.

> **Technician's Notes**
>
> Petroleum jelly (Vaseline) is not recommended for use as a lubricant because it is not water-soluble and is not easily rinsed from instruments.

REFERENCES

Altman, R.D., Dean, D.D., Muniz, O.E., et al.: Therapeutic Treatment of Canine Osteoarthritis with Glycosaminoglycan Polysulfuric Acid Ester. Arthritis Rheum. 32:10, 1989.

Boothe, D.M.: Nutraceuticals in Veterinary Medicine. Part I. Definitions and Regulations. Compend. Contin. Educ. Prac. Vet. 19(11):1248-1255, 1997.

Fascetti, A.J.: Nutraceuticals and Food Faddism. [World Wide Web document, 1998] http://www.avma.org/noah/default.asp

Plumb, D.C.: Veterinary Drug Handbook, 3rd ed. Iowa State University Press, Ames, 1999.

■ Review Questions

1. A 2-year-old beagle is presented with clinical signs of lead toxicity and a history to support the diagnosis. Which agent would be the drug of choice for treating this condition?
   a. Yohimbine HCl
   b. 2-PAM
   c. Calcium EDTA
   d. Methylene blue

2. A client calls and says that she has been giving her cat Tylenol for a limp, and now the cat is breathing fast, its face is swollen, and it is not active. You should tell the client to:
   a. Give the cat hydrogen peroxide orally
   b. See whether she can get the cat to eat
   c. Bring the cat to the hospital to start treatment with hydrogen peroxide
   d. Bring the cat to the hospital to start treatment with acetylcysteine

3. Yohimbine HCl is a reversal agent for:
   a. Rompun
   b. Acepromazine
   c. Pentothal
   d. Oxymorphone

4. Penicillamine should be administered
   a. With food
   b. On an empty stomach
   c. With antacids
   d. With copper

5. Name four drugs that naloxone effectively reverses.

   _____
   _____
   _____
   _____

6. BAL has been administered to a 4-year-old mixed-breed dog for arsenic poisoning. Results of which of the following laboratory tests should be monitored closely?
   a. Packed cell volume (PCV)
   b. Blood urea nitrogen (BUN)
   c. White blood cell count (WBC)
   d. Alanine aminotransferase (ALT)

Common Abbreviations Used in Veterinary Medicine

AD	right ear
ad lib.	freely, as wanted (ad libitum)
A.L.	left ear (auris laeva)
A.M.	morning
AMA	against medical advice
ASAP	as soon as possible
A.U.	each ear (aures unitas)
b.i.d.	twice daily (bis in die)
bol.	large pill, bolus
Bute	phenylbutazone
c̄	with (cum)
caps	capsule
cc	cubic centimeters
cwt.	hundredweight
DDx	differential diagnosis
DES	diethylstilbestrol
DMSO	dimethyl sulfoxide
DS	dose or days not acceptable
D/S or D-S	dextrose in saline
D_5W or D5W	5% dextrose with water
Dx	diagnosis
e.o.d.	every other day
g or gm	gram
gal	gallon
GI	gastrointestinal
gtt.	drops (guttae)
GU	genitourinary
h or hr	hour
IM	intramuscular

IP	intraperitoneal	q4h	every 4 hours (quaque quarta hora)
IV	intravenous		
IVP	intravenous pyelogram	q.d.	every day (quaque die)
K	potassium	q.h. or o.h.	every hour (quaque hora)
l or lt	left	q.i.d.	four times a day (quater in die)
l or L	liter	q.o.d.	every other day
LA	long acting	R or rt	right
lb	pound	Rx	take thou of (prescription)
LRS	lactated Ringer's solution	s̄	without (sine)
mcg or μg	microgram	SC or SQ	subcutaneous
mEq	milliequivalent	s.i.d.	once a day (semel in die)
mg	milligram	sig.	directions, instructions
mm	millimeters	SOB	shortness of breath
Na	sodium	SR	sustained release
non repetat.	do not repeat (non repetatur)	stat.	immediately (statim)
NPO	nothing by mouth (nil per os)	Sx	surgery
O	pint	T, Tbs, Tbsp	tablespoon
O.D.	right eye (oculus dexter)	t, tsp	teaspoon
O.S.	left eye (oculus sinister)	Tab	tablet
O.U.	both eyes (oculi unitas)	t.i.d.	three times a day (ter in die)
oz	ounce	TLC	tender loving care
p.c.	after meals (post cibum)	TR	trace
per os or PO	by mouth, orally	Tx	treatment
Phos	phosphorus	U	unit
p.r.n.	as needed (pro re nata)	UG	urogenital
PTA	prior to administration	μl	microliter
pwd	powder	ung.	ointment
q2h	every 2 hours (quaque secunda hora)	Ut dict.	as directed (ut dictum)
		V-D	vomiting/diarrhea
		×	times, multiply

Weights and Measures

TABLE OF LIQUID MEASURES

  1 cup = 8 ounces
  2 cups = 1 pint   = 16 ounces
  2 pints = 1 quart = 32 ounces
4 quarts = 1 gallon = 128 ounces

Metric	Approximate Apothecary Equivalent
1000 milliliters (ml or cc)	= 1 quart
500 ml	= 1 pint
30 ml	= 1 ounce = 8 drams

WEIGHT EQUIVALENTS

Metric	Approximate Apothecary Equivalent
30 grams	= 1 ounce
4 grams	= 60 grains
1 gram	= 15 grains
60 milligrams	= 1 grain

TABLE OF AVOIRDUPOIS WEIGHT

   16 drams = 1 ounce
   16 ounces = 1 pound
  100 pounds = 1 hundredweight (cwt.)
2000 pounds = 1 ton
2240 pounds = 1 long ton

TABLE OF APOTHECARIES' WEIGHT

20 grains = 1 scruple
3 scruples = 1 dram
8 drams = 1 ounce
12 ounces = 1 pound

TABLE OF TEMPERATURE EQUIVALENTS

$F = (C \times \%) + 32$
$C = (F - 32) \times \%$

Fahrenheit	Celsius
98.6	37.0
99.0	37.2
100.0	37.7
101.0	38.3
102.0	38.8
103.0	39.4
104.0	40.0
105.0	40.5
106.0	41.1

TABLE OF WEIGHT EQUIVALENTS

kilogram (kg) = pound ÷ 2.2
pound (lb)　 = kilogram × 2.2

pound	kilogram
5	2.27
10	4.5
15	6.8
20	9.0
25	11.4
30	13.6
35	15.9
40	18.2
45	20.5
50	22.7
55	25.0
60	27.3
65	29.5
70	31.8
75	34.1
80	36.4
85	38.6
90	40.9
95	43.2
100	45.5

Emergency Drugs

DRUG NAME	DOSE
Apomorphine	40 µg/kg
Atropine (0.5 mg/ml)	0.02 mg/lb IV
	0.1 mg/lb intratracheal diluted in 3 to 10 ml of sterile saline or water; repeated at 5-minute intervals
Dexamethasone	1.8-2.7 mg/lb
Epinephrine (1:1000)	0.1 mg/lb IV
	0.2 mg/lb intratracheal diluted in 3 to 10 ml of sterile saline or water; repeated at 5- to 10-minute intervals
Lidocaine 2% (20 mg/ml)	Dog, 2 to 4 mg/kg IV
	Cat, 0.5 mg/kg IV
	8 mg/kg intratracheal diluted in 3 to 10 ml of sterile saline or water
Mannitol 20% (200 mg/ml)	130 mg/lb IV; give over a 10-minute period
Solu-Delta-Cortef 100 (use 500-mg bottle for dogs over 40 lb)	2.5 to 5 mg/lb IV; may be repeated at 1-, 3-, 6-, or 10-hour intervals as needed
Sodium bicarbonate (1 mEq/ml)	0.25 mEq/lb IV; give slowly

Controlled Substances Information Summary

The Comprehensive Drug Abuse Prevention and Control Act was passed by Congress in 1970 and became effective in May 1971. This law placed narcotics and other drugs with potential for abuse into schedules and called for the registration of professionals who administer or prescribe these drugs in their practices. In 1973, the Drug Enforcement Administration (DEA) was established through the merger of the Bureau of Narcotics and Dangerous Drugs with other agencies. The DEA was established to control the abuse of dangerous drugs through prevention and enforcement.

The drugs that are under the control of the controlled substances act are placed into five schedules, or classes, according to their potential for abuse. The schedule is designated by a C with a Roman numeral (I, II, III, IV, or V) inside the C.

Schedule I substances have no (or controversial) accepted medical use and a high potential for abuse. LSD, heroin, crack cocaine, marijuana, and peyote are substances in this class.

Schedule II drugs have accepted medical uses but have a high potential for abuse. A partial list of schedule II drugs includes morphine, meperidine, codeine, cocaine, oxymorphone, amphetamines, and pentobarbital.

Schedule III substances have less potential for abuse than those in schedule II and include Hycodan, paregoric, barbiturates such as thiamylal or thiopental, and anabolic steroids.

Schedule IV drugs have lower abuse potential than those in schedule III. Included in this class are phenobarbital, diazepam, and pentazocine.

Schedule V drugs are the lowest on the scale of abuse potential and include mostly antidiarrheal and anticough medications. Lomotil and Robitussin with codeine are in this schedule.

Any veterinarian who administers, dispenses, or prescribes a controlled substance must be registered with the DEA. A registry number issued to the veterinarian is used when ordering controlled substances. Schedule II drugs also require a special order form (DEA form 222). Registry must be renewed every 3 years. Registration may be suspended or revoked for noncompliance with the Comprehensive Drug Abuse and Control Act.

An inventory of all controlled substances on hand must be taken on the date that the registered veterinarian first begins the practice and every 2 years thereafter. The inventory should include the following:

1. The name, address, and DEA registration number
2. The date and time the inventory is taken
3. The inventory information
4. The signature of the person taking the inventory

The inventory records of schedule II drugs must be kept separate from all other records in the practice. Schedule III, IV, and V drug records must be kept separate or must be readily retrievable. All inventory records must be kept 2 years.

Controlled substances should be kept in a locked, substantially constructed cabinet.

More detailed information about the Comprehensive Drug Abuse and Control Act may be found in *Veterinary Pharmaceuticals and Biologics* (Veterinary Medicine Publishing Company) or in the *Veterinary Drug Handbook* (Pharma Vet Publishing).

Conversion of Body Weight in Kilograms to Body Surface Area in Meters for Dogs

kg	m²	kg	m²	kg	m²	kg	m²
0.5	0.06	13.0	0.55	26.0	0.88	39.0	1.15
1.0	0.10	14.0	0.58	27.0	0.90	40.0	1.17
2.0	0.15	15.0	0.60	28.0	0.92	41.0	1.19
3.0	0.20	16.0	0.63	29.0	0.94	42.0	1.21
4.0	0.25	17.0	0.66	30.0	0.96	43.0	1.23
5.0	0.29	18.0	0.69	31.0	0.99	44.0	1.25
6.0	0.33	19.0	0.71	32.0	1.01	45.0	1.26
7.0	0.36	20.0	0.74	33.0	1.03	46.0	1.28
8.0	0.40	21.0	0.76	34.0	1.05	47.0	1.30
9.0	0.43	22.0	0.78	35.0	1.07	48.0	1.32
10.0	0.46	23.0	0.81	36.0	1.09	49.0	1.34
11.0	0.49	24.0	0.83	37.0	1.11	50.0	1.36
12.0	0.52	25.0	0.85	38.0	1.13		

The conversion table is based on the following formula: $\dfrac{kg^{0.67}}{10} = m^2$

From Ettinger, S.J.: Textbook of Veterinary Internal Medicine, Vol 1. Philadelphia, W.B. Saunders Company, 1975.

Bibliography

Allen, T.A.: Managing complications of renal failure: A pharmacological update. In Managing Renal Disease and Hypertension. Harmon Smith, 1991.

Bell, F.W., Osborne, C.A.: Maintenance fluid therapy. In Kirk, R.W. (ed.): Current Veterinary Therapy X: Small Animal Practice. W.B. Saunders Company, Philadelphia, 1989.

Bennett, K. (ed.): Compendium of Veterinary Products. North American Compendiums, Port Huron, MI, 1991.

Bonagura, J.D. (ed.): Current Veterinary Therapy XII: Small Animal Practice, W.B. Saunders Company, Philadelphia, 1995.

Boon, G.D., Rebar, A.H., Stickle, J.: Veterinary Values, 3rd ed. AgResources, New York, 1987.

Booth, N.H., McDonald, L.E.: Veterinary Pharmacology and Therapeutics. Iowa State University Press, Ames, 1982.

Boothe, D.M.: Nutraceuticals in veterinary medicine. Part I. Definitions and regulations. Compend. Contin. Educ. Prac. Vet. 19(11):1248-1255, 1997.

Bourne, H.R., Roberts, J.M.: Drug receptors and pharmacodynamics. In Katzung, B.G. (ed.): Basic and Clinical Pharmacology. Lange Medical Publications, Norwalk, CT, 1987.

Bradley, T.: Guide to fluid therapy for veterinary technicians. In Nursing Care in Veterinary Practice. Veterinary Learning Systems, Trenton, NJ, 1993.

Brennan, J.J., Aherne, F.X., Nakano, T.: Effects of glycosaminoglycan polysulfate treatment on soundness, hyaluronic acid content of synovial fluid and proteoglycan aggregate in articular cartilage of lame boars. Can. J. Vet. Res. 51:394-398, 1987.

Calvert, C.A.: Heartworm disease: New concepts in diagnosis and treatment. Veterinary Product News, May/June 30, 1993.

Carter, G.R., Chengappa, M.M.: Essentials of Veterinary Bacteriology and Mycology, 4th ed. Lea & Febiger, Philadelphia, 1991.

Chadwell, John: Ciba unveils new weapon in the flea control wars. Veterinary Product News, February, 1995.

Curren, A.M., Munday, L.D.: Math for Meds, 6th ed. Wallcur, San Diego, 1990.

Deglin, J.H., Mull, V.L.: Calculating drug dosages. In Dosage Calculations Manual. Springhouse Publishing Company, Springhouse, PA, 1988.

Densford, L.E.: Study underscores Adequan's effectiveness in treating degenerative joint disease. Veterinary Product News, January, 1991.

DiBartola, S.P.: Introduction to fluid therapy. In DiBartola, S.P. (ed.): Fluid Therapy in Small Animal Practice. W.B. Saunders Company, Philadelphia, 1992.

Dorland's Pocket Medical Dictionary, 23rd ed. W.B. Saunders Company, Philadelphia, 1982.

Ellefson, D.: Large Animal Veterinarian: Autogenous Vaccines. Watt Publishing Company, Mt. Morris, IL, 1993.

Ettinger, S.J.: Pocket Companion to Textbook of Veterinary Internal Medicine. W.B. Saunders Company, Philadelphia, 1993.

Fascetti, A.J.: Nutraceuticals and Food Faddism [World Wide Web document]. URL: http://www.avma.org/noah/default.asp

Ford, R.B.: Vaccines and vaccinations: Issues for the 21st century. Suppl. Compend. Contin. Educ. Prac. Vet. 20(8C): 19-24, 1998.

Frandson, R.D.: Anatomy and Physiology of Farm Animals, 5th ed. Lea & Febiger, Philadelphia, 1992.

Frye, F.L.: Reptile Care, Vol. I. T.F.H. Publications, Neptune City, NJ, 1991.

Gelatt, K.N.: Textbook of Veterinary Ophthalmology. Lea & Febiger, Philadelphia, 1981.

Gilson, S.D., Page, R.L.: Principles of oncology. In Birchard, S.J., Sherding, R.G. (eds): Saunder's Manual of Small Animal Practice. W.B. Saunders Company, Philadelphia, 1994.

Giovanoni, R., Warren, R.G.: Principles of Pharmacology. Mosby, St. Louis, 1983.

Grundy, H.F.: Pharmacokinetics. In Yoxall, A.T., Hird, J.F. (eds.): Pharmacological Basis of Small Animal Medicine. Blackwell Scientific Publications, Oxford, 1979.

Henke, G.: MedMath, 6th ed. J.B. Lippincott Company, Philadelphia, 1991.

Hodgson, B.B., Kizior, R.J.: Saunders Nursing Drug Handbook. W.B. Saunders Company, Philadelphia, 1999.

Hustead, D.: Large Animal Veterinarian: Vaccines: What's Ahead? Watt Publishing Company, Mt. Morris, IL, March/April 1990.

Hustead, D.E., et. al.: Vaccination Issues of Concern to Practitioners [World Wide Web document]. URL: http//:www.avma.org/noah/members/scientific/vaccination/vacissues.htm

Jenkins, W.L.: Pharmacological principles in therapeutics. In Ettinger, S.J. (ed.): Textbook of Veterinary Internal Medicine: Diseases of the Dog and Cat. W.B. Saunders Company, Philadelphia, 1983.

Katzung, B.G.: Basic and Clinical Pharmacology, 3rd ed. Appleton & Lange, Norwalk, CT, 1987.

Kirk, R.W. (ed.): Current Veterinary Therapy VII: Small Animal Practice, W.B. Saunders Company, Philadelphia, 1980.

Kirk, R.W. (ed.): Current Veterinary Therapy X: Small Animal Practice. W.B. Saunders Company, Philadelphia, 1989.

Kirk, R.W.: Current Veterniary Therapy XII: Small Animal Practice. W.B. Saunders Company, Philadelphia, 1998.

Kirk, R.W., Bonagura, J.D. (eds.): Current Veterinary Therapy XI: Small Animal Practice. W.B. Saunders Company, Philadelphia, 1992.

Kohn, C.W., DiBartola, S.P.: Composition and distribution of body fluids in dogs and cats. In DiBartola, S.P. (ed.): Fluid Therapy in Small Animal Practice. W.B. Saunders Company, Philadelphia, 1992.

Legendre, A.M.: Itraconazole: A New Antifungal Drug. 6th ACUIM Forum. Washington, D.C., 1993.

Lobe, S. (Executive Director, Editorial): Peripheral IV therapy. In Medication Administration & IV Therapy Manual, 2nd ed. Springhouse Corporation, Springhouse, PA, 1990.

McCurnin, D.M.: Clinical Textbook for Veterinary Technicians, 4th ed. W.B. Saunders Company, Philadelphia, 1998.

McIlwraith, C.W.: Seminar notes from the California and Nevada Veterinary Medical Associations' Joint Scientific Seminar & Exposition. Reno, NV, October 1991.

Meleo, K.A.: Veterinary Forum: Immunotherapy. Forum Publications, Fairway, KS, 1994.

Muir, W.W., DiBartola, S.P.: Fluid Therapy. In Kirk, R.W. (ed.): Current Veterinary Therapy VIII: Small Animal Practice. W.B. Saunders Company, Philadelphia, 1983.

Muller, G.H., Kirk, R.W., Scott, D.W.: Small Animal Dermatology, 4thed. W.B. Saunders Company, Philadelphia, 1989.

Olgesbee, B., Bishop, C.: Avian infectious diseases. In Birchard, S., Sherding, R. (eds.): Saunders Manual of Small Animal Practice. W.B. Saunders Company, Philadelphia, 1994.

Plumb, D.C.: Hormonal, endocrine, and reproductive drugs. In Plumb, D.C. (ed.): Veterinary Drug Handbook. Pharma Vet Publishing Company, White Bear Lake, MN, 1991.

Plumb, D.C.: Veterinary Drug Handbook, 3rd ed. Iowa State University Press, Ames, 1999.

Reece, W.O.: Physiology of Domestic Animals. Lea & Febiger, Philadelphia, 1991.

Rice, J.: Principles of Pharmacology for Medical Assisting, 3rd ed. Delmar Publishers, Albany, NY, 1999.

Roberson, E.L.: What internal parasiticides make sense for your practice? Pet Vet. 3(1):18-28, 1991.

Roche, J.E.: Growth promoters. In Roche, J.P. (ed.): Veterinary Applied Pharmacology and Therapeutics, 5th ed. Bailliere Tindall, London, 1991.

Schmall, L.M.: Fluid and electrolyte therapy. In Robinson, N.E. (ed.): Current Therapy in Equine Medicine. W.B. Saunders Company, Philadelphia, 1992.

Swaim, S.F., Gillette, R.L.: An update on wound medications and dressings. Compend. Contin. Educ. Prac. Vet. 20(10): 1133-1145, 1998.

The path to approval: How research discoveries become federally licensed products. Top. Vet. Med. 4:10-15, 1993.

VanKampen, K.R.: Recombinant technology. Suppl. Compend. Contin. Educ. Prac. Vet. 20(8):28-32, 1998.

Wilson, J.F.: A Practitioners Guide to the Thorough Irrigation of Ears.

Wingfield, W.E., VanPelt, D.R., Quirk, P.E.: Fluid Therapy Symposium, Proceedings of the Eastern States Veterinary Conference. Orlando, FL, January 1990.

Zajac, A.M.: Giardiasis. Comp. Cont. Educ. Pract. Vet. 14(5):604-608, 1992.

Answers

Answers to Chapter 1

1. a. An agonist is a drug that has affinity for a receptor and stimulates the receptor to action.

   b. A contraindication is a reason not to use a drug in a particular situation.

   c. Efficacy is the degree to which a drug produces its desired effects in a patient.

   d. An over-the-counter drug is one that may be purchased and used without a prescription from a veterinarian.

   e. A prescription drug is one that must be used under the supervision of a veterinarian.

   f. A receptor is a group of specialized molecules on or in a cell that binds with a drug to cause an effect.

   g. The therapeutic index expresses the relationship between a drug's therapeutic and harmful effects.

   h. The withdrawal time is the amount of time that must elapse between the end of drug therapy and the elimination of that drug from the patient's tissues or products.

   i. The veterinarian-client-patient relationship is the relationship that must exist between the veterinarian, his or her patient, and the patient's owner before prescription drugs may be dispensed.

2. Four sources for veterinary drugs are animal products, plant materials, minerals, and synthetic products.

3. A drug regimen includes the dose, the route of administration, the frequency of administration, and the duration of administration.

4. For a valid veterinarian-client-patient relationship to exist, (1) the veterinarian must assume responsibility for making clinical judgments in relation to the health of the animal, (2) the veterinarian must have recently seen the animal and be acquainted with its care, and (3) the veterinarian must be available for follow-up care of the animal.

5. It is a technician's responsibility to carry out the veterinarian's orders correctly. The technician should read the drug label three times to ensure that the proper drug is being administered and should take care to administer the correct dose by the correct route. The technician should also be aware of the expected effects and potential adverse side effects in order to be able to monitor the patient in a responsible way. In

■ **Answers to Chapter 1—cont'd**

the large animal practice, the technician should be aware of withdrawal times and potential residue problems.

6. A drug is first absorbed (or directly placed) into the bloodstream. In the blood, the drug may bind with a plasma protein or exist in the free state. The circulating blood distributes the drug to the capillary level, where the drug leaves the circulation and enters the interstitial fluid. The interstitial fluid bathes the cell and allows the drug to enter the cell or bind with surface receptors. The drug then exits the cell (or its surface), moves back into the interstitial fluid, re-enters the circulation, and is then transported to the liver for metabolism. After it is metabolized, the metabolite is transported to the kidneys for excretion.

7. (1) The oral route provides a simple route of administration. Many factors may influence the rate of absorption, and the oral route may not be appropriate if the animal is vomiting.
(2) Subcutaneous administration of drugs is usually a simple procedure. Absorption from subcutaneous sites may be slow, and hypertonic solutions should not be given by this route.
(3) The intramuscular route produces faster absorption than the subcutaneous route, but care must be taken with many drugs not to inject them into blood vessels.

(4) The intravenous route allows immediate access to the bloodstream and the dilution of irritating drugs. A toxic or allergic reaction can be a side effect.
(5) The intraperitoneal route may be used to administer fluids and some other solutions when other routes are not available. Absorption from the peritoneal cavity is slow, however.
(6) The intra-arterial route is a seldom-used route that may produce seizures or death.
(7) The intracardiac route is used primarily for administering emergency drugs or for euthanasia.
(8) The intramedullary route may be used to administer fluids or blood to small animals or those with damaged veins.
(9) The inhalation route is used to administer drugs to the respiratory system. Special equipment may be required.
(10) The topical route may be used to place drugs on skin or mucous membranes and may be facilitated by using carrier substances in some instances.
(11) The intradermal route is used primarily for allergy testing and for diagnosing tuberculosis.

8. The absorption of a drug may be influenced by (1) the method of absorption, (2) the pH of the drug and its ionization status, (3) the absorptive surface area, (4) the blood supply to the area, (5) the solubility of the drug, (6) the dosage form, (7) the sta-

tus of the gastrointestinal tract, and (8) interactions with other drugs.
9. b. Liver
10. a. Kidneys
11. Receptors
12. Proprietary/trade
13. The six items that must be on a drug label are the drug names (generic and trade), the drug concentration and quantity, the name and address of the manufacturer, the controlled substance status, the manufacturer's control or lot number, and the drug's expiration date.
14. The government agencies that regulate the development, approval, and use of animal health products include the FDA, EPA, and USDA.
15. Many veterinary clinics dispense rather than prescribe drugs because of the profit earned from selling the products.
16. Veterinary pharmaceuticals may be purchased directly from the manufacturer, from distributors, or from generic mail-order companies. In some instances, drugs may be sold under one label to graduate veterinarians and under another as an over-the-counter product.
17. The Green Book
18. FARAD provides resources concerning the avoidance of drug residues in animals.
19. AMDUCA (Animal Medicinal Drug Use Clarification Act)
20. Compounding refers to the diluting or combining of existing drugs.

■ Answers to Chapter 2

1. Tablets are the most common dosage form of oral medications.

2. The technician should document the time at which the medicine was given, what drug was given, how the medicine was administered, who gave the medicine, and any observations about the patient's progress.

3. The date, owner's name, patient's name, drug name, amount administered or dispensed, technician's name, and veterinarian's name should be written in the controlled substance inventory log.

4. Right patient, right drug, right dose, right route, and right time and frequency.

5. An insulin syringe is divided into units and does not contain a dead space. A tuberculin syringe is divided into tenths of 1 ml and has a dead space.

6. Some drugs are unstable in solution and require reconstitution with sterile water or other diluent before they can be administered.

7. The technician may educate clients about how a medicine should be administered, why it has been prescribed, and what adverse reactions may occur.

8. The eyes produce a constant flow of tears and rapidly remove any foreign substances, including medications.

9. Clipping the hair makes it easier to apply medication to the skin and allows better absorption.

Answers to Chapter 3

PROBLEMS USING RATIOS AND PROPORTIONS

Ratios

1. 1:4; 0.25
2. 75:100; $\frac{75}{100}$
3. 4:1000; $\frac{4}{1000}$
4. $\frac{1}{80}$; 0.0125
5. 9:1000; 0.009
6. $\frac{1}{32}$; 0.031

Proportions

1. 50
2. 8
3. 2.5
4. 5
5. 200 mg
6. 37.5 mg
7. 31.25 ml
8. 118.25 ml
9. 5 ml
10. 1.25 tablets

PROBLEMS USING THE METRIC SYSTEM

1. 0.15 g
2. 2000 ml
3. 2.25 g
4. 5000 mg
5. 3 L
6. 2000 g
7. 500 g
8. 0.005 kg
9. 0.00125 g
10. 4 mg
11. 2.05 mg
12. 0.01 g
13. 500 ml
14. 0.75 L
15. 0.3 mg
16. 2500 μg

PROBLEMS USING THE APOTHECARY AND HOUSEHOLD SYSTEMS

1. 3 pt
2. 1.5 gal
3. 1 Tbsp
4. 12 cups
5. 6 pints
6. 4 Tbsp
7. 128 oz
8. 16 oz
9. 3 qt

PROBLEMS COMBINING BOTH SYSTEMS

1. 480 ml
2. 30 ml
3. 15 ml
4. 16 oz
5. 0.013 pt
6. 25 tsp
7. 45 ml
8. 33 lb
9. 0.52 pt
10. 150 ml
11. 15.9 kg

PROBLEMS MEASURING ORAL MEDICATIONS

1. 2 tablets
2. 1.5 tablets
3. 4 tablets
4. 2.5 tablets
5. 1.5 tablets; 7.5 tablets
6. 20 tablets
7. 200 mg; 100 mg; 50 mg/ml; 4 ml; 2 ml; 44 ml
8. 2.5 tablets; 25 tablets
9. 0.25 tablet; 5.25 tablets
10. ½ tablet (0.5); 4.5 tablets
11. 6.8 kg; 68 mg; 0.75 tablet; 31.5 tablets
12. 120 ml mebendazole; 5 oz Combot
13. 100 oz or 3.125 qt (containing 3 oz powder per quart of water)
14. 0.5 tablet; 7 tablets
15. 66.67 mg; 17.7 ml

Answers to Chapter 3—cont'd

PROBLEMS MEASURING PARENTERAL MEDICATIONS

1. 0.4 ml
2. 3.7 ml
3. 17 ml
4. 1.5 ml
5. 525 mg; 1.75 ml

6. 2 ml
7. 15 mg
8. 0.74 m^2; 0.37 mg; 0.37 ml
9. 2500 mg; 25 ml; 2.5 bottles
10. 54 mg; 0.54 ml

11. 3.5 ml
12. 0.1 ml
13. 47.5 mg; 1.9 ml
14. 30 ml
15. 1.5 ml

INJECTION PROBLEMS

1. 2 ml
2. 5 ml
3. 1.5 ml
4. 3.75 ml

5. 0.25 ml
6. 2 ml
7. 0.75 ml

8. 7.5 ml
9. 0.6 ml
10. 0.22 ml

PREPARING SOLUTIONS

1. $V1 \times C1 = V2 \times C2$
   $V1 \times 100 = 100 \times 10$
   $V1 \times 100 = 1000$
   $V1 = 10$
   10 ml 37% formaldehyde +
   　　　　　　90 ml water

2. $V1 \times C1 = V2 \times C2$
   $V1 \times 50 = 1000 \times 5$
   $V1 \times 50 = 5000$
   $V1 = 100$
   100 ml $D_{50}W$ +
   　　　　900 ml 0.9% NaCl

3. $V1 \times C1 = V2 \times C2$
   $V1 \times 50 = 100 \times 5$
   $V1 \times 50 = 500$
   $V1 = 10$
   10 ml $D_{50}W$ + 90 ml water

4. $V1 \times C1 = V2 \times C2$
   $V1 \times 0.9 = 500 \times 0.45$
   $V1 \times 0.9 = 225$
   $V1 = 250$
   250 ml 0.9% NaCl +
   　　　　250 ml D_5W

5. $V1 \times C1 = V2 \times C2$
   $V1 \times 50 = 2000 \times 2.5$
   $V1 \times 50 = 5000$
   $V1 = 100$
   100 ml $D_{50}W$ + 1900 ml
   　　　lactated Ringer's solution

6. $V1 \times C1 = V2 \times C2$
   $V1 \times 50 = 50 \times 5$
   $V1 \times 50 = 250$
   $V1 = 5$
   5 ml $D_{50}W$ + 45 ml water

7. $V1 \times C1 = V2 \times C2$
   $V1 \times 50 = 500 \times 2.5$
   $V1 \times 50 = 1250$
   $V1 = 25$
   25 ml $D_{50}W$ + 475 ml
   　　　　　　0.45% NaCl

8. Remember: 10% solution =
   100 mg/ml packets containing
   50 gm = 50,000 mg
   　　$V1 \times C1 = V2 \times C2$
   $V1 \times 50,000 = 1000 \times 100$
   $V1 \times 50,000 = 100,000$
   　　　　$V1 = 2$
   2 packets of 50 g GG powder +
   　　　　　　1000 ml water

9. Remember:
   8% solution = 80 mg/ml
   One 5 g vial contains 5000 mg
   　　$V1 \times C1 = V2 \times C2$
   $1 \times 5000 = V2 \times 80$
   　$5000 = V2 \times 80$
   　　$62.5 = V2$
   62.5 ml needs to be added to
   one 50 g vial to prepare an 8%
   solution

■   **Answers to Chapter 3—cont'd**

10. Remember:
    2% solution = 20 mg/ml
    $V1 \times C1 = V2 \times C2$
    $V1 \times 100 = 5 \times 20$
    $V1 \times 100 = 100$
    $\qquad V1 = 1$
    1 ml of Sandimmune (cyclo-
    sporine) + 4 ml virgin olive oil

11. Remember:
    37% formaldehyde = 100%
    formalin
    $V1 \times C1 = V2 \times C2$
    $V1 \times 100 = 50 \times 2$
    $V1 \times 100 = 100$
    $\qquad V1 = 1$
    1 ml 37% formaldehyde +
    $\qquad\qquad$ 49 ml water

PROBLEMS CALCULATING IV DRIP RATES

1. 42 gtt/min or approximately
   0.69 gtt/sec
2. 60 gtt/min or 1 gtt/sec
3. 30 gtt/min or 1 gtt/2 sec
4. 0.15 ml/min or 9 gtt/min
5. 0.5 ml/min or 30 gtt/min

Answers to Chapter 4

1. An agonist is a drug that combines with a receptor to bring about an action, whereas an antagonist combines with a receptor and blocks the action.
2. A neurotransmitter is a chemical substance released by a nerve ending at the synapse; it acts on the adjacent neuron to stimulate, inhibit, or change its activity.
3. b. Thalamus
4. Interrupting the generation or conduction of nerve impulses; interfering with
5. Epinephrine or norepinephrine
6. Mimicking neurotransmitters, interfering with neurotransmitter release, blocking the attachment of neurotransmitters to receptors, and interfering with the breakdown of neurotransmitters
7. To control vomiting, to treat urinary retention, to stimulate gastrointestinal activity, to treat glaucoma, and to aid in the diagnosis of myasthenia gravis
8. Cholinergic blocking agents (anticholinergic)
9. Adrenergic (sympathomimetic)
10. d. Beta blocker
11. Bradycardia and hypotension may be antagonized by using atropine; respiratory depression or excessive CNS depression may be antagonized by using yohimbine.
12. Thiobarbiturates are very soluble in fat, which acts like a sponge to take the barbiturate out of the circulation and away from the CNS. Thin animals have reduced fat levels, which means that more of the thiobarbiturate remains in the bloodstream and may cause excessive depression of the CNS.
13. Analgesia, increased muscle tone maintenance of pharyngeal/laryngeal reflexes, muscle tremors, and loss of the blink reflex
14. Respiratory depression, cardiac depression, agitation, excitement, or seizures
15. Naloxone and nalorphine
16. Because of its tendency to precipitate out of solution when stored
17. Doxapram (Dopram) may be administered on or under the tongue, into the umbilical vein, or by intramuscular injection
18. Some pentobarbital euthanasia agents have a red dye added to distinguish them from pentobarbital agents, which may be used for anesthesia. Since these agents are easily identified as euthanasia agents, they have less potential for abuse.
19. Neurotransmitter
20. Burning
21. Propofol
22. GABA
23. Diazepam
24. Clomicalm
25. Anipryl

■ Answers to Chapter 5

1. Nostrils, nasal cavity, pharynx, larynx, trachea, bronchi, and bronchioles
2. The four functions of the respiratory system are oxygen–carbon dioxide exchange, regulation of acid-base balance, body temperature regulation, and voice production.
3. Structures in the nasal passages filter, warm, and humidify inspired air. The cough, sneeze, and reverse sneeze attempt to remove foreign material that has entered the respiratory system. The mucocilliary mechanism also removes foreign material from the respiratory system. Macrophages and immunoglobulins inactivate or destroy invasive organisms.
4. The three important principles of respiratory therapeutics are control of secretions, control of reflexes, and maintenance of normal airflow.
5. Productive
6. Through the breakdown of disulfide chemical bonds
7. Acetylcysteine is administered by nebulization.
8. Through depression of the cough center in the brain
9. Schedule V
10. Release of acetylcholine, release of histamine, and blockade of beta-2–adrenergic receptors
11. Epinephrine and albuterol
12. Phosphodiesterase
13. Treatment of insect bites and treatment of heaves in horses
14. -amine
15. Treatment of respiratory depression associated with anesthesia and stimulation of respiration in newborn animals
16. 22.7 kg $\times$ 0.22 mg/kg = 4.9 mg 5-mg tablets are available. Dispense 14 tablets.

■ Answers to Chapter 6

1. The urinary system is composed of the kidneys, ureters, bladder, and urethra.

2. The urinary system regulates the body's water balance, acid-base balance, osmotic pressure, electrolyte levels, and concentration of many plasma substances. It eliminates many drugs and toxins from the body and forms urine.

3. During tubular reabsorption, needed substances are filtered from the tubules and returned to the body. Tubular secretion rids the body of unneeded substances and helps to control blood pH.

4. Renal failure may impair the drug's absorption from the administration site or affect the drug's distribution in the body.

5. Renal damage may be categorized as prerenal, renal, or postrenal. It may be differentiated as acute or chronic according to certain parameters common to each condition.

6. A diuretic removes excess extracellular fluid by increasing urine flow and sodium excretion and reduces hypertension.

7. Loop diuretics inhibit tubular reabsorption of sodium and increase the excretion of chloride, potassium, and water. Examples include Lasix and Edecrin.

    Osmotic diuretics promote diuresis by exerting high osmotic pressure in the kidney tubules and limiting tubular reabsorption. Examples include mannitol and glucose.

    Thiazide diuretics inhibit reabsorption of sodium, chloride, and water and increase potassium excretion. Examples include Diuril and Hydro-DIURIL.

    Potassium-sparing diuretics antagonize aldosterone, increase the excretion of sodium and water, and reduce the excretion of potassium. An example is Aldactone.

    Carbonic anhydrase inhibitors produce a bicarbonate diuresis and promote the excretion of sodium, potassium, and water. An example is Diamox.

8. Cholinergic agents mimic the stimulation of the parasympathetic nervous system and promote the function of acetylcholine. An example is Urecholine. Anticholinergic agents are parasympatholytic because they block the action of acetylcholine at receptor sites in the parasympathetic nervous system. Examples include Pro-Banthine and Buscopan.

9. The technician should advise the client that while feeding the diet, no acidifiers, salt, vitamin or mineral supplements, or any other food items should be given to the patient.

10. Struvite uroliths—acidifying agents; ammonium acid urate uroliths—alkalizing agents; calcium oxalate uroliths—alkalizing agents; cystine uroliths—alkalizing agents.

■ Answers to Chapter 7

1. The right atrium and right ventricle serve functionally as one pump for ejecting blood to the lungs, and the left atrium and left ventricle pump blood to the systemic circulation.

2. Syncytium (interconnected mass)

3. Sodium (Na^+), calcium (Ca^{2+}), potassium (K^+)

4. Refractory period

5. *Chronotropic* refers to the rate of contraction, whereas *inotropic* refers to the force or strength of contraction.

6. Preload is the volume of blood in the ventricles at the end of diastole (the amount of blood that must be pumped out). Afterload is the resistance in the arteries that the ventricle must overcome to pump blood.

7. Increasing the heart rate, increasing the stroke volume, increasing the efficiency of the heart muscle, and heart enlargement

8. Control rhythm disturbances, maintain or increase cardiac output, relieve fluid accumulations, increase the oxygenation of blood, and provide oxygen/sedatives

9. Beneficial effects include improved cardiac contractility, decreased heart rate, antiarrhythmic effect, and decreased signs of dyspnea. A toxic effect is vomiting.

10. Stimulation of cardiac contraction in cardiac arrest

11. Conditions that cause hypoxia; electrolyte imbalances; increased levels or sensitivity to catecholamines; certain drugs such as digitalis, barbiturates, and others; and cardiac trauma or disease

12. Class IA—quinidine; class IB—lidocaine; class IC—flecainide; class II—propranolol; class III—bretylium; class IV—diltiazem

13. Hydralazine—arteriolar dilator; nitroglycerin—venodilator; prazosin—combined; enalapril—combined

14. Lasix is called a *loop diuretic* because it inhibits reabsorption of sodium in the loops of Henle.

15. Potassium

16. Sodium restriction and control of debilitation

17. Bronchodilation, oxygen therapy, sedation, aspirin, and centesis

Answers to Chapter 8

1. Entry of food and fluid into the body, absorption of nutrients, and excretion of waste products
2. Dogs, cats, and primates
3. Ruminants have a system of forestomachs, including the reticulum, rumen, and omasum, which allows them to digest coarse plant material, as well as a true stomach (abomasum).
4. Regurgitation is a normal process of ruminants that permits them to bring up partially digested foodstuff for rechewing. Vomiting is the forcible expulsion of gastric contents and is generally considered to be pathologic.
5. Microorganisms in the rumen
6. The autonomic nervous system, hormonal control, and chemical (histamine, prostaglandin, and others) control
7. Bacterial endotoxins may increase the permeability of intestinal blood vessels, resulting in increased fluid loss. They may also induce fever and initiate shock.
8. Chemical substances (digitalis compounds, urea, ketone bodies, and others) and impulses from the inner ear
9. Centrally acting—apomorphine and xylazine; peripherally acting—syrup of ipecac and mustard
10. Antiemetics
11. Reducing the secretion of hydrochloric acid by gastric mucosal cells
12. Cimetidine and ranitidine
13. Peristalsis (a wave of contraction) and segmentation (a mixing action)
14. Withholding food for 12 to 24 hours
15. Rats and horses
16. By retaining water osmotically in the gut, these agents cause softening of the stool.
17. Psyllium
18. By mimicking the effect of acetylcholine
19. Metronidazole
20. C.E.T., Nolvadent, Oral Dent, and Oxydent

■ Answers to Chapter 9

1. Releasing factors (RFs) are messengers made by the hypothalamus in response to its detection of hormone levels in the blood. RFs send messages to the pituitary to stimulate this gland to manufacture trophic hormones. Trophic hormones, in turn, stimulate a specific tissue or gland to produce the hormone in question.

2. The major endocrine glands are the pituitary, the thyroid, the ovaries, the testicles, the adrenals, and the pancreas.

3. To correct a deficiency and to obtain a desired effect

4. In the body; external

5. The pituitary gland is located at the base of the brain ventral to the hypothalamus, and its primary function is to control the activity of the other endocrine glands.

6. A negative feedback mechanism occurs when the hypothalamus senses a high level of a specific hormone in the blood and, in response, reduces the amount of releasing factor (RF) for this hormone. A reduced amount of RF causes a decreased amount of trophic hormone to be produced by the pituitary, and this results in decreased production of the hormone by the target organ.

   A positive feedback mechanism occurs when the hypothalamus senses a low level of the hormone in question and increases its production of RF. Increased RF causes an increase in trophic hormone and a resulting increase in activity of the target organ.

7. Neurohormonal reflex

8. Gonadotropin

9. Progestins

10. Estrus synchronization, to induce abortion, and to induce estrus

11. Pregnant; asthmatics

12. Estrogen and progesterone

13. The reproductive tract has been examined for blockage or torsion.

14. Triiodothyronine (T_3) and tetraiodothyronine (T_4)

15. Soloxine and Synthroid

16. Short acting (regular/Semilente), intermediate acting (NPH/Lente), long acting (PZI/Ultralente)

17. Regular/Semilente

18. NPH/Lente

19. Weakness, ataxia, shaking, and seizures

20. Breeding purposes

21. Because of the potential for abuse by human athletes

Answers to Chapter 10

1. Topical agents are absorbed more readily into the anterior chamber than the posterior chamber. Drugs with both lipid-soluble and water-soluble properties provide maximum corneal penetration.
2. The eye continuously secretes tears that wash away foreign material, including medication.
3. Mydriatics cause dilation of the pupil. Miotics cause contraction of the pupil. Cycloplegics paralyze the ciliary muscle.
4. These drugs are contraindicated in the treatment of glaucoma and keratoconjunctivitis sicca.
5. Corticosteroids are contraindicated in the presence of a corneal ulcer or after intraocular surgery.
6. It may be necessary to clip the hair from the inside of the pinna and to cleanse the ear canal to remove excess wax and debris.
7. Aminoglycosides are contraindicated in the presence of a ruptured eardrum and should not be used with other drugs that may induce ototoxicity. Patients should be monitored for signs of ototoxicity during treatment with aminoglycosides.
8. Because of the life cycle of the ear mite, the treatment of ear mites should last at least 3 weeks.
9. Drying agents may be indicated to reduce the presence of excess moisture.
10. A common flushing solution is a mixture of warm water and chlorhexidine surgical scrub diluted 1:100.

Answers to Chapter 11

1. The skin layers have several functions, including protection, temperature regulation, storage, immunoregulation, sensory perception, secretion, and vitamin D production.
2. Antiseborrheics act as keratolytics and keratoplastics and are used in the treatment of seborrhea oleosa and seborrhea sicca.
3. Bath oils help to normalize the development of keratin and provide relief for dry skin associated with seborrhea sicca.
4. They provide temporary relief of itching and have a safe, beneficial effect.
5. Astringents precipitate proteins and cause contraction after administration. They are most commonly used to treat moist dermatitis and weeping skin wounds.
6. Common topical antiseptics include alcohol, propylene glycol, chlorhexidine, acetic acid, iodine, and benzalkonium chloride.
7. Stage I—Inflammation begins and hemorrhaging is limited; serum leaks into the wound to provide clotting elements, enzymes, proteins, antibodies, and complement. Stage II—Neutrophils and monocytes migrate to the wound to phagocytize bacteria and necrotic debris. Stage III—Granulation tissue is formed.
8. For the patient, these factors include age, nutritional status, rest, environment, and good general health. For the wound, these factors include size, location, environment, infection, inflammation, and contamination.
9. Topical corticosteroids may be used to provide relief from itching, burning, and inflammation.
10. Wound protectants are contraindicated in the presence of deep or puncture wounds.
11. 1. Rubefaction—A reddening of the skin indicating mild irritation accompanied by an increase in blood congestion in the skin.
    2. Vesication—Occurs by applying irritating substances under a bandage, resulting in severe irritation with capillary damage.
    3. Blistering—Occurs as a result of vesication.
12. Counterirritants are applied to the skin of horses to produce local irritation and inflammation and are used in the treatment of chronic inflammatory conditions of tissues below the skin surface. Caustics destroy granulation tissue (proudflesh), superficial tumors, or horn buds.

Answers to Chapter 12

1. Bacteria are commonly classified as either gram-positive, gram-negative, or acid-fast bacilli.

2. The susceptibility of an organism to an antibiotic on an agar diffusion test is determined by the zones of inhibition.

3. The minimal inhibitory concentration is the lowest concentration that macroscopically inhibits the growth of the organism.

4. Some bacteria produce beta-lactamase I (penicillinase), which reduces the effectiveness of the penicillin by converting the penicillin into inactive penicilloic acid.

5. If tetracycline is administered to a pregnant animal, permanent staining of the offspring's teeth can occur. Administered to a juvenile, tetracycline can cause permanent staining of the teeth, and the development of growing bones can be slowed.

6. Aminoglycosides can cause serious side effects such as nephrotoxicity, ototoxicity, and neuromuscular synaptic dysfunction.

7. Nephrotoxicity due to aminoglycosides may be monitored by obtaining a pretreatment serum creatinine level and then measuring the level periodically during treatment.

8. Amphotericin B is diluted in 5% dextrose and administered intravenously.

9. Disinfection time refers to the time for a particular agent to produce its maximum effect.

10. The disinfection time varies between different products and is affected by factors such as the type of material being disinfected, the amount of soil and microbial contamination, the concentration of the disinfectant, and the germicidal potency of the disinfectant.

■ Answers to Chapter 13

1. Internal and external parasites should be controlled because they affect the well-being of an animal and can cause economic loss in food-producing animals.

2. A technician's role may include client education in choosing products and showing how to use the products. Most importantly, a technician must become familiar with each product, its uses, and any possible adverse effects.

3. Today's products are more effective, cause fewer side effects, and many provide different dosage forms for easy administration.

4. Approved products for the prevention of heartworm disease in dogs include products containing ivermectin, milbemycin oxime, diethylcarbamazine citrate (DEC), moxidectin, or selamectin. Approved products for the prevention of heartworm disease in cats include products containing ivermectin or selamectin.

5. An IGR helps to stop the natural development of flea larvae and increases a product's efficacy by interrupting the life cycle rather than just providing treatment against adult fleas.

6. The label must be carefully read before using any product to ensure proper use and handling of the product.

7. Any product that acts as a cholinesterase inhibitor, such as other organophosphates, carbamates, phenothiazine derivatives, and succinylcholine, should not be used with organophosphates.

8. Signs of organophosphate poisoning may include excessive salivation, muscle twitching, miosis, vomiting, diarrhea, and dyspnea.

9. Nematodes, cestodes, trematodes, and protozoa are commonly treated in clinical practice.

10. Examples of nematodes are roundworms, heartworms, lungworms, and kidney worms. Examples of cestodes are tapeworms. Examples of trematodes are liver flukes. Examples of protozoa are coccidia and *Giardia*.

Answers to Chapter 14

1. a. Analgesia is the absence of the sensation of pain.

   b. Deep pain is pain arising from deep receptors in the periosteum, tendons, and joint structures.

   c. Histamine is a chemical mediator of the inflammatory response that is released from mast cells. Histamine causes dilation and increased permeability of small blood vessels, constriction of small airways, and increased secretion of mucus.

   d. Inflammation is a series of events that occur in response to tissue injury and is manifested by redness, heat, swelling, and pain.

   e. Prostaglandin is a chemical substance synthesized by cells from arachidonic acid. It serves as a mediator of inflammation and has other physiologic functions.

   f. Pyrogen is a substance that causes fever.

2. C

   A delta

3. Cerebral cortex

4. The NSAIDs relieve pain by inhibiting the enzyme cyclooxygenase, which in turn reduces the amount of prostaglandin (pain mediator) produced.

5. Acetaminophen causes the conversion of large amounts of an abnormal form of hemoglobin called *methemoglobin,* which results in anemia, cyanosis, liver damage, and death in this species.

6. Potential adverse side effects associated with the NSAIDs include gastrointestinal ulceration, bleeding tendencies, nephrotoxicity, and bone marrow suppression.

7. Antihistamines inhibit the inflammatory response by combining with histamine receptors (H_1) or by displacing histamine from the receptors.

8. H_2 receptors are found in the gastric mucosa, and they control the secretion of hydrochloric acid.

9. Myositis, intervertebral disk syndrome

10. Glucocorticoids and mineralocorticoids

11. The release of natural corticosteroids is controlled through the hypothalamic-pituitary-adrenal axis. When the level of cortisol in the blood is lowered, the hypothalamus senses this and sends a chemical messenger called *corticotropin-releasing factor* (CRF) to the pituitary gland, telling the pituitary to release adrenocorticotropic releasing factor (ACTH). ACTH is carried by the bloodstream to the adrenal cortex, which is stimulated to release more cortisol. An increased amount of cortisol in the blood is also sensed by the hypothalamus, which decreases the amount of CRF released to lower blood levels of cortisol through this feedback mechanism.

12. Short-term effects of corticosteroid use include polyuria, polydipsia, polyphagia, and delayed healing. Long-term effects include thinning of the skin, gastric ulcers, osteoporosis, and iatrogenic Cushing's disease.

13. Local anesthetics prevent generation and conduction of nerve impulses by peripheral nerves.

14. Local anesthetics are used for infiltrating into local areas for suturing wounds, for nerve blocks (lameness examinations), for antiarrhythmic effects, for topical use, and others.

Answers to Chapter 15

1. Hyperkalemia is an excess of potassium in the blood.
2. b. 5%
3. A fluid solution is balanced if it resembles extracellular fluid in composition.
4. mEqL, mOsm/L, and g/100 ml
5. c. 300
6. Sensible losses are primarily represented by urine losses. (In a research setting, fecal losses might be considered sensible because they can be measured.) Insensible losses include fecal, sweat, and respiratory losses.
7. Obese animals
8. 500, 1000
9. Hydration deficit, maintenance requirement, and ongoing losses
10. 2520 ml
11. 26 gtt/min
12. First check the bag to ensure that the solution is clear. Inspect the container's insertion port cover to make sure that it is intact and then remove the cover, being careful not to contaminate it. Close the flow clamp on the administration set and remove the cover from the set spike. Wipe the port with an alcohol swab and insert the spike into the insertion port. Hang the bag and fill the administration set line, clearing all the bubbles in the process. Close the flow clamp and attach the line adapter to the intravenous catheter using sterile technique. Open the flow clamp and adjust the flow rate.
13. Draw 50 ml from the bottle of 50% dextrose solution and add it to 450 ml of water.
14. Lactate is added to help correct acidosis in a patient. Lactate is converted to bicarbonate (alkaline) by the liver.
15. An esophageal feeder is used to provide oral electrolytes to neonatal calves. It consists of a tube (with a hollow ball on its end) attached to a heavy plastic bag. Oral electrolytes are placed in the bag, and the tube is passed into the esophagus of the calf. The ball on the end of the tube prevents entry into the trachea.
16. Hypertonic

■ Answers to Chapter 16

1. Iron compounds
2. Chronic renal failure; erythropoietin
3. Because a patient's response to hematinics does not occur quickly enough
4. EDTA
5. Because of the existence of an intrinsic clotting mechanism
6. A silver nitrate stick; by coagulation of blood proteins
7. Vitamin K_1; SC or IM
8. A fibrinolytic agent such as streptokinase
9. G_O, resting; G_1, presynthesis preparation; S, DNA synthesis; G_2, RNA production; and M, mitosis
10. Alkylating agents—cyclophosphamide; antimetabolites—methotrexate; plant alkaloids—vincristine; antibiotics—Adriamycin; hormonal—prednisolone; and miscellaneous—biologic response modifiers
11. Canine lymphoma monoclonal antibody
12. Treatment of autoimmune hemolytic anemia, treatment of lymphocytic-plasmacytic enteritis, treatment of rheumatoid arthritis, and treatment of lupus erythematosus
13. Because most antineoplastic drugs are very irritating to tissue and may cause sloughing
14. Designate a specific location for handling. Wear non-permeable latex gloves when handling. Cover work surfaces with a disposable, plastic-backed sheet. Wear an appropriate laboratory coat and mask. Reconstitute all materials carefully to avoid aerosolization. Clean reconstituted material of any contamination, and properly mark and date it. Dispose of contaminated material in leak-proof, puncture-resistant containers. Wash hands thoroughly.

■ Answers to Chapter 17

1. The response of a patient is determined by several factors such as the health and age of the patient, the type of vaccine given, the route of administration, concurrent incubation of infectious disease, exposure to an infectious disease before complete immunity is reached, and drug therapy.

2. Inactivated vaccines contain organisms that are treated by chemicals to kill the organism but produce very little change in the antigens that stimulate protective immunity.

   Live vaccines are prepared from live microorganisms or viruses that may be fully virulent or avirulent.

   Modified live vaccines contain organisms that undergo a process to lose their virulence so that when introduced to the body they cause an immune response instead of disease.

3. Live vaccines may cause disease in humans as a result of accidental injection, ingestion, or exposure through a cut or the mucous membranes.

4. An antitoxin neutralizes toxins produced by microorganisms, and an antiserum kills living, infectious antigens.

5. Intramuscular and subcutaneous administration are the most common, but some vaccines are administered intranasally or by the intraocular route.

6. Mixing vaccines may cause antigen blocking, resulting in one component's interfering with the action of another so that the animal does not receive adequate antigen to promote an effective immune response. It can also increase the chance of an allergic response.

7. Vaccine failure usually occurs because of improper handling, storage, or administration.

8. Epinephrine

■ Answers to Chapter 18

1. c. Calcium EDTA
2. d. Bring the cat to the hospital to start treatment with acetylcysteine.
3. a. Rompun
4. b. On an empty stomach
5. Oxymorphone, Torbugesic, Talwin-V, and Nubain
6. b. Blood urea nitrogen (BUN)

Index

A

NOTE: Page numbers in *italics* refer to illustrations; page numbers followed by t refer to tables.

375